TREATING SURVIVORS OF CHILDHOOD ABUSE AND INTERPERSONAL TRAUMA

Treating Survivors of Childhood Abuse and Interpersonal Trauma

STAIR Narrative Therapy

SECOND EDITION

Marylene Cloitre
Lisa R. Cohen
Kile M. Ortigo
Christie Jackson
Karestan C. Koenen

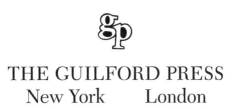

THE GUILFORD PRESS
New York   London

The authors have checked with sources believed to be reliable in their efforts to provide information that is
complete and generally in accord with the standards of practice that are accepted at the time of publication.
However, in view of the possibility of human error or changes in behavioral, mental health, or medical sciences,
neither the authors, nor the editors and publisher, nor any other party who has been involved in the preparation or
publication of this work warrants that the information contained herein is in every respect accurate or complete,
and they are not responsible for any errors or omissions or the results obtained from the use of such information.
Readers are encouraged to confirm the information contained in this book with other sources.

Library of Congress Cataloging-in-Publication data

Names: Cloitre, Marylene, author.
Title: Treating survivors of childhood abuse and interpersonal trauma : STAIR narrative therapy /
    Marylene Cloitre [and four others].
Other titles: Treating survivors of childhood abuse.
Description: Second edition. | New York : The Guilford Press, 2020. | Revision of: Treating survivors
    of childhood abuse / Marylene Cloitre, Lisa R. Cohen, Karestan C. Koenen. c2006. |
    Includes bibliographical references and index. |
Identifiers: LCCN 2020008162 | ISBN 9781462543281 (paperback) | ISBN 9781462543298 (hardcover)
Subjects: LCSH: Adult child sexual abuse victims—Treatment. | Psychotherapy.
Classification: LCC RC569.5.A28 C48 2020 | DDC 616.85/83690651—dc23
LC record available at *https://lccn.loc.gov/2020008162*

To our clients,
who have inspired us with their courage in coming to treatment,
confronting their traumas,
and daring to hope for the possibility of different lives
from the ones they have known

A survivor ultimately has two psychological possibilities: to shut down or to open up. Usually the survivor does both. . . . The protean self opts for opening out. . . . This includes the basic satisfaction, even joy, in being alive, in not having died, along with the sense of having undergone an experience that is illuminating in its pain. Survival also implies persevering, holding on, maintaining one's existence . . . a physical and mental strength. That sense of victory over destruction is evident in gatherings of survivors . . . where one hears clearly the words, even if actually unspoken: "We are here! We're alive! We have won!"

—ROBERT JAY LIFTON (1993, pp. 81, 82)

About the Authors

Marylene Cloitre, PhD, is Associate Director of Research in the National Center for PTSD Dissemination and Training Division, Palo Alto VA Health Care System; Clinical Professor (Affiliate), Department of Psychiatry and Behavioral Sciences, Stanford University; and Research Professor, Department of Psychiatry, NYU Langone Medical Center. Dr. Cloitre's primary clinical and research interests are the developmental consequences and treatment of childhood abuse in adults and adolescents. She is the recipient of the Award for Outstanding Contributions to Practice in Trauma Psychology from Division 56 of the American Psychological Association, is past president of the International Society for Traumatic Stress Studies, and was a member of the World Health Organization's ICD-11 working group on trauma spectrum disorders.

Lisa R. Cohen, PhD, has maintained a private practice in clinical psychology in New York City since 2001. Dr. Cohen specializes in the treatment of trauma and stress-related disorders, as well as co-occurring anxiety, mood, eating, and substance use disorders. Previously, she was a Research Scientist at the New York State Psychiatric Institute at Columbia University Medical Center, where she focused on developing, evaluating, and disseminating evidence-based psychotherapies for PTSD and substance use disorders.

Kile M. Ortigo, PhD, is Program Director in the National Center for PTSD Dissemination and Training Division, Palo Alto VA Health Care System. He leads a national initiative to evaluate and implement webSTAIR, an online program based on STAIR. Dr. Ortigo's research and writing have largely focused on personality, trauma, adult attachment, and lifespan developmental models of self. He has a private practice at the Center for Existential Exploration, which he founded, in Palo Alto, California. He serves as the lead editor for Psychedelic Support, an online resource and directory of clinicians.

Christie Jackson, PhD, is Director of Clinical Training for webSTAIR, an online program based on STAIR. Since 2005, Dr. Jackson has maintained a private practice in clinical psychology in New York City. She formerly served as Director of the PTSD Clinics at the Manhattan and Honolulu VA Medical Centers. She has worked with Marylene Cloitre since 2007 on numerous projects to evaluate and disseminate STAIR within the VA and in the community. She currently serves as Lead Trainer for the STAIR Institute.

Karestan C. Koenen, PhD, is Professor of Psychiatric Epidemiology at the Harvard T. H. Chan School of Public Health. She uses a developmental approach to understanding the epidemiology of trauma exposure and stress-related mental disorders such as PTSD and depression. Dr. Koenen is a recipient of the Award for Outstanding Contributions to the Science of Trauma Psychology from Division 56 of the American Psychological Association and the Robert S. Laufer, PhD, Memorial Award for Outstanding Scientific Achievement from the International Society for Traumatic Stress Studies. Dr. Koenen also advocates for survivors of violence and trauma.

Preface

What Is the Interrupted Life?

When the first edition of this book was published in 2006, we focused on the "interrupted life" of those who had experienced childhood sexual or physical abuse. We noted that abuse interrupted the development of an individual's emotional, social, and intellectual capacities, and accordingly, their growth as a capable and confident person. We created Skills Training in Affective and Interpersonal Regulation (STAIR) Narrative Therapy in large part as a "resource rehabilitation" program, intended to connect survivors of abuse with an enriching learning environment that they did not experience during their childhood.

Over the 20 years that we have delivered the treatment and trained other mental health providers, we have realized that there are many other circumstances in which the development of key life resources can be interrupted. These circumstances include emotional abuse or neglect in any of its varieties, such as inadequate nutrition, inconsistent parenting, or inappropriate supervision. Even more remarkably, we have observed that individuals whose predominant traumas occur in later life, such as domestic violence and exposure to genocide, terrorism, combat, or sustained civil war, also benefit from "resource rehabilitation" of emotional and relational capacities. Long periods of exposure to trauma can and usually do cause deterioration in these capacities. Furthermore, many populations who confront systematic discrimination and social prejudices (e.g., ethnic minorities, LGBTQ individuals) experience a kind of chronic stress that, when combined with other forms of trauma, leads to similar depletion of internal and external resources.

For all these reasons, we now recommend the treatment described in this book as relevant to survivors of all kinds of severe and/or chronic interpersonal traumas, such as childhood sexual abuse, domestic violence, and community violence. The conceptual frame of the book remains focused on the impact of chronic interpersonal traumas, but does so through a broad model of resource loss and then a more specific model of resource loss when trauma occurs during the developmental years (Chapters 2–3). The rationale for the treatment (Chapters 4–7), the assessment strategies and guidelines for implementation (Chapters 8–9), and the actual application of the treatment (Chapters 10–26) are appropriate for survivors of a wide range of traumas.

The program presented in this book, STAIR Narrative Therapy, comprises two modules. The first module, STAIR, has been explicitly developed to generate and strengthen social and emotional resources for effective living in the present (Chapters 10–19). A treatment for trauma, however, would not be complete if it did not in some way address the equally profound and widely recognized problem of traumatic memories. Because the emotions associated with traumatic memories—terror, humiliation, and betrayal—are extremely painful, the memories are often avoided. As a result, the traumatic memories are not assessed or integrated in any meaningful or coherent way into one's understanding of oneself or the world. But the emotional power of the memories remains, driving their expression through intrusive reexperiencing and reenactments of the trauma, all of which interfere with the capacity to live meaningfully and fully in the present. The inability to experience oneself as coherent and existing through time is another way in which life is "interrupted" for the survivor of trauma. The second module of the treatment, Narrative Therapy (Chapters 20–26), thus focuses on reviewing a range of traumatic memories, for the purposes of making meaning of these experiences and integrating them into the context of the individual's life story to help provide a coherent sense of self.

Narrative Therapy provides a structure and strategy for approaching, managing, and organizing traumatic experiences that have been unaddressed but are still quite alive with emotional power. Narrative Therapy begins with the emotional processing of fear memories via traditional imaginal exposure techniques (see Chapters 22 and 23). However, we have extended this work in two ways. First, we have developed and systematically employed "contextualization" strategies, grounded in recent models of autobiographical memory, to organize and construct a "narrative of self." Second, through these strategies, the client and therapist can safely explore and effectively organize a sense of self around another two critical affective themes that often burden the survivors of chronic interpersonal trauma: shame and betrayal (Chapter 24) and loss and grief (Chapter 25).

We have described two ways in which chronic trauma interrupts life. It disrupts the development of (or causes substantial deterioration in) important emotional and relational capacities that support effective living. It also disrupts a sense of coherence and continuity in personal identity. Given these pernicious effects, we have chosen the phrase "STAIR Narrative Therapy for the interrupted life" to describe our treatment approach, because it conveys a message of hope. It recognizes the importance and possibility of repair to the damaged self. We also propose the possibility that treatment may extend an individual's capacities beyond what should have been developed or maintained if not for trauma. In regenerating important life skills and a coherent and revitalized sense of self, we hope that clients can, in essence, resume the realization of hidden potential.

WHO CAN BENEFIT FROM THIS BOOK?

This book provides an evidence-based treatment for mental health care providers who work with survivors of interpersonal trauma. The treatment was originally developed for survivors of childhood abuse (i.e., all people who have experienced sexual abuse, physical abuse, or neglect as children). The treatment was also originally developed for women. However, it has also been successfully used with men and gender-diverse clients, and with clients of varied ages (including children and adolescents) who have experienced maltreatment in early life and/or many other forms of interpersonal violence (see Chapter 8). For this reason, we have broadened the language of this book to be more gender-neutral (e.g., "they" and "them" when a specific gender identity is not specified or relevant) and to use person-first language that emphasizes the person behind the trauma and the clinical presentation, rather than a disorder or negative characteristic (e.g., a "survivor of child abuse" rather than "an abused child"). We hope these changes reflect our growing awareness (and that of societies and the profession as a whole) of the benefits of inclusivity, diversity, and empowerment.

THE TREATMENT PHILOSOPY

The orientation of the treatment is a blend of principles from the cognitive-behavioral and the attachment–interpersonal–object relational traditions evolving from the work of Bowlby (1988). The intervention techniques rely heavily on those from the cognitive-behavioral therapy (CBT) tradition. These include, for example, interventions that help individuals acknowledge and appraise the meaning of their traumatic experiences (exposure and cognitive reappraisal). They also include strategies for identifying the implicit interpersonal schemas that guide beliefs, feelings, and behaviors, and revising them through reappraisal processes and the use of role play to facilitate new learning and behavioral changes. They also adhere to a philosophy implicit in CBT: that with practice, new ways of behaving, feeling, and thinking are possible. In this way, CBT is a remarkably practical and optimistic psychotherapeutic tradition.

The theoretical framework of the treatment falls squarely within the interpersonal tradition, particularly as it has evolved from the work of Bowlby. The use of this framework emphasizes the importance of early life attachments and the long-term consequences that disturbances in caregiving relationships have in adult functioning. The cognitive-behavioral strategies are the means by which the client identifies these problems and works toward change. For example, problems in relationships related to early abuse are described through the attachment concept of "internal working models of relating." This concept is operationalized in the practical form of the Relationship Patterns Worksheets—tools that could easily fit into many cognitive therapies and are used here to assess and change ideas about the self and others.

HOW TO USE THIS BOOK

This book is intended to provide therapists with the skills, competence, and confidence to treat survivors of chronic interpersonal trauma. We have provided a session-by-session guide to a treatment that is grounded in theory, has been tested in its benefits, and has been refined over 20 years with feedback from our clients. The book provides practical, "nuts-and-bolts" guidance for all the technical aspects of the treatment. Equally important, the book is organized and written to highlight the rationale for the treatment and the primary goals behind each intervention, so that a therapist can use STAIR Narrative Therapy guided by the principles of the treatment as they fit a particular client, rather than feel compelled to follow the modules, sessions, and interventions in a lockstep fashion.

The book is divided into three parts. Part I characterizes the effects of chronic trauma in the context of a resource loss model and an attachment–developmental framework; Part II describes the theoretical and empirical bases for the treatment rationale and outcome data reporting the benefits of the therapy; and Part III provides session-by-session descriptions of the treatment preceded by assessment and treatment guidelines. The book as a whole is intended to convey *a way of thinking* about survivors of interpersonal trauma that can facilitate effective therapy. Theory, research, and clinical service are unified under the theme that recovery from such trauma requires recognition and redress of a life history in which terrible things have happened—and, equally important, recognition and redress of a life history in which many important normative events and experiences have been absent or diminished.

In Part III, the STAIR module (Module I) targets the generation of social and emotional resources (a focus on the present), while the Narrative Therapy module (Module II) aims to resolve symptoms related to traumatic memories (a focus on the past). Many survivors of trauma will have both types of problems and so will benefit from the use of both treatment components. But a therapist can consider using only one or the other, as suits the needs of a particular client at a particular time. Such judgments are aided by a review of treatment guidelines (Chapter 8), strategies for evaluating when to make the transition from skills training to narrative work (Chapter 20), and a review of the session summaries provided in Part III (the summary is the first box in each chapter from 10 to 19 and from 21 to 26). These "at-a-glance" summaries identify what matters most in the sessions (e.g., the development of emotional awareness) and why it matters. This is intended to liberate the therapist from the assumption that, in order to be successful, a session must be completed as described. Rather, the theme of any given session should prompt the therapist to ask: "How significant is this problem for my client? How skilled is my client in each of these activities? Which of these strategies address my client's current problems?" Ideally, the therapist and client will work together to answer these questions. The selection of the interventions and the choice of specific goals to be targeted are the results of a collaborative effort.

It is well known that the therapeutic alliance influences the benefits of any treatment, and this finding is particularly true for survivors of abuse (see Cloitre, Stovall-McClough, Miranda, & Chemtob, 2004). For this reason, discussions of the nature and role of the therapeutic alliance are integrated into several chapters of the book. Chapter 8 provides an overview of the value of the therapeutic relationship and strategies for building a good working relationship, particularly in the context of potential ruptures common in work with survivors of trauma. Several sessions identify specific therapist attitudes and behaviors that support and facilitate effective implementation of the session interventions—for example, those related to emotional awareness (Chapter 11) and narratives of shame and loss (Chapters 24 and 25).

Finally, we have written with awareness of the need for therapists to manage their own mental and physical health, and have highlighted the importance of therapist self-care (see Chapter 8). We hope that the philosophy and guidelines for treatment we have set out provide compassion and understanding for their clients' condition, and in doing so protect and empower therapists in their work.

Acknowledgments

We wish to thank Ashley Bauer, Lori Davis, Chetali Gupta, Shaili Jain, Annabel Prinz, and Brandon Weiss, who contributed as students, postdoctoral fellows, and colleagues to the development, adaptations, and evaluation of this treatment. We would also like to thank those individuals who have been especially important in our professional development and personal growth, and who have provided inspiration, enthusiasm, and support for us during the writing of this revised edition: Jerilyn Brownstein, Eugene Canotal, George and Susan Cohen, David and Joyce DeArman, Caleb Ferguson, Maximilian Greer, Denise Hien, Marc Horowitz, Alice Jackson, Nick Jollymore, Kathleen Koenen, Carol and Arvil Ortigo, Verna and Ted Ortigo, Lorcan Purcell, David Schroeder, and Thea Stone.

Contents

PART I

Theoretical Frameworks

CHAPTER 1

A Resource Loss Model

Childhood abuse is not a diagnosis but a life experience.
—FRANK W. PUTNAM (2004)

The treatment described in this book is the result of more than two decades of listening and responding to the needs and concerns of clients with histories of childhood abuse and other interpersonal trauma experiences. When the first edition of this book was published, Skills Training in Affective and Interpersonal Regulation (STAIR) Narrative Therapy was the first demonstrably effective treatment developed specifically for survivors of childhood abuse. It has undergone rigorous empirical evaluation and has been demonstrated as efficacious, feasible, and (most importantly) acceptable to survivors. The motivation for the first edition of this book was derived from the observation that mental health services were not providing programs for survivors of childhood abuse. Fortunately, this is no longer the case; many health care systems are striving to provide trauma-informed services, including the use of STAIR Narrative Therapy.

This new edition reflects the results of more than a decade of work with both survivors of childhood abuse, as well as other survivors of complex interpersonal trauma, including refugees and veterans of combat. We came to understand that the treatment was applicable and valuable to these populations. We also learned that individuals presenting with adulthood interpersonal trauma, such as first responders to the September 11, 2001, terrorist attacks, could develop a complex trauma symptom profile, depending on how horrendous the exposure had been and the degree to which they had social and emotional resources to support them in the recovery process. We realized that STAIR Narrative Therapy was applicable, and indeed could be successfully delivered, to these populations with little adaptation (Levitt, Malta, Martin, Davis, & Cloitre, 2007). The current chapter describes the principles of STAIR Narrative Therapy within the framework of a resource loss model. This model is applicable to individuals who have experienced trauma as children or adults. Chapters 2 and 3 focus specifically on attachment-related resource losses that occur as results of abuse and neglect during childhood.

TRAUMA AND A NEW DIAGNOSIS: COMPLEX PTSD

Community studies indicate that trauma is common, with over 70% of the global population reporting exposure to at least one traumatic event, and 30% reporting exposure to four or more such events (Benjet et al., 2016). Traumatic experiences include those that are interpersonal and often involve violence perpetrated by one person on another, such as physical assault, rape, and combat; they also include other types of experiences, such as serious accidents and natural or human-made disasters. The majority of interpersonal traumas, which include sexual and physical violence, occur before the age of 18 (Kessler et al., 2017). Thus the most devastating traumatic experiences occur to those least developmentally able to cope with them. Childhood abuse and neglect or other maltreatment (all of which are types of interpersonal trauma) are particularly common; more than one in four persons have experienced abuse by a caregiver by the age of 17 (Finkelhor, Turner, Shattuck, & Hamby, 2013).

Since the first edition of this book appeared in 2006, childhood abuse specifically and trauma broadly have been recognized as major public health problems (Teicher & Samson, 2013). Evidence for the long-term adverse mental and physical health effects of childhood trauma in particular has been recognized by the American Heart Association (Suglia et al., 2018). Persons with histories of childhood abuse have an earlier age at onset of psychopathology, greater symptom severity, more comorbidity, a greater risk for suicide, and poorer treatment response than those with no history of abuse who have the same diagnoses (Teicher & Samson, 2013).

The impairment and psychic suffering caused by childhood abuse are enormous. In 2018, the World Health Organization (WHO) identified the particularly complex nature of the effects of childhood abuse and other chronic and sustained interpersonal traumas through the introduction of a diagnosis, complex posttraumatic stress disorder (CPTSD), into the 11th revision of the *International Classification of Diseases and Related Health Problems* (ICD-11; WHO, 2018). ICD-11 is the official diagnostic system used worldwide, including (finally) in the United States. The diagnosis includes not only the traditional symptoms of posttraumatic stress disorder (PTSD), but also the effects that trauma can have on emotion regulation, self-concept, and relational capacities. When the first edition of this book was published, the diagnosis of PTSD as presented by the *Diagnostic and Statistical Manual of Mental Disorders,* fourth edition, text revision (DSM-IV-TR; American Psychiatric Association, 2000), was the dominant formulation of the psychological effects of trauma. At that time, we discussed problems we observed among survivors of childhood abuse that extended beyond DSM-defined PTSD, particularly regarding emotion regulation, interpersonal functioning, and negative self-concept, but that were not officially recognized. Such symptoms are now addressed in DSM-5 (American Psychiatric Association, 2013), which has added a symptom cluster of "negative alterations in cognitions and mood" that references negative beliefs about self and others, as well as feelings of detachment from others. It has also added a "with dissociative symptoms" subtype of PTSD that identifies one type of emotion regulation difficulty (hypoactivation). However, the inclusion of the CPTSD diagnosis in ICD-11, which provides a coherent and empirically supported profile of symptoms typically associated with complex trauma, makes the problems typically seen among survivors of childhood abuse easier to recognize, assess, and treat. We discuss the specific symptom profile associated with ICD-11 CPTSD, as well as its assessment, in Chapters 8 and 9.

The purpose of this book is to provide a treatment guide for individuals who have experienced childhood abuse and other interpersonal traumas that result in a wide range of symptoms, including those found in ICD-11 CPTSD. We believe that this book is now needed more than ever, as a result of the addition of CPTSD to the diagnostic nomenclature. However, we recognize that not all of the problems that survivors of childhood abuse and other severe interpersonal traumas experience are captured by this diagnosis. Accordingly, it is our intention to provide a conceptual framework and a treatment program that address the *experience* of chronic interpersonal trauma, rather than a diagnosis. The formulation of the effects of trauma as a resource loss provides an explanatory frame for PTSD and CPTSD, as well as for other disorders and psychological problems that can result from various types of interpersonal trauma. The treatment program presented in this book, STAIR Narrative Therapy, addresses all problems represented in the diagnosis of CPTSD. It can also address other problems, once these are understood in the context of resource loss and resource rehabilitation. The remainder of this chapter describes trauma as a resource loss phenomenon. This includes specifically the types of losses resulting from trauma that occurs during childhood, particularly at the hands of caregivers; the ways in which these losses are represented in the CPTSD diagnosis; and the rationale for STAIR Narrative Therapy as a resource rehabilitation program.

ALL TRAUMAS AS RESOURCE LOSS EVENTS

Resource loss is a critical and universal feature of all traumas: Life after a trauma is diminished. Depending on the trauma, the resource loss may be psychological (such as a person's sense of security, optimism, and social support), material (such as a home, family, schooling or employment, and a community within which to prosper), or both. In addition, certain types of traumatic events and their harshest consequences befall those who are already in circumstances with limited resources. Trauma often comes to people with fewer financial resources. For instance, persons who cannot afford to live in areas outside of hurricane paths and floodplains experience more hurricanes and floods, and more devastating consequences from those natural disasters. Similarly, those who have fewer physical and psychological resources to protect themselves, such as children, elderly individuals, and injured persons, are likely to experience interpersonal violence. Forcible rape among females, for example, is not randomly distributed across the lifespan, but occurs predominantly in the vulnerable years of childhood and adolescence; as noted above, over half of sexual and physical assault occurs by the age of 18 (Kessler et al., 2017).

In addition, those who are most vulnerable to trauma because of limited resources will have more difficulty recovering. The irony of trauma is that recovery requires the presence of resources greater than those the victim often had in the first place. Rebuilding a house destroyed by a hurricane requires more than bricks, mortar, and the owner's own toil; it also requires a team of roofers, bricklayers, plumbers, and painters. Just as the homeowner's own resources are not enough, the resources of a survivor of trauma are often insufficient without additional investment from the outside. This is particularly true of persons who have been traumatized as children. Childhood is a time when an individual is vulnerable to victimization, and once victimization occurs, the child has even fewer psychological and social resources than before with which to negotiate a recovery process.

Lastly, the traumatized state is not static. If resource regeneration does not occur, the result is not stasis, but rather continued resource loss and degeneration (see Hobfoll, Mancini, Hall, Canetti, & Bonanno, 2011). The unrepaired or partially repaired house will be buffeted by wind, risk further decay, or be entirely destroyed in the onslaught of another hurricane. Similarly, without resource recovery, the psychological and social trajectory for a survivor of trauma will be vulnerable to the vicissitudes of both ordinary life stressors and additional traumas. The risk of a downward trajectory is particularly relevant and evident among those traumatized in childhood. The mandate of childhood is growth—physical, psychological, and social. Trauma reduces the resources necessary not only for recovery, but also for the developmental tasks integral to childhood. As a result, the achievement of such tasks is often compromised, with impairments evident in poor life functioning and accumulating into adulthood.

The resource loss model thus informs our understanding of trauma recovery. Trauma recovery requires resource recovery (Hollifield et al., 2016). Accordingly, the principle of intervention to which this program adheres is one of recovery of resource losses—in particular, the rehabilitation of the psychological, emotional, and social capacities whose development has been interrupted by trauma.

PSYCHOLOGICAL TRAUMA AS A RESOURCE LOSS

"Trauma" has been defined in medicine as a circumstance in which some part of the body has been suddenly damaged by a force so powerful that the body's natural protections are unable to prevent injury and the body's natural healing abilities are inadequate to resolve the injury without medical assistance (*Stedman's Medical Dictionary*, 2000). The word "trauma" is, in fact, derived from the Greek for "wound." As noted by Chris Brewin (2003), Freud (1920/1955) was the first to define the term "psychic injury" by analogy to physical injury. Freud described psychic trauma as an event that "penetrates a kind of mental skin designed to protect a person from excessive external forces; trauma [is] essentially a 'breach in an otherwise efficacious barrier'" (Brewin, 2003, p. 4). The breach is the result not only of the strength and impact of the external force, but of the inability of the organism or affected area to deflect, absorb, neutralize, or compensate for the injury.

Following this analogy, we describe psychological trauma as a circumstance in which an event overwhelms or exceeds a person's capacity to protect their psychic well-being and integrity. It is a collision between an event and a person's resources, where the power of the event is greater than the resources available for effective response and recovery. Deterioration in functioning occurs, and intervention or resources beyond those the individual has available are required for recovery. Psychological trauma, like physical trauma, represents a complex relationship between an event and a response. The objective characteristics of a potentially traumatic event—its force, strength, or "dose"—can be quantified, but the impact of the event cannot be determined without taking into account the resources and vulnerabilities of the particular individual who sustains the injury.

CHILDHOOD MALTREATMENT TRAUMA AS A RESOURCE LOSS

This analysis has significant implications for our understanding of childhood abuse or neglect as a major trauma. To continue the medical analogy, it is well known that certain toxic chemicals and environmental pollutants have a significantly greater impact on children than on adults, even when the amount of exposure or "dose" is the same. Children's immature development makes them particularly vulnerable to the effects of such toxins. The impact on their bodily systems is more potent than that experienced by adults, and the effect of a toxin on one system has negative effects on other related and vulnerable developing systems.

Now let us consider, for example, sexual abuse as a powerful physical and psychological toxin to the child because of their immature development. "Sexual abuse," by definition, is physical contact with a child for sexual purposes without the child's meaningful consent. This act is one in which the perpetrator takes ownership of the child's body, which, by definition, is the essential and basic territory of the self. Furthermore, sexual abuse often, if not typically, co-occurs with physical abuse (e.g., Kim, Mennen, & Trickett, 2017). Thus a typical picture of childhood abuse is one in which there are repeated exposures to multiple forms of violence to the body. An effective response to this circumstance requires internal and external resources of a kind and quantity not typically within a child's grasp.

The internal or personal resources with which children can protect themselves are limited by the simple fact of their life stage. Their levels of cognitive, affective, and physical development place significant limits on their capacity to recognize, avoid, or escape perpetrators. Explicit or implied suggestions that sexual activity with a caregiver or other adult is good, or that physical abuse or neglect is deserved, are difficult for children to oppose or resist. They tend to be naive or confused by the threat hiding behind the blandishments and compliments of perpetrators of sexual abuse. Their small size also makes them easy targets for physically abusive adults.

In addition, children's external resources are far more limited than those of adults. When adults experience a trauma such as a rape or motor vehicle accident, or when they witness violence, they are more likely to have a place of safety to recover and/or a social support network on which to rely on for care as needed. In contrast, children have little choice about where they live or on whom they depend. Their home, the traditional source of safety, is also often the source of what most threatens them. The caregivers on whom the children depend are frequently those who are committing the transgressions against them. The necessary alternative in this situation—telling someone about a caregiver's abuse or neglect—can be frightening in its implication of loss of home and caregiver, or attendant sense of betrayal, regardless of the danger posed by the abuse. Even getting access to agencies and institutions that aim to protect children is difficult or impossible for a child to do alone, as it legally requires the accompaniment or aid of other adults.

The resource limitations of children confronted with maltreatment lead us to define such maltreatment as a trauma in all of its essential characteristics. In particular, children who are abused are individuals who are helpless in the face of repeated, unavoidable, and inescapable transgressions against their bodies. A child's resources are no match for the immediate and consistent threat of physical or sexual assaults by an adult, particularly when that adult is a parent or other caregiver.

SPECIFIC RESOURCE LOSSES ASSOCIATED WITH CHILDHOOD MALTREATMENT

The resource limitations a child experiences in confronting the trauma of maltreatment are defined by their life stage and yield a circumstance in which the child rarely succeeds in warding off or neutralizing sexual or physical threats or neglect. In addition, once the trauma occurs, its presence creates a cascade of resource losses that continue during its typically chronic course and have significant consequences long after the abuse ends.

The most immediate consequences of childhood abuse or neglect are the losses of physical safety and physical integrity. Less evident, but equally profound and perhaps unique to childhood maltreatment, are the losses of many psychological and social-developmental opportunities and advances, which are diminished or negated as either direct or indirect results of the maltreatment. Childhood abuse or neglect is a trauma perpetrated by an adult, usually an important caregiver upon whom a child depends significantly for psychological and material resources. It occurs during a time of life when many developmental tasks, involving the growth of emotional and social competencies, are being completed; these tasks require sustained contributions by caregivers, family members, and the community. Under conditions of maltreatment, these necessary resources are often deficient or disturbed, compromising the child's ability to complete these tasks successfully. Lastly, it is critical to note that recovery from the effects of maltreatment, like recovery from all traumas, requires the investment of additional "repairing" resources. But for a child or adolescent, this investment often requires the initiative of the caregiver—and if the caregiver is the perpetrator of the trauma, they are motivated to ignore, hide, or deny the maltreatment. This aspect of abuse or neglect, the silence and stigma associated with it, adds to further resource loss (i.e., the support and intervention of the community). All of these losses and the absence of intervention in a time of development conspire to create substantial functional impairment among adult survivors of childhood maltreatment.

Acknowledging all these circumstances, we have catalogued the potential resource losses that childhood maltreatment engenders in both the short and long term. They include (1) loss of healthy attachment and healthy sense of self, (2) loss of effective guidance in the development of emotional and social competencies, and (3) loss of support and connection to the larger social community.

Loss of Healthy Attachment and Healthy Sense of Self

One of the most devastating aspects of childhood abuse or neglect is that the perpetrator of the trauma is almost always a parent or other important caregiver. The implications of this circumstance as a resource loss are staggering. The attachment of a child to a parent or other primary caregiver creates the base for learning about the essentials of living. This attachment is a resource from which springs the evolution of effective agency, self-definition, and autonomy. It is intended to provide sufficient safety and security for the child to explore and learn about the world, and to grow in confidence and autonomy. Ideally, a caregiver provides a secure base or home for "refueling" of resources to explore the world. This secure base involves the caregiver's availability to act as a facilitator to the child's growing capacities in self-management and effective interaction with the social and physical environment. The power of the parent as a source of safety was documented during World War II. Child psychiatrists in London noted that that children were better off staying with parents during bombings than being separated from the parents for the "safety of the countryside"; indeed, children did rather well if their parents did well by them and were psychologically healthy themselves (Carey-Trefzer, 1949). Children look within their immediate environment, and particularly to their caregivers, to gauge safety and interpret the level of threat in a particular situation.

Children use their parents as anchors or reference points to understand the meaning of traumatic events, understand cause and effect, experience safety and support, obtain comfort, and receive guidance in effective coping. Maltreatment is essentially a betrayal of the assumption of care by a parent for a child (DePrince et al., 2012), and in every aspect of the betrayal of parenting responsibilities, there is a definable loss.

There is a profound loss of a sense of security and personal safety; associated with this is a restricted capacity for curiosity and exploration about the world. There is also the loss of a healthy trajectory of affective organization. The developing capacity for self-soothing is challenged by physical and sexual violations in particular, and guidance from the abusing caregiver is often absent, irregular, or deviant. Moreover, there is significant disturbance in the development of a sense of autonomy and agency. Rather than recognize and protect the necessary but vulnerable authority of the child as an agent of their own experience, the maltreating caregiver acts in such a way that the child becomes an extension of the caregiver's own sexual and aggressive impulses. The betrayal of the attachment bond often leads to loss of trust in intimate relationships, with long-term consequences in the management of future interpersonal relationships.

Lastly, childhood maltreatment leads to loss of the capacity for self-love and positive self-regard. Healthy attachment includes expressions by the caregiver of positive regard for the child, which the child internalizes. Under circumstances of abuse and neglect, the child still absorbs the messages communicated by the caregiver, but they are negative: "You are bad," "Look what you made me do," "I should give you away," "I will give you away if you tell anyone." These messages establish a working model of a self-identity as "bad" that is often not consciously formulated and can be difficult to identify and change in later years.

Moreover, neglect or sexual and physical abuse often elicit feelings of shame and guilt that are integrated into the child's self-identity, leading to feelings of shame and guilt about who they *are* versus what *was done to them*.

Loss of Opportunities for Social and Emotional Development

Childhood maltreatment derails the development of important life skills, particularly emotional and social competencies that lead to effective self-management and interpersonal relationships. Children who are maltreated often come from families in which parents or caregivers often were maltreated themselves as children, are limited in emotional expression and interpersonal functioning, and often suffer from PTSD and other mental health problems themselves (Anderson, Edwards, Silver, & Johnson, 2018; Widom, Czaja, & DuMont, 2015); thus they are less than ideal role models for learning such skills.

In addition, maltreatment within the home setting creates paradoxical and conflicting information about acceptable and effective rules for living. For example, standard rules of sexual and physical behavior are applicable in general, but not in the home. These inconsistencies, often unexplained, can create inappropriate social behaviors that lead to peer rejection and loss of confidence in the survivor's own perceptions and judgments about social realities. The diminished emotional and social competencies associated with maltreatment are further exacerbated or result in continued social and emotional injury and loss in the larger social environment during both childhood and adolescence. For example, compared to their peers, children who have been abused have greater difficulty socializing with peers and managing conflict, are more uncomfortable with high levels of emotion, expect little social support from adults in resolving social difficulties, are less confident, and report lower self-esteem (Naughton et al., 2013; Perepletchikova & Kaufman, 2010). In adolescent years, those with abuse histories are more likely than their peers to develop mental health problems (McLaughlin et al., 2012), drop out of school, engage in substance abuse and delinquent behaviors, and experience interpersonal violence both as victims and as perpetrators (Amstadter et al., 2011; Carliner, Gary, McLaughlin, & Keyes, 2017).

In adulthood, individuals with a history of childhood abuse often report a profound sense of lost opportunities in realizing desired goals in both their work and personal lives. Widom, in her work following a cohort of children who experienced abuse and are now grown up, reports individuals with histories of childhood abuse are more likely than their peers without such histories to fall short in achieving expectable life milestones, including achieving fewer years of education, having more criminal arrests (Horan & Widom, 2015), living in less desirable neighborhoods, and engaging in illicit drug use (Chauhan, Schuck, & Widom, 2017; Chauhan & Widom, 2012). Childhood abuse also has long-term effects on emotion processing that persist into adulthood (Young & Widom, 2014), and such persons suffer from increased rates of depression and anxiety throughout their lives (Jaffee, 2017; Li, D'Arcy, & Meng, 2016). Perhaps, as the ultimate behavioral expression of all that ails them, person with abuse histories are more likely to attempt suicide than are their peers without such histories (Liu et al., 2017).

Loss of Perceived Support of the Community

It has become clear that welcoming children into the larger community enhances their development, including self-esteem, social skills, and physical well-being. The support of the community is expressed in the explicit valuing of children as community members. This is demonstrated by acknowledgment of their presence in the community, concern about their experiences, expression of positive regard, and active efforts to provide them with appropriate roles. Children who have been maltreated often do not experience full and positive engagement in the community. This can occur in many ways and for many reasons. Children who have been maltreated may be hampered in integrating themselves if their emotional resources are primarily absorbed by the demands of the home environment (i.e., managing maltreating parents and experiences). Their lesser social and emotion regulation skills, as described above, may make them less attractive to peers, teachers, coaches, religious leaders, or other important figures of influence. Furthermore, silence about the maltreatment may create feelings of alienation and a loss of any authentic sense of relating to peers, teachers, or other members of the community.

Lastly, the stigma of maltreatment and general discomfort about recognizing its presence may keep community members at a distance from a maltreated child or youth. The tendency to "blame the victim" emerges from the distress that is elicited by recognizing and responding to victimization. It forces recognition of malfeasance toward a vulnerable person, and in the case of childhood maltreatment, adult malfeasance toward an innocent person. Children who have been maltreated can make adults uncomfortable, because they challenge the belief system that the world is benevolent and that we are all competent to take care of ourselves. The desire to maintain this illusion leads us to expect an unrealistic level of competence in children to defend themselves (Langton, Berzofsky, Krebs, & Smiley-McDonald, 2012).

The alternative to "blaming the victim," which is to recognize the existence of maltreatment, leads to other kinds of difficulties. There may well be confusion and uncertainty about how to intervene, and reluctance to do so. Indeed, data indicate that while the majority of Americans view childhood maltreatment as a serious problem, it is rarely reported ("How America Defines Child Abuse," 1999). The impulse to intervene in the activities of a family where a child is being victimized by a parent or other caregiver conflicts with traditional beliefs about the integrity and autonomy of the family unit. Strategies for intervention have been developed through family courts and the development of agencies that monitor the safety of children, but there is a sustained tension between these interventions and beliefs about the privacy and authority of the family unit and its potential superiority as a context for caring for children.

Finally, as exemplified by the development of safety-monitoring agencies, children who have been maltreated, like all persons who have experienced trauma, require the extension of social and community resources. Such resources include money, time, and effort. If such resources become scarce, sympathy for these children may yield to feelings of resentment or indifference. Those with more resources may lose patience with those who have fewer of them. Thus the consequences of childhood maltreatment as a resource loss ripple out to the community in which a maltreated child lives and needs to be supported. Reactions to the diminution of resources often lead to conflict and reduced integrity of the community and its members. The integration of a maltreated child into the community is strained. Stigma remains, and the child still feels alienated and out of the mainstream. The alienation generated by the silence is transformed into alienation generated by resentment.

SUMMARY AND IMPLICATIONS FOR TREATMENT

This chapter has described the myriad ways trauma during childhood results in developmental losses regarding the effective growth of emotional, cognitive, behavioral, and social capacities. The treatment philosophy described in this book affirms that recovery from childhood trauma requires the rehabilitation of resources and life skills that were derailed or denied in the skirmish to survive in a chronically abusive environment. Our treatment is at heart a resource recovery program, with an emphasis on reclaiming and building emotional and social competencies. We adhere to the notion that resources above and beyond those necessary for basic survival must be recruited and accumulated in order to recover from the damages inflicted by a trauma. In addition, like many other researchers, therapists, and survivors, we have found that emotional processing of the trauma is a powerful if not a critical component in trauma recovery.

Accordingly, we have developed a two-module treatment program in which the development of resources and emotional processing of the trauma are equal and balanced partners. The first treatment module, STAIR, is dedicated to building emotional and social competencies as resources. The second treatment module, Narrative Therapy, involves the emotional processing of the traumatic events in the context of a safe and supportive environment. The ordering of the components is purposeful. Resource development precedes the trauma-processing work because skills in emotion regulation and social connection not only help improve functioning in day-to-day life, but can support the effective use of Narrative Therapy. Although we encourage flexibility in the ordering of treatment modules so that they are sequenced to meet the needs and preferences of individual clients, empirical support for the benefits of this particular sequence is provided in Chapter 4.

We have proposed that in the course of a life that includes childhood maltreatment or exposure to other chronic traumatic events, the development of CPTSD is the result of insufficient resources with which to heal from the trauma. In the same way, we propose that in the course of therapy, confronting the pain of multiple traumatic memories requires the presence of emotional and interpersonal resources to be successful and healing. The treatment is in essence a recapitulation of the appropriate order of development in the ideal case: The fortunate person is provided with the advantage of the accrual of multiple and diverse resources as they face their life challenges.

CHAPTER 2

Attachment

When Protector and Perpetrator Are One

> Attachment theory starts from the power of adults to protect and provide security for their children. In abuse, this fundamental biosocial contract between adults and children is ruptured: adults use their power for their own ends rather than those of the child.
> —JEREMY HOLMES (2001, p. 95)

THE POWER OF THE ATTACHMENT BOND

A child's parents (or other primary caregivers) are the child's most important resources by far. Parents provide safety. They provide instruction on how the world works and how to function in it. They stand between the child and the vicissitudes of life until the child is ready to face these independently. Parents extend the child's awareness of external resources to those in the larger world, and oversee the child's ability to use these resources on their own behalf: in maintaining safety, in solving problems, in finding friends and a supportive environment, and in experiencing pleasure and joy. Parents also build the child's internal resources. A parent helps a child develop a sense of competence through regular instruction and feedback. More importantly, the parent mirrors back not only success in a learned skill, but something more ineffable and more valuable: pride in the child's accomplishment. The infrastructure of the child's self is built on the parent's internalized view of the child: that of being well regarded and valued. These perceptions are the foundations of self-esteem, self-confidence, and self-love, which allow the developing child to do well. This positive view of self provides the child with the capacity to confront new situations with the expectation of doing well, and to meet new people with the expectation of being well regarded. It also allows the child to approach difficulties with the belief that solutions can be found and that personal limitations can be managed.

Perhaps it is inevitable that the proximity of a child to a caregiver, intended to secure the child's continued growth, is also an Achilles heel: The primary sources of injury and harm to children are their caregivers. For example, reviews of nearly 3 million cases of documented child abuse in a single year in the United States indicated that 80% of the sexual abuse perpetrators were parents (Golden, 2000). Such circumstances pervert the resource relationship between parent and child. The child's need for physical proximity to the caregiver, and dependence on the caregiver for safety, result in experiences of physical transgressions. The bond with the caregiver becomes an affective and cognitive contradiction: The source of safety is also a source of danger. The explanations for effective functioning in the world at large are suspended, irrelevant, or contradicted at home. The person responsible for building the child's self-regard also breaks it down with physical intrusions or assaults. The parent who creates bridges between the child and the social world also severs those connections with secret sexual transgressions. As a result, the child's feelings of safety and control, positive regard, competence, and connection to the larger world are compromised.

The attachment literature has demonstrated that the connection between caregiver and offspring is a critical dynamic that supports the survival and growth of the child. In this design of care, it is expected that threats to safety are generated beyond the shadow of the caregiver, and that when threatened, the child returns to the safety of home base. Evolution of the fight-or-flight reaction is viewed as consistent with a system of safety in which protection is anchored to a home base. The fight-or-flight response is effective for refueling in the short term and for longer-term resource building in the affiliative/protective network of home base. But this arrangement is not a "fail-safe" system, as demonstrated by circumstances in which parents/caregivers themselves become threats via physical abuse, sexual abuse, and/or neglect of their offspring. The consequence of such circumstances is that for at least some period of time, a child inevitably experiences a relationship in which perpetrator and care provider are one.

The power of the attachment bond remains apparent, even in the context of maltreatment by caregivers. This has been demonstrated in several research literatures. For example, among nonhuman species, offspring will remain in physical proximity to their parents or designated caregivers, even when contact with the caregivers is associated with significant physical pain and aversive experiences (see Perry, Blair, & Sullivan, 2017; Santiago, Aoki, & Sullivan, 2017). The evolution of this circumstance is presumably related to the biosocial net cost of such relationships: Any caregiver is better than none, particularly when the offspring have little capacity to function independently. Among humans, the rate of maturation is relatively slow and the dependence of children on adult caregivers is sustained, with several years of guardianship required to monitor and support the children's constant cognitive, social, and emotional growth.

One of the more perplexing consequences of maltreatment in early life is that attachment to an abusive/neglectful caregiver can be more powerful than that which occurs within nonabusive bonds. Although this is a devastating consequence, it is not difficult to understand once the dynamics of childhood maltreatment are understood. As Freyd (1996, p. 71) notes, "The child is charged by life" to sustain the attachment to parents, and so to sustain the self. A vicious cycle that begins with the child's inherent dependence on the parent is established. In healthy circumstances, development progresses with increasing autonomy and the prerequisite resources to succeed in this independence, all of which are supported by the caregivers. However, autonomy is stymied in circumstances of maltreatment, because injury and diminished capacity actually increase rather than decrease dependence. Research with nonhuman species has shown that maltreatment actually *increases* attachment, because the more an individual is injured or terrorized, the stronger the person's need becomes for protection and comforting. Allen (1995, p. 157) describes the bond in terms of a three-part cycle: The worse the injury, the greater need for care and security, and so the tighter the bond.

This dynamic operates with children under circumstances of intrafamilial trauma. The children grow more helpless and less competent. Typically living in relative social isolation and naïve to alternatives, the children continue to turn to their parents for help. In addition, children assume that their parents have their best interests in mind, despite the maltreatment. Frightened and confused, they are seeking safety and security; the provision of any shred of care, affection, or attention will draw them closer to their parents.

ABUSE-GENERATED RELATIONSHIP MODELS

One of the most alarming legacies of childhood abuse is repeated victimization (Coid et al., 2001; Desai, Arias, Thompson, & Basile, 2002). This includes relatively high rates of bullying and scapegoating experiences in childhood (e.g., Shipman, Zeman, Penza, & Champion, 2000), of sexual assaults and date rape among adolescent girls and young women (e.g., Gidycz, Hanson, & Layman, 1995; Krahe, Sheinberger-Olwig, Waizenhofer, & Koplin, 1999), of domestic violence among women (Messman & Long, 1996; Polusny & Follette, 1995), and of particularly high rates of repeated sexual assaults among women with significant psychiatric illness (Cloitre, Tardiff, Marzuk, Leon, & Portera, 1996).

Recent research has identified that multiple factors mediate the relationship between childhood abuse and adult revictimization, including dissociation (Zamir, Szepsenwol, Englund, & Simpson, 2018), substance misuse (Messman-Moore, Ward, & Zerubavel, 2013), depression, and expectations about sexual behaviors (Miron & Orcutt, 2014). We propose that these factors function as coping strategies for emotion dysregulation (distress management) and habitual modes of interpersonal relating that are actually based on a healthy impulse to engage in and maintain relationships. We propose that the affective and interpersonal strategies by which attachments develop are based on the experiences of abuse, which create substantial risk for revictimization. Engaging with other people and staying in relationships are learned behaviors. When significant learning experiences come from an abusive context or abusive people, the resulting interpersonal expectations and social behaviors are likely to have features that maintain abusive interpersonal dynamics. One goal of the present treatment is to help survivors maintain the desire for connection, but to change their behavioral patterns of relating and the people with whom they relate.

The treatment uses the notion of a "relationship model," derived from the work of John Bowlby and other attachment theorists, as an explanatory construct for understanding how healthy impulses go wrong. The identification of relationship models within an attachment model is theoretically very important, because it provides a value-neutral explanation of revictimization within the context of general principles of interpersonal behavior.

SOME ASPECTS OF ATTACHMENT THEORY

Bowlby (1969) and others have suggested that several biologically based mechanisms support the propensity to maintain closeness to the available caregiver and function to maximize survival. Their nature and complexity are in accord with the point at which they emerge during the course of behavioral, cognitive, and affective development. One mechanism is the development of "relationship models." These models, sometimes also called "interpersonal schemas," have been described as information-organizing cognitive–affective structures that, based on experience, specify and anticipate the contingencies for maintaining relatedness to the caregivers (Safran, 1990a, 1990b; Safran & Segal, 1990). Multiple models develop through time, based on differing interpersonal events of consequence with different important people. Relationship models are also amenable to revision as a result of changing circumstances. There is some evidence, however, that the first and oldest of relationship models, formed within the context of attachment relationships, play a central role in shaping future thoughts, feelings, and behaviors in the interpersonal domain (see Cicchetti & Toth, 2015; Doyle & Cicchetti, 2017).

Among the earliest and prototypical models are those pertaining to specific behaviors that will elicit the approach or proximity of a caregiver. Under advantageous circumstances, this proximity yields a response of care and concern. In turn, the caregiver experiences the expression of care elicited by the child as intrinsically satisfying. However, the relationship model that emerges in an abusive caregiving setting will deviate from this proposed dynamic of mutual satisfaction. For example, in a physically assaultive home, proximity—a condition for care—may also elicit physical assault. Thus care and physical assault become paired. In sexually abusive homes, proximity can elicit sexual activity. Such contingency experiences, whatever their particulars, may lead to the following models of interpersonal relatedness: "To be interpersonally engaged means to be abused" and "Abuse is a way to be connected."

THE SELF-FULFILLING NATURE OF RELATIONSHIP MODELS

Because relationship models are assumed to be the underlying templates that guide future expectations and behaviors, it is easy to see how negative patterns set down in childhood can guide one toward repeating activities that are maladaptive in adulthood. The model suggests that reliance on past experiences to anticipate the future is a typically adaptive strategy for living, and that the resultant tendency to repeat one's history is normative. Indeed, for those who have had positive attachment experiences, the self-fulfilling aspect of models works to their advantage: Expectations of positive regard tend to elicit positive responses. For survivors of abuse, however, reliance on past experiences means reliance on deviant patterns of relating. This tends to lead the survivors to function in social environments in ways that elicit similar deviant patterns, or to find that abuse-adapted patterns for relating are no longer effective in healthier social contexts.

The first time we observed this principle in action with disastrous results concerned a case of a female soldier in the Army who had been sexually assaulted by a fellow soldier. The two had been romantically involved. When the woman decided to break off the relationship, her boyfriend responded with rage and physically assaulted her. He also threatened to make her life miserable for the duration of their time on the base. Fearful of continued physical reprisal from him, she bought groceries and sundries from the post exchange and brought them to him at his barracks. His response was one of outrage: He sexually assaulted her and enlisted the help of a bunkmate in this act, which was repeated several times. During this woman's first visit at our clinic, the interviewer asked, in a gentle, supportive, but curious way, why she had gone to the boyfriend's barracks. She answered with surprise, "Why, this is what I knew to do when I got beat." It had always worked to save her from trouble before. The child of severely abusive parents, this woman had learned that the most effective way to appease her brawling parents was to take over household tasks—to go for groceries, do the cooking, and clean the house.

The woman was acting in a way that was intended to protect herself. However, the actions that had previously worked well now, in a changed environment, failed her; in fact, they contributed to the repetition of an old scenario she was trying to escape. The rules guiding effective living in an abusive environment needed to be changed, now that she had left it.

DIMENSIONS OF ABUSE-RELATED RELATIONSHIP MODELS

Our empirical inquiry (see Cloitre, Cohen, & Scarvalone, 2002a) into the general characteristics of abuse-related relationship models has been derived from a well-established system of categorizing types of self–other interactions (Kiesler, 1983; Leary, 1957). It is a model intended to capture the full range of potential interpersonal interactions as based on two independent dimensions that are assumed to be present in all human interactions: an affective/affiliative dimension (warm to cold) and a control dimension (high to low). We compared the interpersonal expectations of women with histories of childhood abuse, women with childhood abuse and adult revictimization experiences, and women who had never experienced abuse or other forms of interpersonal victimization. When asked to recall the responses of their caregivers to them in a variety of emotional and social circumstances, the survivors described their caregivers as predominantly cold—and, among those survivors with repeated victimizations in adult life, cold and highly controlling. In contrast, the never-abused group reported their caregivers' reactions to them as warm and responsive to their situation and as respectful of their autonomy.

When asked to think about an important person in their lives now (e.g., their current best friend), the most common type of interpersonal attitude and behavior expected was, for each of the study groups, a match to the type described for the caregiver. The group who had never experienced trauma had the largest number (60%) of women who expected those in their current lives to behave in ways similar to their caregivers—that is, as warm, responsive, and open to them, and as willing to follow their lead. In contrast, the majority of those with abuse histories described their current relationships as cold, and their significant others as emotionally unresponsive, controlling, and domineering. The self-fulfilling prophecy thus appeared to operate among both the traumatized and the nontraumatized respondents, with the only difference between the groups being the particulars of their life experiences and expectations.

These results are consistent with relational models of behavior, which describe generalization from predominant relationship models as a basic human cognitive–affective tendency. It also supports our analysis of revictimization as a consequence of a general principle of functioning, rather than as a pathological behavior associated with survivors of abuse. Still, the implications for the two groups differ. Among those who are not traumatized, routine model-driven actions may be an effective strategy for living, as the expectation for positive interactions creates a bias toward positive outcomes. In contrast, survivors of trauma are burdened with the necessity of recognizing and changing their patterns of relating if they are to improve their functioning and escape their traumatic past.

WHEN THE PROTECTOR FAILS TO PROTECT

Most epidemiological studies of childhood abuse (see Finkelhor, 1994; Russell, 1983; Wyatt, Loeb, Solis, & Carmona, 1999) indicate that sexual abuse is most often perpetrated by males in caregiving roles or positions of authority. Still, we know from the theory and research of Bowlby and other attachment specialists that the capacity for relatedness is modifiable, and that the presence of "even just one" positive care figure can produce a "protective shield" around a child and mediate negative outcomes (Lieberman & Amaya-Jackson, 2005). This leads to the question of the role of the mother or other critical caregivers in a child's system of care as a factor mediating or contributing to the child's immediate or long-term outcome. The topic is remarkably complex (Tener & Murphy, 2015). For example, research on disclosure of abuse suggests that telling a mother or someone else with power to intervene about the abuse is not related to symptom status in either the short or long term (e.g., Blieberg, 2000; Wyatt, Guthrie, & Notgrass, 1992). Disclosure may be positive only when the telling leads to a protective and supportive response. Responses of agitation, denial, and even upheaval in the family system may negate any benefit that might accrue (see Alaggia, 2002; Heriot, 1996). Similarly, disclosure to friends or social community leads to negative as well as positive impact on the survivor (Andalibi, Haimson, De Choudhury, & Forte, 2016).

Among survivors of abuse who seek treatment, we have found either that they have typically experienced abuse from multiple caregivers, or that nonabusing caregivers are neglectful, are absent, or simply deny or avoid recognition of the abuse. In our study (Cloitre et al., 2002a), sexual abuse was perpetrated most often by a male family member (88%), and abuse of some kind (physical, verbal, or sexual) by the mother was reported in half of the sample. The characterizations of the paternal and maternal caregivers did not differ: Both father and mother figures were reported as either cold and distant or cold and controlling, and there were no significant discrepancies between the abuse characteristics and relationship models for the two types of figures.

Research on the topic of the parent who is a witness to abuse rather than an active agent of it suggests that passivity in the face of abuse is itself harmful as a form of betrayal of trust, or what is now called "betrayal trauma" (Platt & Freyd, 2015). Indeed, our clinical experience suggests that the failure of a parent to care for and safeguard a child appears to have its own specific impact on the interpersonal beliefs and attitudes of survivors (e.g., "When I am in trouble, I know I need to take care of things myself"). This is most salient in clients' narratives about a passive or neglectful parent figure who turns a blind eye to the presence of physical or sexual abuse in the home. Anger and a sense of betrayal are directed toward the parent who did not intervene: the father who silently watched the mother batter their children, or the mother who denied the sexual intrusions of the father, stepfather, or boyfriend.

Steven Gold (2000) makes the important point that the significant impact of a parent who is a passive bystander is often overlooked:

> It is not unusual to hear therapists voice the conviction that resentment directed toward non-offending parents of others who did not prevent or stop the abuse is undeserved, or represents displaced hostility that, in actuality, is related to the perpetrator. This follows logically from a trauma model framework which assumes that the abuse itself is cardinal in its impact. However, this viewpoint negates a child's fundamental need to be valued and cherished enough to be protected, supported, and affirmed, particularly by parental figures and other caretakers . . . the anger toward non-offending parties may also reflect the fact that failing to stop the abuse was just one of the myriad of ways in which parents and other caregivers abrogated their responsibilities to nurture, validate, and safeguard the client in childhood. (p. 31)

Consistent with this perspective, we view the parent who neglects a child as representing a variation of a disturbed attachment relationship. The primary function of the attachment relationship is to ensure the safety of the child. The absence of this simple but essential dimension from the child's relationship with the parent/caregiver is an instance of a separate and independent psychological trauma. An attachment compromised by neglect, inconsistency, or hostility/distance also has a significant impact on a child's capacity to manage abuse, even when the abuse is not perpetrated by the primary caregiver; indeed, it may create vulnerability to sexual abuse by other adults in the child's larger system of care (see Chapter 3).

SUMMARY AND IMPLICATIONS FOR TREATMENT

The overriding theme of this chapter has been the impact of abuse on the capacity for interpersonal relatedness when abuse is perpetrated by a primary caregiver. We have articulated the outcome of this experience through the shorthand of the relationship model "To be connected means to be abused." This shorthand refers to the tendency of survivors' relationships to consist of victim–perpetrator bonds and dynamics. These dynamics are expressed directly in repeated abusive relationships (e.g., date rape, domestic violence) and high rates of revictimization. They are also reflected in chronic and pervasive problems with intimacy: Suspicion, anger, and mistrust erode relationships, leading to patterns of relationships that are short-lived or end badly.

We have also suggested that a sense of self develops in the context of relationships to others. When abuse occurs, both the sense of self and the capacity for relating are disturbed. So feelings of self-love and compassion are in part the results of having been loved and protected, and the capacity to love someone is related to one's own capacity to feel lovable and loving. Feelings of security are instilled by trust-inspiring caregivers, and these in turn allow risk taking in relationships.

All these ideas are realized in the treatment in a practical way through the notion of the "relationship model." The relationship model is a conceptual tool with a specific structure and is included in many of the interventions in our treatment program. During STAIR, therapists and clients work to identify problematic relationship models. These are often variations of "To be attached means to be abused," and, once organized, they reveal and clarify deep-seated beliefs involving feelings and themes of fear, despair, shame, and grief. The models articulate negative beliefs about self and expectations of others, which limit the range of perceptions the clients can have of themselves and of experiences with others. Alternative models and associated experiential exercises are proposed. These alternative models become the basis for exploring, testing, and practicing alternative ways of relating to others and experiencing new personal possibilities.

Relationship model analysis is part of both STAIR and Narrative Therapy and creates a conceptual bridge between the two modules. During the narrative work, therapists and clients identify the core relationship models embedded in the clients' narratives. The abuse-related models embedded in these narratives are contrasted with the newly emerging models that have been proposed in STAIR. This contrast reminds the clients that the old narratives represent contingencies for living that belong to the past and need not be continued in the present. The new models represent the opportunity for living in the present and ideas for shaping a possible future. This contrast helps move clients from a view of themselves as victims with limited options, to a sense of themselves as adults with new resources, new choices, and new ways to think through and plan for the future.

CHAPTER 3

Development in the Context of Deprivation

> Growing up in an abusive household is like
> learning to run under water.
> —AUGUSTEN BURROUGHS (2003)

The context in which a child who is chronically maltreated lives is directly contrary to the kind of environment required for healthy development. The child strives to develop in a setting that lacks the essential resources needed to support growth. The treatment presented in this book is based on the understanding that the reduction, loss, or absence of normative social experiences is a critical feature of chronic childhood trauma, equivalent to and potentially more powerful than the acute traumatic events themselves. The first component of our treatment program provides the opportunity for survivors of childhood abuse and other interpersonal trauma to explore and systematically address specific social and emotional difficulties that have a negative impact on their functioning, future opportunities, and quality of life. The goal of this treatment component is to help survivors, whose progress was interrupted when resources for appropriate learning were deficient or unavailable, develop emotional and social competencies.

Most people who have experienced trauma, or know someone who has, understand the potent psychological effects such events can have. The successful management of both daily tasks and major life challenges results from having specific emotional and social skills. These abilities include how to know what one feels, communicate those feelings effectively to others, solve problems effectively, recognize the value of practical and emotional social support, and know how to recruit such support when needed. All of these skills grow and are elaborated and reinforced during the childhood years of physical, cognitive, emotional, and behavioral development. Adults who experience trauma but have learned these skills earlier in life can capitalize on them for their posttraumatic healing. The intrusion of trauma and the context of an abusive home in childhood, though, can compromise the development of these skills. We describe below the specific developmental disturbances that have been documented among people who have experienced childhood abuse. Tracing these problems to their origin has helped us understand the particular competencies often compromised by abuse, which in turn has allowed us to formulate a program with interventions and activities to address them.

The compromised competencies can have pernicious effects on abused persons' confidence, particularly in trusting their perceptions and judgments about themselves and about others. They second-guess their own emotional reactions, fearing (sometimes accurately) that they have damaged or disturbed "emotion sensors." Because their learning experiences have deviated from ideal ones, survivors of abuse also often second-guess their appraisals of situations and the motives of others. Fundamentally, at a very deep level, they do trust neither themselves nor others.

One overarching theme in the treatment we have developed for adult survivors is facilitating the rebirth and growth of their confidence in themselves. This confidence generates the freedom to engage effectively and fluidly in day-to-day life, and the belief that they can respond effectively to future hardships.

CHILDHOOD TRAUMA INTERRUPTS DEVELOPMENT

Intrafamilial trauma during childhood creates a burden that both distracts from and distorts the achievement of typical developmental goals in the childhood and adolescent years. A highly traumatized childhood often involves putting energies into strategies for maximizing physical and psychological survival. In the case of childhood sexual and physical abuse, such strategies are often physical activities that reduce the risk of exposure to the assaults, or psychological strategies such as numbing, denial, dissociation, or distorting the meaning of the events when physical escape is not possible. A significant literature exists on the psychological mechanisms children use for coping with chronic intrafamilial abuse (e.g., Shapiro, Kaplow, Amaya-Jackson, & Dodge, 2012). These mechanisms, while possibly adaptive at the time, often divert energies away from fulfilling normative developmental milestones. In contrast, in adulthood, the long-standing consequences of this deprivation and diverted energies continue and can even become more apparent.

Emotional and Sensory Development

Sexual or physical abuse disturbs the development of a coherent and integrated experience of the body. This disturbance occurs, in part, because the immature body of the child is overwhelmed by the unmodulated, uncontrolled, and undifferentiated sensations of arousal that occur during sexual and/or physical abuse. Perhaps more important is that children are almost always abused by parents or other caregivers, and abusive caregivers fail in the fundamental tasks of guiding children in modulating arousal. An effective caregiver modulates a child's emotional arousal by providing appropriate doses of soothing and stimulating activities (Stern, 1985). Doing so does not just maximize comfort and security; it facilitates the child's learning of how to self-soothe and to orient selectively to either the internal or external environment. This learning, in turn, contributes to the accumulation of additional experiences of discrimination and categorization—between self and other, as well as across different kinds of emotions and emotional exchanges (see Gergely & Watson, 1996; Nichols, Gergely, & Fonagy, 2001).

Through a caregiver's nonverbal behavior (e.g., tone of voice) and later through language, the learning of self-soothing and affective discrimination expands. For example, parents ideally contribute to healthy emotional development in their children by accurately labeling feelings the children express. A mother might say to a distressed child, "You're upset because you missed seeing your friend today." This statement gives a label to a feeling, describes the experience, and ideally explains the source of the feeling. A typical report from an adult survivor of childhood abuse describes a scene in which a parent slaps a child and follows the slapping by stating, "That did not hurt." The child experiences a discrepancy between the internal experience and the label. From such events, abused children often experience confusion, distrust of their sensory perceptions, and a limited capacity to describe and accurately differentiate their feeling states.

Furthermore, abusive caregivers are poor guides to emotional modulation because they have limited emotion regulation skills themselves. Parents of abused children are significantly more likely to have histories of drug and alcohol problems, substantial mood disturbance, legal trouble and jail time, psychiatric hospitalizations, and fewer mental health services despite need (Hien & Honeyman, 2000; Sheridan, 1995; Baumann & Kolko, 2002; Haskett, Smith Scott, & Ward, 2004; Kaplan, Sunday, Labruna, Pelcovitz, & Salzinger, 2009; Stith et al., 2009). Such parents are poor role models for "learning by observation." The things their children learn are unlikely to be behaviors and attitudes that lead to effective emotion regulation. Instead, what abused children observe are the relative absence of emotion regulation and the negative consequences of this absence—such as a deteriorating family environment, acrimony in the family, legal difficulties, hospitalizations, and substance-related problems.

Poor affect regulation development in abused children is behaviorally evident as early as the toddler and preschool years (e.g., Cicchetti & White, 1990; Shields & Cicchetti, 1998). For instance, early maltreatment, including both sexual and physical abuse, corresponds to high levels of negativity and anger in toddlers and lack of self-control in preschoolers (Erickson, Egeland, & Pianta, 1989). In the preteen and adolescent years, those with abuse histories are much more likely to engage in impulsive behaviors, including sexual and drug-related activities and reactive aggression (Lipschitz et al., 1999a, 1999b; Lipschitz, Rasmusson, Anyan, Comwell, & Southwick, 2000; Kilpatrick et al., 2003).

In adulthood, difficulty with emotion regulation is one of the primary reasons for seeking mental health treatment (Levitt & Cloitre, 2005). Several researchers have identified these individuals' central clinical concern as problems with modulating feeling states. Some researchers describe this clinical population as "emotion-phobic" (van der Kolk, 1996) or even "alexithymic" (Frewen, Dozois, Neufeld, & Lanius, 2008); others note significantly higher levels of hostility and anxiety compared to other clinical samples (Zlotnick et al., 1996), as well as chronic problems with mental health, suicidality, and medical conditions (Maniglio, 2009; Norman et al., 2012).

In sum, survivors of childhood abuse learn the negative consequences of unregulated feelings. What they do not learn is that emotional states can be experienced and managed in healthy ways, can support relationships, and can even be a source of pleasure. Our treatment helps address this deficit by introducing the feeling and management of emotions as positive, life-affirming, and essential to the human experience.

Cognitive Development: Experience of Agency

As early as 12 months of age, infants demonstrate an understanding of cause and effect, and integral to this development is the experience of the self as an agent or cause of events (see Gergely, 2004; Gergely & Watson, 1996). Caregivers play a critical role in this process. They draw out connections of cause and effect through movement and tone of voice, as well as by directing children's attention to changes in the environment that are causally related. In particular, a caregiver draws attention to a child's actions as having consequences in the environment, including effects on that most important and powerful figure of the social world—the caregiver. The child's sense of agency develops and is reinforced by the caregiver's directed responses to the child's expressed needs. The child then experiences the self as an initiator of action or the cause of an effect (i.e., "If I do something, I get a response").

Conversely, caregivers diminish children's sense of agency by remaining unaware of, neglecting, or ignoring the children's signals. In fact, caregivers who sexually or physically abuse children nullify their experience of agency, since these events occur without regard to their needs or despite their protests. An abused child is given the message "You don't exist," or "You don't count."

One experiences a sense of agency in part through expressions of feelings. A child cries, and the caregiver responds; the child stops crying, and the caregiver changes behavior once again. This type of experience contributes to the child's sense of ownership of and authority over feelings. It also encourages feelings to become valid reference points from which the child initiates action with some expectation of success. Abuse by caregivers includes the experience of having feelings ignored, dismissed, or distorted. Survivors of chronic abuse often not only lack awareness of their own feelings, but also do not expect their feelings to matter or to be respected. They do not use their feelings as points of initiative or justification for action (e.g., "I feel this way, so I better do something about it").

One also creates a sense of agency and vitality through interpersonal experiences—particularly experiences of recognition by a caregiver who follows and supports the child's actions and responds to them in a complementary fashion (Ammaniti & Ferrari, 2013). These responses happen in play or in "mirroring-back" behaviors, where the caregiver reflects back, amplifies, or elaborates the child's actions. For example, a child may slap a hand down on a table, creating a smacking sound and look to the caregiver, who responds by clapping with delight, simultaneously reinforcing and praising this instance of cause ("My hand clapping . . .") and effect (". . . makes noise"). Abuse undercuts the self-enhancing power of experiences in which the child takes initiative and experiences reinforcement by the caregiver. Abuse expresses the perpetrator's power to initiate and sustain action, regardless of the child's will or intention. The overwhelming power of the abusive caregiver denies the child's recognition of the self as an autonomous being and may convey to the child that they are merely an extension of the abuser's will. As adults, survivors often report feelings of incipient "annihilation" during experiences of conflict. These experiences may result from lapses in recognizing the survivors' agency and transgressions of their autonomy during their abusive childhoods. It is thus not surprising that survivors often struggle with power dynamics in interpersonal relationships—sometimes feeling overly dependent and passive, and other times exerting great effort to be "in control" of a relationship.

Our program's interventions help clients become better at identifying feeling states and more effective in interpersonal relationships. In many of the Part III chapters describing Module I of the treatment (STAIR; see Chapters 10–19), the therapist instructions include not only how to teach clients a particular skill, but also what attitude to bring to the task and how to give feedback, so that the therapist acknowledges clients' experiences in a supportive, affirming, and accepting manner. We hope that in this emotionally corrective process, clients will not stop at learning just the names of their feelings. Ideally, they will also experience themselves as the authors of their own feelings and agents of their meaning and use, and in the task of adopting new interpersonal positions and responses with the therapist, they will experience "being seen" by the therapist as persons in their own right.

Interpersonal Development

As implied above, interpersonal development incorporates the management of feelings in relation to others. Interpersonal development across childhood and adolescence involves at least three key tasks: learning and implementing interpersonal models for establishing relationships; learning how to resolve conflicts; and developing flexibility in interpersonal expectations and behaviors. As adults, individuals can revisit these tasks and update their understanding based on new experiences.

Relationships with parents, other caregivers, and siblings establish the first models for relating to others, which act as templates to guide expectations and prime behaviors in developing relationships that follow. These first relationships are essentially characterized by the reliance of the young on elders, particularly primary caregivers, as sources of safety and nurturance. This domain of development is that of Bowlby's (1969) attachment system. Over many years of clinical practice and research, we have found that people abused in childhood adopt interpersonal frameworks ("internal working models," as Bowlby called them) assuming that relationships are essentially adversarial or unreliable, that vulnerability leads to exploitation, and that intimacy leads to pain and betrayal. These assumptions become most evident in important relationships and at times of conflict, when differences between individuals can threaten a survivor's sense of safety, control, autonomy, and recognition of needs.

Social-observational studies of maltreated preschool and school-age children have found an association between abuse and maladaptive internal working models of attachment, particularly for those associated with disorganized attachment (Carlson, Cicchetti, Barnett, & Braunwald, 1989; Main, Kaplan, & Cassidy, 1985; Solomon, George, & DeJong, 1995). In addition, such internal working models are associated with aggressive and fearful relationships with peers and externalizing symptoms in school-age children (e.g., Lyons-Ruth, Alpern, & Repacholi, 1993). Although empirical investigations of the role of specific internal working models and behavioral problems among children and youth with histories of abuse continue, the presence of interpersonal and social impairment among such children and youth is well established. Childhood victimization is associated with social behaviors such as peer rejection and bullying in the school years (Shields & Cicchetti, 1998; Schwartz & Proctor, 2000). Among adolescents, it is associated with increases in both aggression and social avoidance, as well as significant increases in criminal and delinquent behaviors and early sexual activity (Giaconia et al., 1995; Horowitz, Weine, & Jekel, 1995; Malmquist, 1986; Pynoos et al., 1987).

Experiences of early trauma, unfortunately, can continue to affect adult relationships, often at least partially through their impact on attachment and internal working models of self and others (McCarthy & Maughan, 2010; O'Dougherty Wright, Crawford, & Del Castillo, 2009; Ortigo, Westen, DeFife, & Bradley, 2013; Riggs, Cusimano, & Benson, 2011). Consistent with these observations, adult survivors of child abuse report significant interpersonal problems. In a large study of the effects of childhood physical and sexual abuse on adult women, 91% of the respondents described significant problems in relationships (van der Kolk, Roth, Pelcovitz, & Mandel, 1993). The most frequent difficulties were sensitivity to criticism, inability to hear other viewpoints, difficulty in standing up for themselves, and a tendency to quit jobs and relationships without negotiation. Our own research corroborates these findings: Among treatment-seeking women, the majority reported significant problems with intimacy, being too controlling, acting too submissive, being inappropriately assertive, and being insufficiently sociable (Cloitre, Scarvalone, & Difede, 1997; see also Chapter 4).

Taken together, these studies suggest that central difficulties arise in emotion-laden situations involving the management of conflict or balance of power in relationships. These behaviors are quite understandable when viewed from the perspective of the lessons learned about relationships in abusive homes. The hypersensitivity to conflict reported by adult survivors is a legacy of these experiences. The interpersonal schemas that survivors of abuse most frequently rely on reflect expectations that others will respond to them in a cold, controlling, hostile, or distant manner (Cloitre et al., 2002a). Their current behaviors may, in part, be preemptive maneuvers to avoid the negative outcomes they expect—or, alternatively, reenactments of familiar interpersonal roles or dynamics.

The interpersonal schema study discussed in Chapter 2 (Cloitre et al., 2002a) also found that the schemas of survivors of abuse tended to be limited in number and fairly rigidly applied across different people and different situations. For example, when these survivors reviewed hypothetical situations in which the behavior of another person was most likely to be warm and inviting, the survivors still responded with expectations of the other to be cold, hostile, and controlling. In addition, the particular relationship with the significant other did not seem to make a difference to the expectations of the survivors: They responded to situations involving a mother, father, significant other, and best friend in the same way, regardless of the expectations' appropriateness for each person in these situations.

Part of the normative trajectory of social development involves refining and adding interpersonal rules for relating, depending on the contexts and the individuals involved. For example, children learn when aggressive behaviors are appropriate (e.g., on the basketball court) and when they are not (e.g., with a toddler sibling); when obedience to an adult is appropriate (e.g., with a teacher in the classroom) and when it is not (e.g., with a stranger in an elevator); and so on. Parents help guide this knowledge with specific teaching about diversity in interpersonal expectations within and beyond the family, and they provide children with opportunities to explore their emotional reactions as they experience these different interpersonal scenarios. Our data suggest that this sensitivity and flexibility does not fully develop among treatment-seeking survivors of abuse. Moreover, rigidly applying a negative schema–behavior dynamic to new situations only serves to reinforce further the "truth" ascribed to the negative expectations. The self-reinforcing nature of these self-fulfilling prophecies impedes natural healing that may occur with safe others (Wachtel, 1997).

The treatment program we have developed and refined over the years includes a strong emphasis on expanding the number and kind of interpersonal schemas a client has available for consideration. We propose models of interaction (schemas) in which the client's overtures of warmth can be met with warmth, and overtures of appropriate assertiveness can be met with recognition and respect. Furthermore, we ground the development of these new models in an understanding of their context-sensitive nature—that is, the concept that different types of relationships (work vs. romantic vs. parenting relationships) require different expectations and/or different actions and reactions. Key goals of the treatment involve helping the client develop alternative ways of relating to people from those that emerge from abuse, and develop sensitivity to the diversity in the nature, character, and context of relationships.

INFLUENCE OF POOR CAREGIVING ON ABUSE FROM OUTSIDE THE HOME

Individuals who as children experience sexual and physical abuse from outside the family often still have primary caregivers who have impaired parenting skills and do not or cannot effectively respond to their attachment mandates. This situation is clearly the case when caregivers perpetrate the abuse. However, clinical experience and substantial research suggest that individuals who come to treatment with a history of abuse outside the home often report parenting or environmental difficulties that predate or are separate from the abuse experiences. Many researchers (e.g., Conte, Wolfe, & Smith, 1989; Gold, 2000; Finkelhor, 1980; Gapen et al., 2011) have suggested or found that beyond the fact of abuse itself, the presence of problematic attachment, disturbed parenting behaviors, and certain types of living environments and neighborhoods create vulnerability to abuse and other types of interpersonal trauma outside the home. On top of that, their presence in general makes recovery more difficult.

A substantial literature indicates that problematic attachment can occur with a nonabusing parent because the parent is too preoccupied, distant, or distressed to be reliably responsive and nurturing (van IJzendoorn & Kroonenberg, 1988). Other factors might include the presence of psychiatric problems, including ones stemming from the caregiver's own trauma history, such as PTSD or depression. The intergenerational transmission of trauma is, sadly, a well-known phenomenon (Bowers & Yehuda, 2016), and it corresponds with Bowlby's (1984) original ideas of how familial violence affects both the attachment and caregiving systems. Environmental pressures, such as limited income and poor health or injury among family members, may also contribute to the caregiver's difficulties. In such circumstances, the caregiver may not have the ability to provide a sufficient, reliable "secure base" for the child, effective guidance in developing socioemotional competencies, protection from significant threats, or the nurturing capacity to help the child recover from traumas.

In addition, the families of survivors of abuse have certain similar characteristics, regardless of whether the abuse occurs inside or outside the home. Studies have found shared characteristics of high levels of rigid behavioral control, and low degrees of adaptive emotional expressiveness (Nash, Hulsey, Sexton, Harralson, & Lambert, 1993; Ray, Jackson, & Townsley, 1991). Translated into terms of daily living, relationships among family members tend to be circumscribed within specific roles (often of an authoritarian nature), with little flexibility or range in expression of emotions. Moreover, the experience of limited and rigid relationship roles tends to limit children's ability to learn the subtle but critical life lesson that different people and different contexts require diverse ways of relating and different sets of interpersonal expectations.

In his book on treating survivors of child abuse, Gold (2000) suggested that the typical characteristics of these families are likely to produce or mold expectations and behaviors in children that leave them vulnerable to exploitation and abuse by predatory adults. For example, a caregiving environment that is cold, unaffectionate, and unresponsive to a child's emotional needs may result in a child who hungers for warmth, recognition, support, and validation. Such a child may be particularly vulnerable to the attentions, blandishments, and flattery of a child molester. In DSM-5 (American Psychiatric Association, 2013), disinhibited social engagement disorder is a sad and extreme but prime example of this outcome of indiscriminate trust after severe neglect or abuse. Family systems that are high in authoritarian and controlling behaviors toward children may elicit and shape interpersonal styles marked by either unassertiveness, deference, and appeasement, or "trigger-finger" rebelliousness and disengagement. The first adaptation creates an interpersonal dynamic that allows a child to be easily intimated and coerced by demanding adults. The second creates dynamics of power struggles, isolation, and even bullying of others. A family that is low in organization, cohesion, and expressiveness can reduce clarity about appropriate adult behaviors and reduced confidence in perceptions of threatening behavior, further reducing the likelihood of a child's avoiding or escaping from adult intrusions (see Gold, 2000). These patterns, sadly, often continue into adulthood.

In our own clinic population, parents are the primary perpetrators of abuse in 80% of cases (e.g., Cloitre, Miranda, Stovall-McClough, & Han, 2005). The remainder of clients (those whose abuse has been perpetrated by someone outside the family) report some form of maltreatment in the home—typically verbal abuse and neglect, or some combination. These statistics and our own clinical experiences have led us to surmise that negative family contexts, and cold and distant relationships with caregivers in particular, are associated with victimization outside the home. Children seek out and sometimes feel comfort by the presence of alternative caregivers—in the form of babysitters, coaches, teachers, religious or community leaders, or more generally individuals who make themselves available to give attention to neglected children. Some of these adults are good models and lead the survivor to a path of resilience. Not all of these adults, however, are trustworthy, which can lead to continuing instances of trauma inflicted by other adults who were not the original perpetrators.

In fact, larger trends on attachment are not encouraging about the likelihood of moving toward security without direct clinical intervention. In a cross-cultural meta-analysis of infant attachment styles (van IJzendoorn & Kroonenberg, 1988), studies reported an average of 65% of infants as securely attached, 21% as insecure-avoidant, and 14% as insecure-resistant. For adults in the general population, a large review by Bakermans-Kranenburg and van IJzendoorn (2009) found that 58% had an adult attachment style described as secure, 23% as dismissing, 19% as preoccupied, and 18% as unresolved due to loss or trauma (roughly akin to disorganized attachment in infants). Another meta-analytic review of adults in the general population confirmed this trend toward less attachment security over time (Konrath, Chopik, Hsing, & O'Brien, 2014). To address these trends at both individual and larger societal levels, we must consider the role of trauma at all stages of life.

In short, a survivor of childhood abuse has almost always grown up in a family that provides little in the way of skills necessary for adaptive or even adequate socioemotional functioning. The difficulties in emotion management and interpersonal relating described above are known to emanate most often from intrafamilial abuse, but they can also serve as risk factors creating vulnerability to further abuse and additional types of trauma outside the home even into adult years

SUMMARY AND IMPLICATIONS FOR TREATMENT

In this chapter, we have noted that difficulties in emotion regulation and interpersonal relationships are present at each developmental stage among those abused in childhood, including toddlerhood, the middle years, and adolescence. These data suggest that the similar problems seen in adults who come to treatment may have their origins in the developmental years. They also suggest the entrenched and enduring nature of such difficulties.

One critical goal of the STAIR component of our treatment program is that in providing clients with a clear analysis of their problems, we also respond to gaps in their socioemotional competence by building and reinforcing emotion management and social skills. In this way, we conceptualize the treatment as the provision or rehabilitation of basic and life-enhancing social and emotional competencies with which survivors of abuse often have not had sufficient experience.

One cannot overstate the role of poor emotion management in interpersonal difficulties. The reasons for interpersonal conflict are often readily identified as emerging from distressing and unmanageable feelings. Anger leads to words that are later regretted, to strained or ruptured friendships, and sometimes to physical violence. Feelings of anger, hurt, sadness, and humiliation are often out of proportion to the events that elicited them. Even when justified, such feelings may be expressed in ways that do not lead to a satisfactory conclusion or a sustained human connection. Alternatively, emerging positive feelings such as happiness, pride, or pleasure can also feel overwhelming or destabilizing to survivors' ability to function in a situation; the survivors may have learned to distrust positive emotions or feel that these are followed by punishment or despair. The consequence may be that all emotionally intense feelings and situations are avoided, leading to social withdrawal and isolation.

We have developed STAIR with the view that individuals communicate powerfully if not primarily through the expression of feelings—verbal or nonverbal, intended or not. As a result, the interpersonal interventions exercise clients' awareness of and behaviors related to the expression and modulation of emotion. Simply put, feelings are often about others or about the self in relation to others. STAIR aims to help clients develop an expanded repertoire of emotional expressiveness so that they can more effectively and adaptively communicate with others. As adults, they can awaken to their own inner power and agency, and can heal from the wounds that have kept them impaired for so long.

PART II

Foundations of Treatment

CHAPTER 4

Treatment Rationale

Psychotherapy is not really about symptom relief;
its essential purpose is to help a person function
in the world, and ideally, to function well.
—ANONYMOUS

There are now several effective treatments for PTSD, with those identified as most effective focusing predominantly on confronting and working through the traumatic memories (International Society for Traumatic Stress Studies [ISTSS], 2019a). However, we propose that although such treatments are effective in treating PTSD related to past traumatic exposure, they do not optimally address clients' range of problems in the present, which interfere with effective functioning. The clients who come to mental health services seek help for long-standing and pervasive problems in emotion management, in relationships, and with work and career goals. Often clients acknowledge the presence of PTSD symptoms when asked, but do not identify them as their primary reason for entering therapy. Others report that they have hit "rock bottom" and can no longer deny the level of functional impairment in their lives. These clients are often unemployed or working at jobs far lower than their education or abilities warrant, have lost one or more jobs per year for several years, and/or have intimate partners who are threatening to leave or who have already left.

These problems are not random assortments of life difficulties. Rather, they reflect specific and enduring disturbances in emotion regulation and interpersonal capacities. The common sources of these problems in daily functioning appear to be limited emotional and social competencies. Such clients do not know how to manage emotional distress effectively or deal with fluctuations in negative emotional states. Similarly, the many failed relationships they report are often the results of limited expectations that relationships can involve mutual trust, respect, and support; of limited skills in creating such relationships (including the selection of appropriate partners and friends); and of limited skills to maintain healthy relationships and end unhealthy ones. All these limited competencies are consistent with the characteristics of "derailed development" as predicted by attachment theory.

Our goal in developing STAIR Narrative Therapy has been to create a treatment program that supports recovery from the full range of difficulties resulting from exposure to interpersonal trauma in the developmental years. The formulation and testing of STAIR Narrative Therapy have been based on evidence emerging from the clinical, trauma, and developmental literatures. This chapter describes the systematic empirical investigation that yielded the rationale for this treatment, as well as the empirical outcomes of the treatment. Our goal in providing this historical review is to allow readers to critically evaluate what makes sense to them, and to effectively adapt the strategies described in Part III of the book in an informed way that is governed by the particular needs of individual survivors.

WHAT DO CLIENTS REALLY WANT?

The first empirical effort in our initiative was to determine what survivors were most concerned about and what they wanted from treatment. In order to answer these central questions, members of our clinical staff conducted a phone survey of 98 survivors of childhood abuse (Levitt & Cloitre, 2005). As Table 4.1 shows, they found that the most common reasons for seeking services were interpersonal problems (67%), emotion management problems (31%), and symptoms of PTSD (59%).

It clearly did not seem sufficient to provide treatment for the one set of problems for which we had effective therapy—the PTSD symptoms. Nor did we wish to assume that targeting this one problem set would automatically resolve the other two. Indeed, this seemed unlikely. Certainly, PTSD symptoms do disrupt functioning; for example, sexual intimacy can be quickly disturbed when certain touches or sensations are traumatic reminders of sexual abuse and trigger flashbacks, acute physical discomfort, and fear. But many of the observed emotion management and relationship problems seemed to derive from other aspects of the experience of childhood trauma—particularly disturbances in emotional and social learning experiences. We wished to provide treatment that would directly respond to the most evident needs expressed by survivors of childhood abuse beyond those of PTSD.

WHAT MAKES CLIENTS' DAILY FUNCTIONING SO DIFFICULT?

We were committed to the ideal that good treatment requires attending to our clients' complaints and taking seriously the factors having the greatest apparent impact on their

TABLE 4.1. Reasons for Seeking Treatment

Reason for seeking treatment	Percent
Interpersonal problems	67%
PTSD symptoms (any)	59%
Mood problems	31%
Other kinds of problems	
Suicide attempt (lifetime)	45%
Substance abuse	33%

Note. n = 98. Data from Levitt and Cloitre (2005).

day-to-day functioning. Indeed, one traditional way to identify the presence of significant mental health problems is to assess the impact of the problem on a client's functional status. DSM-5, for example, the current compendium of formally accepted psychiatric disorders in the United States, stipulates that functional impairment must be associated with symptoms as a requirement for a psychiatric diagnosis (American Psychiatric Association, 2013).

In an effort to organize a trauma treatment around functional capacity, our team analyzed the data from the face-to-face assessment interviews of the first consecutive 167 treatment-seeking women with a history of childhood abuse. We conducted a series of statistical analyses to determine to what extent each of the three symptom sets—PTSD symptoms, emotion management problems, and interpersonal problems—made a significant contribution to functional impairment. The importance of this task was reinforced by the treatment literature on the mood and anxiety disorders, which indicated that while various treatments were successful in resolving disorder-specific symptoms, significant functional impairment persisted (e.g., Agosti & Stewart, 1998; Coryell et al., 1993; Rapaport, Endicott, & Clary, 2002; Serretti et al., 1999). These data were taken to suggest that functional impairment not only is a direct result of diagnostically defined symptoms, but also has other sources.

The results of our own investigation indicated that functional impairment was related not only to PTSD symptoms, but also to emotion regulation difficulties and interpersonal problems (see Cloitre, Miranda, Stovall-McClough, & Han, 2005). Analyses were conducted conservatively, maximizing the opportunity for PTSD symptoms to be associated with functional status. To the extent that PTSD and the other symptom sets shared the predictive weighting of functional status, the predictive weighting was credited only to PTSD. After age and other sociodemographic factors were accounted for, PTSD symptoms accounted for 20% of functional impairment. Emotion regulation difficulties alone accounted for an additional 4%, and interpersonal problems for yet another 18% of functional impairment (see Figure 4.1). In sum, emotion regulation and interpersonal difficulties combined accounted for essentially the same proportion of functional impairment as PTSD symptoms did. This finding indicated an important organizing framework for developing the treatment. In order to improve functional outcomes among survivors of trauma, we needed a treatment that focused on ameliorating emotion regulation and interpersonal difficulties as well as PTSD symptoms.

The extent to which these three factors together accounted for functional impairment—a total of 42% of impairment—gave us confidence in advocating for resources of time, money, and effort to be spent on developing an intervention that would directly address each of these domains. To put the relative explanatory power of this model into perspective, we considered the translation of statistical results into funding resources for physical health problems salient to women. For example, researchers' investigations into the causes of breast cancer have found that family history accounts for 10% of breast cancer cases (e.g., Yang et al., 1998) and is a significant predictor of the disease. Several million dollars have been spent disseminating this information and providing prevention and early detection interventions. By comparison, our research described above has captured a much greater proportion of the sources of the problem of interest. In this context, the results of the study become more compelling.

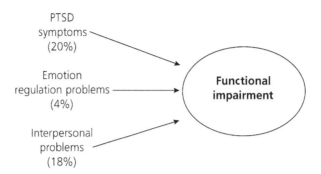

FIGURE 4.1. Contributions of PTSD symptoms, emotion regulation difficulties, and interpersonal problems to functional impairment. Data from Cloitre, Miranda, Stovall-McClough, and Han (2005).

THE CENTRAL ROLE OF EMOTION REGULATION IN HEALTHY LIVING

Having both good emotion regulation and interpersonal skills contribute to good overall functioning. However, it is becoming clear that emotion regulation capacities constitute a powerful driving force that influences the quality of relationships and has an independent influence on several aspects of life, including general mental health and physical health. Developmental studies have found that children's emotion regulation capacity, measured by their ability to manage intense feelings, predicted *2 years later* how well liked they were by schoolmates, how many friends they had, and how well adjusted they were rated by their teachers (Parke, McDowell, Cladis, & Leidy, 2006). Several studies among young adults have shown a similar sequential relationship between emotion regulation capacities and multiple positive outcomes.

For example, Westphal, Seivert, and Bonnano (2010) evaluated the emotion regulation skills of college students in their first year of college, and found a significant relationship between strength of emotion regulation during that first year and good outcomes 3 years later regarding general mental health, physical health, ability to accomplish goals, ability to cope, and quality of social interactions. Moreover, the benefits of good (vs. less good) emotion regulation skills in the first year was most pronounced among those who had experienced high levels of stressors during the intervening years, suggesting that emotion regulation contributes to resilience in difficult times. "Good" emotion regulation comprises several characteristics, among which include being able to express authentic feelings rather than hide or suppress them (Bonnano et al., 2007), being able to express emotions in a way that is appropriate to the social circumstances, and being able to express positive emotions and share positive feelings (Papa & Bonanno, 2008).

All of the data cited above support our decision to organize the STAIR module in such a way that emotion regulation skills precede and lay the foundations for interpersonal skills development. Emotion regulation skills support effective relationship functioning in several ways. The first sessions of STAIR focus on cultivating awareness of feelings, which can lead to more authentic and appropriate self-expression to others, while emotion regulation skills allow an individual to choose when and how to share their feelings. Interwoven through most of these sessions is attention to experiencing positive emotions and engaging in pleasurable or playful experiences. These types of experiences help create a sense of life as worth living, balancing out the pain that many have experienced; can help individuals experience living in the here and now; and, importantly, can act as "glue" strengthening bonds in relationships.

DIFFERENCES BETWEEN CHILDHOOD AND ADULTHOOD TRAUMA

In the previous chapters, we have described scenarios suggesting that limitations in emotion management and interpersonal functioning may have their source in disturbed attachment and social learning. The salience of these early life experiences, their influence on adolescent and later-life emotional and social development, and their cumulative impact over decades suggest that such problems may be more severe among survivors of childhood abuse than among those who have experienced their first significant trauma in adulthood. The most compelling support for this view are studies that have directly compared individuals with childhood-onset trauma to those with adult-onset trauma (e.g., survivors of rape or natural disasters) and found that survivors of childhood abuse are consistently more troubled, particularly in the domains of affect modulation, anger management, and interpersonal relationships (Cloitre et al., 1997; van der Kolk et al., 1993; Zlotnick et al., 1996).

Results from a study by Cloitre et al. (1997) found that while rates of PTSD were similar among women who sought treatment for rape in adulthood versus childhood sexual abuse (70% vs. 75%, respectively), those with childhood sexual abuse as their primary concern reported significantly more affect regulation difficulties and had more significant interpersonal problem profiles. Both groups were compared on these measures to a comparison group of women of similar age and background who reported that they had never been traumatized and had no psychiatric diagnoses (see Figures 4.2 and 4.3). Women who had experienced childhood abuse showed much more pronounced impairments in affect regulation than either of the other groups, while the survivors of rape looked rather similar to the nontraumatized comparison group. Affect regulation was measured by alexithymia (difficulty identifying and labeling feelings) and dissociation. We also included lifetime suicide attempts, following Marsha Linehan's (1993) notion that suicide attempts often represent a way of controlling and ending chronic and acute states of extreme distress—a commonly endorsed reason for suicide attempts among survivors of childhood abuse (see Brodsky, Cloitre, & Dulit, 1995).

A similar pattern was obtained in the assessment of interpersonal problems: Survivors of childhood abuse consistently reported more problems than did either the survivors of rape or the nontraumatized comparison group. Of particular interest was that the survivors of childhood abuse reported significant problems in all aspects of interpersonal functioning examined in the study, including problems with being assertive and with being submissive, as well as problems with being *too* controlling. Although these may look like contradictory endorsements, our work with this population suggests that the reporting is accurate and reflects these survivors' overall problems in managing power dynamics in relationships:

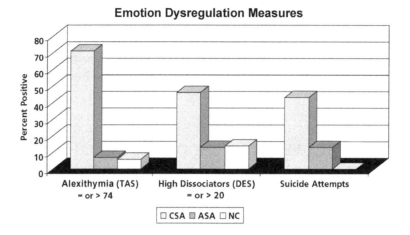

FIGURE 4.2. Differential impact of trauma on emotion regulation depending on life stage: Emotion regulation. TAS, Toronto Alexithymia Scale; DES, Dissociative Experience Scale; CSA, group with childhood sexual abuse; ASA, group with adulthood sexual abuse (rape); NC, never-abused comparison group. Data from Cloitre, Scarvalone, and Difede (1997).

being insufficiently assertive in situations that call for a self-protective response, but being too controlling in situations that do not warrant it. Sustained problems in managing power and control in relationships are also consistent with our research on relationship models among survivors of childhood abuse, which indicated a rigidity in perceptions of power dynamics, reflected in a predominant model of human relationships that is based on control (Cloitre et al., 2002a; see also Chapter 2).

Evidence highlighting the differences between individuals who have experienced a single-event trauma and those who have been exposed to sustained, chronic, or multiple types of trauma, particularly during the developmental years, has been accumulating over

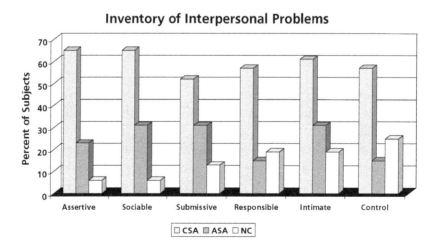

FIGURE 4.3. Differential impact of trauma on interpersonal problems depending on life stage: Interpersonal functioning. CSA, ASA, and NC as in Figure 4.2. Data from Cloitre et al. (1997).

the past decade. A greater number of traumatic exposures is typically associated with more severe and a greater number and types of problems, regardless of whether traumatic exposures began in childhood or adulthood. However, when exposure to repeated or chronic trauma occurs in childhood, the risk for an increasing diversity of problems is greater than when trauma occurs in adulthood (Cloitre et al., 2009), and this is particularly true of problems in the area of emotion regulation, interpersonal functioning, and self-concept (Briere & Rickards, 2007). The evidence that has accumulated is sufficiently substantial that there is now a formal diagnosis of CPTSD in ICD-11 (WHO, 2018), as mentioned in Chapter 1. This new diagnosis explicitly acknowledges the presence of disturbances in emotion regulation, negative self-concept, and interpersonal difficulties as defined symptom domains, in addition to those traditionally viewed as belonging to PTSD (e.g., nightmares and reexperiencing symptoms). We expect that STAIR Narrative Therapy will be effective for survivors of trauma in general, but may be particularly beneficial to those with CPTSD. More details about this diagnosis and its assessment are provided in Chapter 9.

MATCHING INVERVENTIONS TO TARGETED PROBLEMS

The CPTSD diagnosis and the presence of reliable and valid measures will help identify individuals who might be a good match for this treatment. Box 4.1 lists a broad range of symptoms that can result from childhood abuse and neglect. Not all of them are explicitly included in the CPTSD diagnosis, but they are known consequences of childhood interpersonal trauma and can act as "flags" for consideration of whether a treatment such as STAIR Narrative Therapy might be of value.

Given that survivors of childhood interpersonal trauma frequently have both PTSD symptoms and other types of problems, we determined to develop two distinct modules of treatment. The first module of treatment focuses on the development of effective adaptive emotional expression, an enhanced repertoire of interpersonal behaviors, and an improved sense of self. The immediate goals of this module, STAIR, are to vigorously and directly address problems in affect and interpersonal domains, and to help clients improve their self-esteem and capacity for functioning in daily life.

The second module focuses on the emotional processing of the trauma and is intended to resolve the PTSD symptoms. The therapy with the most evidence for the resolution of PTSD symptoms is prolonged exposure (ISTSS, 2019a). We modified prolonged exposure and adapted it to the needs of survivors of abuse (Cloitre, Koenen, Cohen, & Han, 2002b), and we developed a series of interventions wrapped around it called Narrative Therapy. The sequencing of STAIR before Narrative Therapy is intended to enhance the effective use of narrative work through the development of a good relationship with the therapist and through improvement in emotion management skills.

A summary of the interventions for STAIR Narrative Therapy is provided in Box 4.2. Detailed descriptions of the reasoning behind the selection and development of the specific interventions for STAIR and for Narrative Therapy are provided in the next two chapters (Chapters 5 and 6, respectively).

BOX 4.1

General Symptom Profile of Survivors
of Childhood Abuse and Neglect

PTSD SYMPTOMS

- *Reexperiencing symptoms:* Nightmares, flashbacks, intrusive thoughts/images related to the trauma
- *Avoidance and emotional numbing:* Avoidance of thoughts, people, places, or activities that produce reminders of the trauma; loss of interest in things that used to give pleasure; feeling numb
- *Hyperarousal:* Difficulties with sleeping and concentration; exaggerated startle response; irritability

EMOTION REGULATION PROBLEMS

- Emotional reactivity (fear, rage, avoidance) to minor stimuli
- Difficulty in "getting back to baseline" or restoring sense of equilibrium
- Tendency to dissociate under stressful circumstances
- Engaging in self-injurious behaviors (self-cutting, burning)
- Coping through excessive use of alcohol or other substances

NEGATIVE SELF-CONCEPT

- Feeling worthless
- Feeling like a failure
- Feeling "invisible" to others
- Feeling to blame when things go wrong
- Chronic sense of shame or guilt

INTERPERSONAL PROBLEMS

- Difficulty with intimacy and trust
- Sensitivity to criticism
- Inability to hear other viewpoints
- Difficulty in standing up for oneself
- Tendency to quit jobs and relationships without negotiation
- History of repeated victimization (e.g., domestic violence, date rape)

BOX 4.2

Overview of STAIR Narrative Therapy with Symptom Targets

MODULE I: SKILLS TRAINING
FOR AFFECTIVE AND INTERPERSONAL REGULATION (STAIR)

Symptom Targets: Emotion Regulation Difficulties, Interpersonal Problems

- *Emotional awareness:* Identification and labeling of feelings, self-monitoring of emotions; skill of Focused Breathing
- *Emotion regulation:* Psychoeducation on emotional responding in physiological, cognitive, and behavioral channels; skills of Focused Breathing, Thought Shifting, Positive Imagery, Positive Self-Statements; working with fear and anger, pleasurable activities, and positive emotions
- *Emotionally engaged living:* Goal identification; distress tolerance; skill of Pros and Cons; using positive feelings as guide to decision making and action; acceptance of negative emotions

Symptom Targets: Changing Relationship Patterns

- Understanding the self-fulfilling nature of trauma-based relationship models
- Taking an opportunity to change; revising interpersonal expectations
- Agency in relationships; focus on appropriate assertiveness, changing relationship models; practice in role play
- Flexibility in relationships; focus on maintaining respect for self and others, regardless of power balance
- Increase ability to be close to others and stay close despite conflict
- Review of improvements in skills; importance of self-compassion and of practicing it even in difficult times; skill of Self-Compassion Meditation

MODULE II: NARRATIVE THERAPY

Symptom Targets: PTSD Symptoms, Emotion Regulation Difficulties, Interpersonal Problems

- Narratives of traumatic memories with focus on fear, shame, loss
- Using postnarrative grounding strategies to orient client to present
- Identifying relationship models in narratives; contrasting trauma-generated models with alternative and more positive and flexible models based in STAIR work
- Practicing new behaviors, exercising emotional awareness, contrasting the present with the past, redirecting attention and energy to the present

WHY A SEQUENTIAL TREATMENT?

One might consider that skills training could be provided simultaneously with more traditional trauma-focused work, or, alternatively, after the trauma-processing work has been done. But we decided against this for several reasons.

Giving Clients Time to Learn

First, the empirical literature has indicated that when coping interventions and trauma processing were conducted simultaneously within a session, the benefits of the treatment were no greater than the benefits of treatments that just provided one or the other component of treatment. Some treatment researchers (e.g., Foa, Dancu, Hembree, Jaycox, & Meadows, 1999) have suggested that the limits on effectiveness may be the result of "information overload," in which clients cannot absorb the substantial amount of information provided in the limited time typically available for treatment.

Preparing Clients for Narrative Work

Second, we wanted our clients to have a maximal skill set with which to engage in the narrative work. Although many survivors of trauma are able to discuss their traumatic memories in a sustained and emotionally connected way, there is a substantial clinical literature reporting concern that survivors of childhood abuse may come to the work with fewer resources than are optimal for the emotional effort involved. For example, Steven Gold (2000) comments:

> Adults with adequate adaptive skills that have been disrupted by the impact of a single traumatic event enter treatment with an array of personal capacities (e.g., coping skills, judgment, a sense of efficacy) and environmental resources (e.g., social support, financial reserves) that are nowhere near as likely to be accessible to survivors of extended child abuse. The former group, therefore, even if they are highly symptomatic individually, has firmly rooted strength to draw upon that greatly bolster their capacity to face and productively process trauma. The latter group, however, lacks these advantages. Consequently, even the routine stressors of daily adult living tax their capacities and can be destabilizing. It is unreasonable to expect that they are in a substantially better position to productively assimilate traumatic experiences than when those events originally occurred. (p. 58)

Indeed, several clinical reports indicate that clients who have compromised capacities in tolerating distress and difficulty securing good relationships with their therapists may experience symptom exacerbation during the processing involved in exposure-based trauma treatment or drop out of the therapy (Larsen, Stirman, Smith, & Resick, 2016; McDonagh et al., 2005; Scott & Stradling, 1997; Tarrier et al., 1999), or may not obtain as good an outcome as clients without such problems (Foa, Riggs, Massie, & Yarczower, 1995b; Ford, Fisher, & Larson, 1997; Ford & Kidd, 1998; Funari, Piekarski, & Sherwood, 1991).

The implementation of STAIR prior to trauma processing was intended to address these concerns. Data from a study by Cloitre and colleagues (2010), described in the next section, identify the benefits of sequencing treatment in reducing symptom exacerbation and drop-out rates from treatment.

Respecting the Power of the Therapeutic Alliance

Lastly, we were sensitive to the importance of the therapeutic relationship. The working relationship between the therapist and client is the single most important factor predicting good treatment outcome (Horvath & Symonds, 1991; Martin, Garske, & Davis, 2000). This is a remarkably durable phenomenon. It has been observed in interpersonal (e.g., Krupnick et al., 1996), cognitive (e.g., Muran, Segal, Samstag, & Crawford, 1994), and dynamic (e.g., Stiles, Agnew-Davis, Hardy, Barkman, & Shapiro, 1998; Yeomans et al., 1994) therapies, as well as in a range of therapy targets (e.g., alleviating depression or anxiety, treating alcohol or other substance use).

It is clearly important for the therapist and client to develop a rapport and good understanding of each other before engaging in the emotional processing of the trauma. Many trauma therapists have alluded to the difficulties any survivor of interpersonal trauma has in tolerating the interpersonal nature of therapy—that is, "the [need] to . . . trust another person with his or her pain" (Turner, McFarlane, & van der Kolk, 1996, p. 538; see also Pearlman & Saakvitne, 1995; Lindy, 1996). This difficulty would seem further exacerbated in exposure-based treatments, which require a significant and sustained amount of emotional disclosure. We wished to maximize the client's sense of being understood and supported by the therapist—and, just as important, the therapist's and client's mutual recognition that the therapist is familiar with the client's strengths and vulnerabilities and will attend to them accordingly during the narrative work.

BENEFITS OF A SEQUENTIAL TREATMENT

Our research with STAIR Narrative Therapy has supported the notion that a sequential treatment with skills preceding narrative work contributes to good outcome in trauma processing. The first randomized controlled trial (RCT) compared STAIR Narrative Therapy to a minimal-attention wait-list condition (Cloitre et al., 2002b). We found that two characteristics of STAIR significantly influenced the success of the narrative work: a strong and positive therapeutic alliance, and the development of emotion regulation skills. While STAIR produced many positive and important improvements for the clients, such as decreases in anxiety and depression, only improvement in negative mood regulation and the strength of the therapeutic relationship were significantly related to PTSD reduction in the narrative phase (see Table 4.2). These results suggested the relative specificity of the resources that support effective processing work, as well as the value of organizing the treatment components in a chronological fashion.

TABLE 4.2. STAIR Predictors of Success in Narrative Therapy as Measured by PTSD Symptom Reduction

Phase I variables	R	p	Effect size[a]
Therapeutic alliance (WAI)	–.64	.03	Large
Improved negative mood regulation (NMR)	–.47	.03	Medium–large

Note. WAI, Working Alliance Inventory; NMR, Generalized Expectancy for Negative Mood Regulation Scale. Data from Cloitre, Koenen, Cohen, and Han (2002b).
[a]An effect size of 0.10 is small; one of 0.30 is medium; one of 0.50 is large.

Treatment Outcome

The RCT described above was an initial study to assess whether STAIR Narrative Therapy was an efficacious treatment as compared to a wait list. As expected, the treatment resulted in significant reductions in PTSD symptoms. In addition, there were significant improvements in experiencing and modulating emotions (as measured by increased ability to identify and name feelings, improved mood regulation, and decreased dissociation). There was also significant and sustained reduction in three central mood disturbances: anxiety, anger, and depression. Lastly, interpersonal problems were significantly reduced, and role functioning in home, work, and social domains was improved. All of these gains were maintained at 3- and 9-month follow-ups.

A second RCT was completed, which compared STAIR Narrative Therapy to each of its component parts (Cloitre et al., 2010). In one comparison condition, STAIR was replaced with supportive counseling (SC) plus Narrative Therapy to determine whether the active ingredients in STAIR (skills training) were contributing to overall good outcome and might have a positive impact on reducing dropout, as well as preventing the symptom worsening (increase in PTSD and dissociative symptoms) that sometimes occurs in trauma-focused treatment. In the second comparator, Narrative Therapy was replaced with SC to determine whether PTSD symptoms could be improved in the absence of trauma-focused work.

The results indicated that STAIR Narrative Therapy was superior to the SC plus Narrative Therapy condition in the reduction of PTSD diagnosis, while STAIR plus SC fell in the middle. A similar result was observed with self-reported PTSD symptoms: STAIR Narrative Therapy produced greater improvements than the SC plus Narrative Therapy condition and was superior to both treatment conditions in improving interpersonal problems. All treatments showed improvements in each of three main outcomes, and at the immediate posttreatment assessment, it looked as if the results of the three therapies did not differ substantially. However, at the 3-month outcome and then certainly by the 6-month follow-up, STAIR Narrative Therapy was superior on all three outcomes. (See Figures 4.4 through 4.6.)

We hypothesize that the combination of the narrative work and skills work was responsible for these findings. That is, the narrative work helped clients put their traumas in the

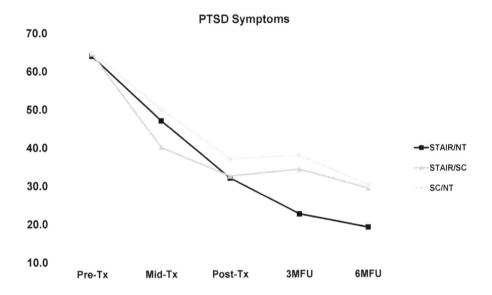

FIGURE 4.4. Reduction in PTSD symptoms (as assessed with the PTSD Symptom Scale Self-Report Version, or PSS-SR). STAIR/NT, STAIR Narrative Therapy; STAIR/SC, STAIR plus supportive counseling (SC); SC/NT, SC plus Narrative Therapy. Data from Cloitre et al. (2010).

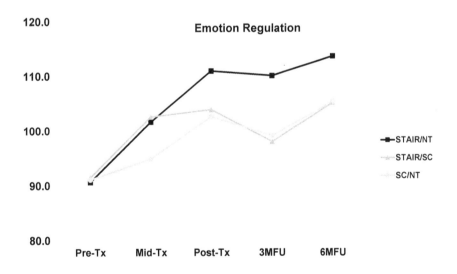

FIGURE 4.5. Improvement in emotion regulation (as assessed with the Generalized Expectancy for Negative Mood Regulation Scale). Abbreviations as in Figure 4.4. Data from Cloitre et al. (2010).

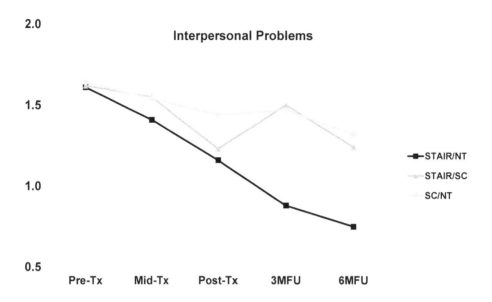

FIGURE 4.6. Reduction in interpersonal problems (as assessed with the Inventory of Interpersonal Problems). Abbreviations as in Figure 4.4. Data from Cloitre et al. (2010).

past where they belonged, while the skills allowed them to do better in daily living through improvements in relationships and functioning, which in turn reinforced the message from the narrative work that the trauma was indeed behind them.

Improving Completion Rates and Reducing Challenges of Trauma Processing

An important goal of the component study was to determine whether introducing skills training before narrative work would have a positive impact on some of the challenges of narrative work that can lead to dropout and increased symptoms. Indeed, the STAIR Narrative Therapy dropout rate was significantly lower than the SC plus Narrative Therapy dropout rate (15.2% vs. 39.4%). There were also significantly lower session-to-session PTSD symptoms during Narrative Therapy when it was preceded by STAIR than it was when not. A similar pattern, though not significant, occurred with the dissociative symptoms. (See Figures 4.7 and 4.8.)

Inspection of the graphs shows that the PTSD symptoms at the beginning of the narrative work (see Session 10) were almost as low when preceded by STAIR (line with squares at assessment points) as when there was no Narrative Therapy happening (line with triangles). This is in contrast with the condition where Narrative Therapy was not preceded by STAIR (line with round circles), in which there was a substantial increase in PTSD symptoms and dissociation. Overall, these results suggest that STAIR Narrative Therapy reduced distress during the very important process of telling about the trauma.

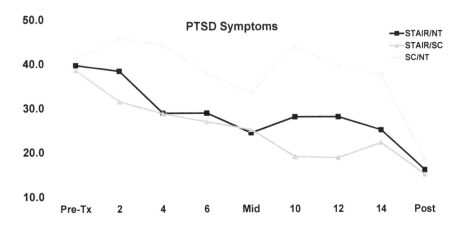

FIGURE 4.7. Session-by-session self-reported PTSD symptoms (as assessed with the PSS-SR). Abbreviations as in Figure 4.4. Data from Cloitre et al. (2010).

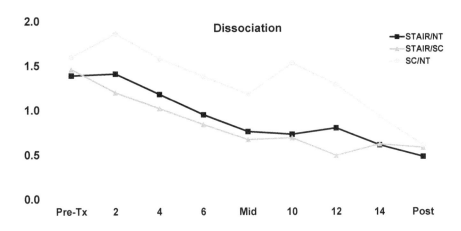

FIGURE 4.8. Session-by-session dissociation symptoms (as assessed with the Trauma Symptom Inventory's Dissociation scale). Abbreviations as in Figure 4.4. Data from Cloitre et al. (2010).

EXPERIENTIAL ASPECTS OF STAIR NARRATIVE THERAPY

As we spent time working with our clients, we came to appreciate an experiential aspect of sequencing skills training before the narrative work, for which we have no data but our own clinical observations. We noted that the skills work, in combination with a positive relationship with the therapist, provided the clients with increased confidence and perceptions of themselves as persons who were competent, well regarded, and esteemed. These new self-perceptions seemed to provide the clients with a way of thinking about themselves that made the confrontation of the past less difficult and overwhelming. The confidence in engaging in the narrative work seemed to come not only from the clients' awareness of their own capacity to manage the feelings the trauma memories engendered, but also from their knowledge that they were no longer exactly the persons they described in their narratives.

The narrative work requires going back to the past and telling about traumatic events with emotional depth and intensity. This process returns clients to their early life histories and often leads to a deeply felt awareness of the far-reaching influence these experiences have had on the trajectory of their lives. This seems more easily acknowledged when the clients have achieved some sense of distance from their past and from the more vulnerable persons they were then. From the position of present strength, the clients are able to feel compassion for the young persons they once were, and for the fear, pain, and disappointment they experienced then. They can also feel more respect for their current achievements both in and out of the therapy.

The completion of the narrative component in turn seems to strengthen the clients' appreciation for the present and their motivation to live well in it. During the narrative work, the clients grapple with the pain generated by the traumatic experiences; with this effort, their emotional lives are often deepened and enriched. The experience can lead to an increased capacity for openness in emotional experiencing and greater authentic connection with others. When clients complete the narrative work, they often return to STAIR skills practice with a deeper appreciation of the emotional and social benefits of this work. The STAIR module provides the clients with tools for behaving, thinking, and feeling in more positive and competent ways, and expanding their reach for positive relationships and self-awareness. The clearest indicator that narrative work has been successfully completed, as well as its greatest benefit, is that the clients "let go" of the past in favor of the present. Recovered survivors find the present a more interesting place to be—and, with the needed skills, a place where they can feel at home.

SUMMARY AND IMPLICATIONS FOR TREATMENT

This chapter has provided a systematic review of the empirical data that generated the formulation of the treatment described in this book—a treatment that includes interventions focused on affective and interpersonal problems particularly for survivors of interpersonal trauma, and that sequences treatment modules so that skills training precedes trauma-focused work. The chapter also identifies data from RCTs describing the benefits of a sequential treatment. These data are intended to give therapists a clear understanding of why they are providing the interventions in this program and the potential benefits of sequencing interventions. Being aware of these data can help therapists feel confident about the work they are doing and why. This information can also be shared with clients, to clarify the rationale for the treatment and to help the clients determine whether the treatment is a good match to their needs.

CHAPTER 5

Building Emotional and Social Resources
Overview of STAIR

Humans have the capacity for change and growth
through the entire life span.
—JEROME KAGAN (1980)

This chapter provides the rationale for the STAIR session topics and for their order. By conscious design, the session topics follow the human developmental trajectory in the maturation of emotional and social competencies, particularly as these competencies contribute to the growth of agency and connection with others. Agency, a sense of oneself as a source of action, originates in the ability to know what one feels and to use feelings as a guide to action. The expression of these feelings aids communication with others and, if effectively done, contributes to connection with them. Sustained connection requires the ability to express one's feelings in a way that can be understood by others and to endure certain amounts of distress in resolving conflict. It also requires the ability to balance self-interests with recognition of the interests of others. Flexibility in expectations of others, depending on their needs and the social context, allows one to have different kinds of relationships. Relationships can range from those with easy-going and fleeting acquaintances to those with long-term or lifelong partners and friends. Diverse kinds of relationships provide one with enriching experiences and resources for living. The STAIR treatment includes skills training in identifying feelings, managing and expressing emotions, enhancing assertiveness, managing power dynamics, optimizing levels of intimacy, and increasing flexibility in relationships, which all build on each other to create emotional and social resources. Lastly, STAIR highlights the importance of cultivating self-compassion through the learning process. Compassion itself may be one of the most important resources for living that exists, and it animates all of the skills and recovery processes described in this book.

The progression of emotional and social skills development described above is reflected in the order of the STAIR sessions. The first sessions address emotional awareness, emotion regulation, and effective emotion-informed planning and action. Session 2 begins with the task of identifying and labeling feeling states. Once feelings are named and their reality is affirmed, the sessions progress to the tasks of discriminating among feelings and communicating about them. The middle sessions (Sessions 3–5) introduce the critical skills of modulation of feelings, including the appropriate and effective expression of these feelings to others, as well as how to use information from feelings to make decisions about whether tolerating distress is worthwhile for larger personal goals and values. The next series of STAIR sessions (Sessions 6–9) makes the transition to matters of interpersonal functioning—in particular, the role of emotional experiencing and expression as central means of creating and maintaining healthy attachments. These include developing assertiveness skills and effectively managing power balances in relationships. These sessions highlight the importance of responding flexibly to a growing range of social circumstances, individuals, and experiences, but always with a sense of respect for oneself and others. Session 9 introduces what may be the most challenging task of those who have experienced interpersonal violence—namely, working toward, achieving, and maintaining healthy levels of intimacy and closeness with others. The final STAIR session (Session 10) explicitly discusses the concept of self-compassion, while reflecting on gains made thus far in their skill development.

The treatment proceeds from the very beginning with the therapist expressing and modeling an attitude of compassion and respect toward the client as they work toward their goals. In the final session, the importance of self-compassion is explicitly discussed as the client prepares either to make the transition to Narrative Therapy or to continue practicing skills on their own. Every person will fail to meet some goals and will experience relapses to problematic behavior at some point. Acceptance of these failures or limitations can paradoxically lead to greater ease in creating change and experiencing growth. Reactions to failures such as self-criticism and anger consume time and emotional energy that could otherwise be channeled into reassessment and change. For those going on to Narrative Therapy, an attitude of compassion for self and others will be helpful as the clients review painful and disappointing experiences.

Although the growth and maintenance of self-regulation capacities and self-compassion constitute a lifelong endeavor, the goal of STAIR is to help each client develop core emotional and social competencies that will provide a foundation for future efforts. Below, we describe the concepts and skills that are introduced in the STAIR sessions, and we provide descriptions and rationales for the specific interventions used to develop those skills. An at-a-glance, session-by-session summary is provided in Box 5.1.

EMOTIONAL COMPETENCIES

"Emotional competencies" are the abilities to identify, monitor, manage, and express emotions for specific functional or adaptive purposes. Chapters 2, 3, and 4 have described the developmental literature on children who have experienced maltreatment, as well as empirical assessments of adult survivors of childhood abuse. The research thus far indicates that many emotional competencies, particularly those influenced by experiences with

BOX 5.1

Building Emotional and Social Resources: Outline of STAIR Sessions (Module I)

Session	Content
Session 1	*The Resource of Hope: Introducing the Client to Treatment.* Treatment overview and goals; introduction to Focused Breathing.
Session 2	*The Resource of Feelings: Emotional Awareness.* Psychoeducation on the function of emotions and importance of emotional awareness. Introduction of Feelings Monitoring Form.
Session 3	*Emotion Regulation: Focus on the Body.* Review of healthy and unhealthy efforts to cope along the body channel. Introduction to skills of Basic Self-Care, Soothing the Senses, and Progressive Muscle Relaxation.
Session 4	*Emotion Regulation: Focus on Thoughts and Behavior.* Review of common healthy and unhealthy efforts to cope in the thought and behavior channels. Selection and practice of skills tailored to each client, which can include the Evidence Technique, Positive Imagery, Take a Break/Time Out, Opposite Action, Seek Support, and Plan Pleasurable Activities.
Session 5	*Emotionally Engaged Living.* Introduction of distress tolerance as an essential set of skills to encourage engaged and/or value-centered living. Introduction of Pros and Cons skill. Organization and practice of skills from all three channels to reach an identified valued goal.
Session 6	*Understanding Relationship Patterns.* Introduction of concept of relationships models as drivers of interpersonal habits. Examples of trauma-generated models are provided. Clients generate examples of their own relationship models.
Session 7	*Changing Relationship Patterns: Focus on Assertiveness.* Psychoeducation on effective assertiveness and basic personal rights; discussion of alternative relationship models; role plays requiring assertiveness; generation of alternative relationship models.
Session 8	*Changing Relationship Patterns: Managing Power and Maintaining Respect.* Psychoeducation on impact of trauma on experience of respect for self and others. Practice in being flexible regarding expectations and behaviors, depending on power balance in relationship. Practice of skills in acknowledging the needs, feelings, and beliefs of others.

(continued)

Session	Content
Session 9	*Changing Relationship Patterns: Increasing Closeness.* Review of different kind of relationship boundaries. Introduction of skills to increase closeness to others, such as skills for repairing a relationship after an argument and beginning a new relationship.
Session 10	*Self-Compassion and Summary of Skills Training.* Review of treatment progress. Reflection on role of self-compassion in recovery; introduction and practice of Self-Compassion Meditation. Discussion of next steps—either self-directed continued skills practice or transition to Narrative Therapy.

caregivers, are disturbed by maltreatment. These disturbances include difficulties in identification and labeling of feeling states, differentiation among different emotions, appropriate danger detection, effective strategies for managing and modifying feelings, and expression of feelings in social and interpersonal contexts. We have organized emotional competencies into three core skills: (1) emotional awareness; (2) emotion regulation; and (3) emotionally engaged living, with a focus on the pursuit of valued goals.

Emotional Awareness

Emotional awareness is a prerequisite to effective emotion modulation and effective living. Whether we are aware of our feelings or not, they guide our decision making and actions. They inform others, and indeed even ourselves, about who we are. Emotions have a powerful and pervasive influence in all aspects of living. Accordingly, awareness of our feelings is a first step toward self-knowledge, self-regulation, and self-direction. Awareness of our emotions allows us to modulate them in a more purposeful, direct, and mindful way than is possible when we attempt to avoid or suppress them, or when we simply experience them as a cascade of undifferentiated sensations. In addition, awareness of feelings gives us greater degrees of freedom in living. Realizing and naming what we are feeling opens up options— the option to modulate a feeling, as well as the options to change it, act on it, accept it, or let it go.

Identifying and labeling feeling states

The task of identifying and labeling feeling states has particular significance for survivors of childhood maltreatment. The social environment of a child who has experienced maltreatment is one in which the labeling of feeling is limited and, in regard to the maltreatment, either highly distorted or altogether absent. Because physical and sexual abuse incidents in particular are hidden from public view and knowledge, and are not typically topics of conversation in the social network, opportunities for correction or reanalysis of "victim blaming" or other distorted labeling is not easily available. In addition, the silence about the reality of the maltreatment in the home is inadvertently reinforced by the silence of the larger social environment. For the survivor, the absence of a descriptive language for a key life experience often leads to feelings of inauthenticity—and, worse, to an internalized vocabulary that is self-blaming ("You deserve what you are getting"), incongruent with the actual experience ("This was good for you in the end"), or full of denial ("Maybe it really didn't happen or was as bad as I remember"). As a result, survivors of childhood trauma are often at a great disadvantage in coming to terms with the impact of their trauma. Feelings arising from the maltreatment remain inaccurately named or even unnamed; moreover, the fear, anger, depression, and aggression related to the abuse are often not connected to the trauma, by the survivors or by anyone around them.

The first intervention in STAIR involves the systematic exploration of feelings—their names, their intensity, and the context in which they occur. This effort is intended to yield clarity about specific feelings, recognition of different kinds of feelings by reference to different events and experiences, and sustained awareness of the presence of feelings in daily life. The opportunity for survivors of interpersonal trauma to name their feelings and describe their emotional experiences is vital to the process of self-discovery and ongoing self-assessment. The naming of things is the first step in each client's discovery of an authentic personal voice. The ongoing expression and organization of feelings throughout the treatment are essential to the creation of a coherent narrative of the client's personal history.

Emotion Regulation

"Emotion regulation" refers to the capacity to modulate emotional reactions and expression. Persons who have problems in emotion regulation experience rapid and intense emotional reactions, with difficulty returning to baseline (Linehan, 1993; van der Kolk, 1996). Marsha Linehan was the first to label such disturbance in ability to manage emotions and to discuss it thoroughly as a problem that many clients bring into treatment. Linehan, a well-known psychologist, has worked many years with clients who present with chronic suicidality. She has observed that suicide attempts are often efforts to terminate either the pain of intense negative emotions as they are occurring in the moment, or the dread of the emotions' relentless and uncontrolled appearance in these clients' lives. Linehan has developed a program called Dialectical Behavior Therapy (DBT), which is shaped by the principle that treatment should provide clients with options for how they might choose to respond to an emotion or experience, rather than being simply carried away by it (Linehan, 1993). This principle is applied to both internal and interpersonal experiences. With this ground-breaking work, Linehan has oriented therapists and researchers to the importance of the study and treatment of emotion management difficulties.

Basic skills in emotion regulation

Difficulties in emotion regulation reflect disturbances in underlying sensory, cognitive, and behavioral systems, rather than problems with one specific type of emotional experience. The research literature has consistently identified the development of these three core coping systems across all ages—from the toddler years through adolescence into adulthood and old age—as contributing to effective emotion management. This literature thus suggests the relevance of these systems in the treatment of clients with emotion regulation difficulties, which are often seen in clients with a history of early and repeated trauma. It also has provided us with a heuristic for organizing the emotion skills training. The three systems, or what we call "channels," of emotional experiencing are described in this treatment as follows: (1) the "body channel," which includes interventions related to physical/ physiological management (e.g., deep breathing, exercise); (2) the "thought channel," which includes cognitive strategies (e.g., self-statements, reframing of upsetting events, attentional control); and (3) the "behavior channel," which includes behavioral efforts at management and/or social support (e.g., taking a time out, calling friends for help, talking with others about feelings).

A client's coping strategies are assessed within each channel, with the goals of strengthening and elaborating existing strategies and training the client in new ones. The overall goal is to create a well-integrated set of coping strategies, so that physical sensations, thoughts, and behaviors influence one another and work together toward well-modulated emotional experiences.

Modulating negative feelings

Fear and anger are often the emotions to which management skills are first applied. The reason for this order of priority is that fear and anger tend to be highly prevalent among survivors of interpersonal trauma and also create immediate and obvious problems in their day-to-day functioning, particularly in monitoring personal safety (inaccurate threat perceptions) and avoiding interpersonal ruptures (anger). The application of emotion regulation skills to feelings like shame and grief tends to occur later in the treatment, as these feelings often first emerge when the trauma history is explored in the development of the life narrative. The emotion regulation skills described above effectively result in reduced difficulties in managing day-to-day experiences; better management of difficult feelings such as anxiety, anger, and depression; and reduction in dissociation. They also contribute, through their application during the trauma processing, to a reduction of PTSD symptoms (e.g., hyperarousal, reexperiencing).

Accepting and modulating positive feelings

Although it seems counterintuitive, the experience of positive emotions can be painful to survivors of interpersonal trauma. Positive feelings are unfamiliar, and their unfamiliarity creates unease. Positive emotions are also threatening because they create the risk of new ways of being "out of control" or may lead to disappointment if the survivors cannot sustain the emotion. Accordingly, clients are introduced to the notion that emotion regulation includes the ability to modulate not only negative feelings, but positive ones. The clients are encouraged to engage in simple pleasures and to practice modulation skills to keep their feelings within bounds that are comfortable to them. The immediate consequence of introducing small pleasures is the satisfaction that the ability to confront and modulate negative feelings carries with it the reward of experiencing positive feelings as well.

However, more importantly, this exercise conveys the true meaning of emotion regulation. It refers not only to the abilities to self-soothe and to reduce negative feeling states, but also to the abilities to raise and sustain positive feelings. It is the capacity to create an "emotional comfort zone" that is neither too intensely high nor too low, and as such allows a person to function, learn, and stay connected with the environment.

Emotionally Engaged Living: Toward the Pursuit of Valued Goals

For many survivors, the only alternatives to living painful and out-of-control lives are emotional avoidance, social withdrawal, limited pleasure in daily activities, and severely limited actualization of their potential. Such clients are encouraged to identify positive goals for themselves—to articulate their desires and wishes, and to consider ways in which they may realize these. Leaving the familiarity of an avoidant lifestyle requires support from the therapist and the development of several skills—making sound judgments about which goals to attempt, pacing goals, and weighing the costs and benefits of any new experience. The concept of "distress tolerance" and the skills associated with it (see Linehan, 1993, 2015) are introduced and practiced repeatedly in the treatment. This process is intended to provide survivors with the skills necessary to control the pace of their gradual reconnection to the emotional and social world.

Distress tolerance

Once survivors are able to identify and manage emotional reactions, they can allow themselves the experience of (well-managed) distressing feelings that serve an important purpose or goal, or are simply an inevitable aspects of certain life experiences. For example, if a client wants to get a job, a job interview is likely, and so is some anxiety. If a client wants to get married or have a long-term relationship, the anxious feelings associated with first meeting someone, coming to know this person, and risking rejection are all inevitable. Interventions for distress tolerance are introduced, so that the client can successfully achieve certain valued goals. This skill also involves weighing a goal against the likely distress it will generate, evaluating one's capacity to manage the distress, and deciding to adjust or delay the goal.

Accepting positive feelings as guides to planning and action

Clients are also introduced to the utility of positive feelings in identifying valued goals. Positive feelings about certain activities, people, or projects are identified as legitimate and valuable guides in decision making. This work builds on the previous interventions in which the clients are introduced to small pleasures and practice in modulating and enjoying positive feelings. In this next step, the clients are introduced to ways to enhance quality of life by engaging in "approach behaviors" to life experiences that are positive or goals that provide intrinsic pleasure.

SOCIAL COMPETENCIES

The majority of survivors of interpersonal trauma are motivated to come to treatment because of self-identified problems in relationships. Inevitably, problems in relationships include problems with emotions: feeling too much, feeling too little, or having a feeling poorly matched with the demands of the situation. Thus the skills developed in the first sessions are directly relevant to improving relationships. In addition, problems in relationships for survivors of child maltreatment emerge from maltreatment-generated interpersonal expectations and patterns of behaviors that are not adaptive in the clients' adult worlds. Problems with starting and maintaining relationships, sustained conflict in intimate relationships, consistent feedback from friends about approach–avoidance patterns of relating, failures in appropriate assertiveness in the workplace or among family members, anger fits in front of their children, and fears of handing down the legacy of their maltreatment to their children all often have their source in trauma-related beliefs and behaviors and are all reasons for entering into treatment.

Identifying Trauma-Related Relationship Models

Chapter 2 on attachment has proposed that working models of relationships, or what we more simply call "relationship models," emerge from experiences with early caregivers or other significant people and are important because they influence the selection, character, and dynamics of relationships that follow. In STAIR, we have adapted the concept of relationship models to define and explore the negative patterns of relating that dominate clients' lives and over which they feel little control. Our research has indicated that the relationship models of survivors of interpersonal trauma represent "self and other" in victim–perpetrator patterns, where the expected contingencies for relationships, abstracted from their particulars, reflect formulations such as "To be attached means to be abused" and "Abuse is one way of attaching."

One of the central tasks in the STAIR treatment is to identify trauma-related relationship models and describe them as the result of a healthy impulse, attachment, which has gone astray because of the malicious environmental context in which the rules for attachment were derived. Both therapists' empathy for their clients and the clients' eventual empathy for themselves are based on the understanding that schemas constitute a built-in "ambush" for survivors in the form of the self-fulfilling prophecies.

Relationship models have a positive function, in that they allow the anticipation of future events on the principle that "The future will be much like the past" or "The past predicts the future." People's behaviors are guided by behaviors that prepare them for *expected* rather than *all possible* outcomes. Such preparations often help create the expected outcomes and close out other possibilities. This process is adaptive among people who have positive expectations or who live in unchanging, stable environments. However, it leads to significant negative consequences for survivors of childhood maltreatment, who have left the maltreating environment but still (and rather inevitably) maintain expectations generated in that environment. For example, a young woman from an abusive family who has developed the understanding that interpersonal relatedness is contingent on sexual behavior is more likely to engage in or initiate sexual activity as a way of emotionally connecting to others, whether or not she is interested in sex and whether or not her partner is actually expecting sex.

We view the identification of relationship models as a critical aspect of treatment. It represents the distillation of central beliefs about self and others that provide clarity about the clients' motivations for action. The clients' behaviors become understandable to themselves and to their therapists. In addition, the sources of the models as they derive from past experience can be explored, and the accuracy of their application to the present can be empathetically challenged. Alternative ways of thinking about self and other can be constructed.

Changing Relationship Models

As just introduced, the second and more difficult aspect of the treatment is to begin proposing and adopting alternative relationship models—ones suggesting that the "glue" of relationships can be found in other behaviors and emotions, such as mutual respect, positive regard, and affection. This work requires moving a client from the realm of expected outcomes to that of imagined outcomes. It requires the therapist to provide guidance, suggestions, and proposals that will prompt the client to think in ways that personal history has not supported and that essentially require an act of imagination and even faith. The therapist is in some ways "reparenting" the client in the possibilities of interpersonal relationships and creating alternative working models—through their own relationship, as well as by explicitly proposing alternative formulations of relationships and putting them to an experiential test.

This effort is supported by each client's inner desire for a more fulfilling life, one not riddled with all of the ongoing negative effects of trauma. The maladaptive nature of trauma-generated relationship models is evident when clients' goals for themselves are disrupted by the activation of these models. For instance, a client may become aware that anger at a past abusive authority figure is getting in the way of forming current relationships with other authority figures. Or expectations of sexual exploitation based on sexual abuse may be creating disturbance and upheaval in current romantic relationships. The discrepancies between feelings/beliefs from the past and current goals sometimes become evident through painful real-world experiences. The treatment attempts to avoid this type of "hard-knocks" learning by using the therapy sessions as a setting in which to practice, via role plays, what clients can feel, say, and do in situations related to goal implementation. Through therapist feedback and the clients' own monitoring of feelings and statements, the clients can revise behaviors and feelings in ways that are more in accord with their identified goals, and can practice these new behaviors in sessions. A session is, in essence, a place to explore—to "try on" and assimilate different attitudes, behaviors, and words that match desired goals for self-expression and effective communication with others.

In STAIR, relationship models are structured as simple contingency statements (i.e., "If . . . , then . . . , " or "When . . . , then . . ."). Clients find that these formulations are easy to use and effectively elicit their implicit interpersonal contingency beliefs. Typical examples include "If I do as I am told, I will be loved," or "When I ask for my needs to be met, then I am rejected." This approach allows therapists to distill clients' "core beliefs" about self and others, to provoke clients' thoughts and reactions, and to help clients develop alternative "trial relationship models" for consideration (e.g., "If I don't ask for my needs to be met, then my friends will never know what I want"). This exercise is repeated from the sixth session of treatment to the later trauma-processing sessions and through to the very end of treatment.

Linking Current Relationship Models to Past Trauma during the Narrative Work

Relationship models are the tools, and model analysis is the strategy for creating change in interpersonal attitudes and behaviors. Several STAIR sessions focus on identifying, proposing, and implementing alternative and more adaptive relationship models. However, even when the narrative work begins, model analysis continues. Relationship models embedded in the narratives of childhood trauma are identified and compared to those that are imagined and tested daily in the present. This activity helps gauge positive changes. It also creates anchors in the implicit development of a life story. This process is valuable for survivors of childhood maltreatment, who often fear that by letting go of their past beliefs, they are betraying or invalidating the reality of their trauma. It suggests that the past will be respected and recognized as part of the clients' evolving life stories and not forgotten or taken for granted, even while new schemas are elaborated in the treatment. Lastly, relationship models function across both the STAIR and Narrative Therapy components of treatment to provide clients with a shorthand method for recollecting the pains of the past, without necessarily feeling those pains in depth during the recovery and change process.

Problems with Power Dynamics: Issues of Assertiveness

We have observed that as survivors struggle to adopt alternative relationship roles, they can often move out of victim roles and into victimizer roles. This shift may occur in evolving relationships where a survivor of maltreatment, in an attempt to be assertive and appropriately "in control" of events in the relationship, becomes utterly rigid and extreme. This rigid response is often related to the relative lack of variety in types of relationship templates with which a survivor is familiar. The victim–victimizer dyad is the template for relating. If the survivor has had few relationships other than the victimizing ones, the client has very little room for maneuvering into new ways of relating.

We use the notion of relationship models to sketch out alternative dyadic relationships that manage power in different, more egalitarian, and mutually respectful ways (e.g., "Having my needs recognized/recognizing those of others is a way to connect"). Because a relationship model often effectively articulates the generalized rules with which survivors have lived, they are quickly embraced as tools for the revision of interpersonal expectations. The new models are often more ideas than realities. Clients are usually stymied in their early efforts to engage in the feelings, behaviors, and language associated with dyads other than the victim–victimizer pairing. For this reason, role plays in therapy sessions are critical, as are carefully selected, well-graduated exercises with others outside the treatment. These exercises provide the real-world "stuff" and experiential evidence of the reality of alternative ways of relating, compared to the introduction of the concept of relationship templates, which is more theoretical and abstract.

Flexibility in Managing Power Dynamics, and the Role of Respect for Self and Others

The generation of alternative relationship models highlights the importance of moving away from the "all-or-nothing" view of power that characterizes victim–victimizer dynamics, and toward a view that relationships can vary in the types of power dynamics that define them (e.g., parent–child, supervisor–supervisee). The application of an egalitarian model across all relationships would lead to poor outcomes, because even that model fails to account for different relationship types and structures. An insistence on maintaining a healthy diet is a reasonable and expected demand by a parent of a child—but it is not generally appropriate with a spouse (with whom decisions concerning what to eat in the household are usually shared), and certainly not with a boss who is discussing their favorite desserts and fondness for sweets.

Nevertheless, a constant in managing the power dynamics of any relationship is that a person experience and maintain a sense of respect for the self and for those with whom they interact. A parent will create a better relationship with a child if they keep in mind that the child deserves understanding and respect for the developmental phase in which the child is growing and experiencing life. The supervisee will do better in managing an exchange with their boss if they remember to respect the burdens, responsibilities, and perspective of being a supervisor. Power dynamics can be difficult for an individual who has experienced interpersonal trauma. Power over another person (be it physical, financial, material, psychological, emotional, or maturational) is exploited to perpetrate maltreatment against another person. Power often is used not only to harm but to demean and diminish the other person. A physically abusive parent may say to a child, "This is what you deserve," or a rapist may tell a victim, "You wanted this," in an effort to humiliate and demean the victim. It is not surprising that survivors of early maltreatment equate power with maltreatment and are fearful of it. This underlying fear leads the survivors to have problematic interactions with those who have power, as well as difficulties when they have power themselves. They may fear falling into a perpetrator role, or may simply not know how to manage power in an effective and appropriate way.

The next step in STAIR moves clients toward recognizing and being comfortable with different relationship power balances. Indeed, research on interpersonal relationships has found that one of the strongest correlates of overall psychological health and life satisfaction is flexibility in interpersonal expectations and behaviors (Hill & Safran, 1994). Relationship models with different power balances are formulated, but each includes awareness of the worth and value of the client as well as the person with whom they are interacting. Developing skills that express an attitude of mutual respect, regardless of the balance of power in the interaction, will facilitate the client's ability to move fluidly and effectively in a larger social landscape.

Problems with Intimacy and Closeness

Difficulty with developing and maintaining close relationships is so pervasive among survivors of trauma that this characteristic is included in definitions of PTSD (DSM-5; American Psychiatric Association, 2013) and CPTSD (ICD-11; WHO, 2018). Survivors fear that their experiences are "out of the norm," and that others will not understand what they have been through—or, worse, will blame or shame them for what they have endured. So they keep a distance from others. Moreover, as suggested above, some believe on the basis of their past experiences that relationships lead to exploitation or pain and are best avoided. Other survivors maintain a defensive, dismissive attitude: They view relationships as unnecessary or worthless, given past disappointment and pain. Ultimately, some survivors have lived so long avoiding relationships that their skills in forging intimacy and closeness have "rusted." Others have really never quite gotten the chance to develop appropriate skills in the first place. During the final sessions of STAIR, beliefs that are barriers to intimacy and closeness are explored, and alternatives are proposed. Skills are introduced to help clients try out the first steps of approaching others and learn how to manage and resolve conflict.

Transition to Narrative Therapy

Relationship models are effective tools for working with multiple relationship difficulties that concern survivors of interpersonal trauma, including repeated negative relationship patterns, pervasive difficulties in managing power dynamics, and problems in establishing alternative ways of approaching and relating to others. In addition, because relationship models characterize both the actions and feelings in an anticipated exchange, they allow the exploration of feelings, particularly the power of feelings in derailing behaviors. In the treatment, a therapist and client develop new schemas to articulate desired interpersonal goals and ways of being. The implementation of the new relationship models is often difficult, because feelings from the past conflict or compete with interpersonal goals of the present. The conflict between feelings from old relationship models and the goals shaped by new models can be clearly brought forward to the client for examination and change. The contrast between old models (based in a traumatic past) and new emerging models are further highlighted during Narrative Therapy, the second module of treatment.

SUMMARY AND IMPLICATIONS FOR TREATMENT

Emotional and social skills are not abilities we humans are born with. They are learned. The limited scope of the abilities that survivors have developed does not represent personal failure or pathology but limited opportunities. These limitations put the survivors at risk for developing problems such as anger outbursts, substance misuse, and risk avoidance, among many other possible negative emotional and behavioral patterns. They also prevent clients from achieving what they want (having secure relationships, doing well at their jobs or careers, being good parents, etc.). For survivors, doing well in life can be a mystery. STAIR provides skills that fill the gaps left by the tumult of trauma. A client completing this module of treatment noted with relief, "It's learning things that everyone else knows." The goal of STAIR is to have the world become a little less mysterious and much more negotiable for such clients. The skills are intended to provide support for the clients to achieve important life goals and have a greater number of life choices.

CHAPTER 6

Working with Traumatic Memories
Overview of Narrative Therapy

> Speaking about the [trauma] . . . provides the possibility of turning
> passivity into activity. In retelling an experience, we voluntarily
> evoke it. Narration is thus like play in that one can assume control
> over the repetition of an event which, in its occurrence, ran counter
> to one's wishes . . . [Here, one moves] from being the helpless victim,
> one becomes an effective storyteller.
> —MARTHA WOLFENSTEIN (quoted by Janoff-Bulman, 1992,
> pp. 108–109)

The goals of the Narrative Therapy component of treatment are to resolve PTSD symptoms through the process of "revisiting" the traumatic memories, and to put the trauma in perspective as one experience or set of experiences within a larger life story. The first goal involves the process of retelling the traumatic events, with the purpose of confronting the feared elements of the experience and dissolving the power of the memory to elicit fear. The second process involves appraising the meaning of the traumatic experiences in the context of an evolving life story. Narratives, in both name and process, convey the message that a life story is composed of a past, present, and future. Telling about trauma creates and reinforces its "pastness." Moreover, narration assumes a chronological structure that not only allows the trauma to be located in the past, but provokes consideration of the present and imagination of a future. The life story that begins to emerge flows from the models or formulations of self and other that are anchored in time and distinguished by differences between present and past realities. Both the repeated narrations and the meaning analyses are intended to free clients from the grip of a traumatic past, so that they can begin living in the present and can have a sense of a future.

In this chapter, we review the rationale and history of imaginal exposure and the updating of memories as interventions to resolve PTSD symptoms. An at-a-glance, session-by-session overview of Narrative Therapy is provided in Box 6.1.

Working with Traumatic Memories:
Outline of Narrative Therapy Sessions (Module II)

Session	Content
Session 11	*Introduction to Narrative Therapy.* Description and rationale for narrative activities; establishing commitment for narrative work; developing a memory hierarchy.
Session 12	*Narrative of First Memory.* Practice with neutral memory. Then conducting first narrative of trauma memory; listening to recording together; exploring beliefs about self and other.
Sessions 13–17	*Narratives of Fear.* Selection of memory for narration, and conducting narrative. Then identifying relationship models embedded in narrative and providing alternative relationship models; identifying current life difficulties and implementing skills.
Sessions 13–17	*Narratives of Shame.* Procedure same as for fear narratives. Also, providing clear response of positive regard following narratives of shame; emphasizing social and personal resources that support positive appraisal.
Sessions 13–17	*Narratives of Loss.* Procedure same as for fear narratives. Also, exploring ways of transforming loss for living in the present.
Session 18	*The Final Session.* Review of gains; planning for next steps; addressing relapse risks; providing resources and referrals.

WHY VISIT THE TRAUMATIC PAST?

It is commonly accepted that a crucial task in resolving PTSD symptoms is the emotional processing of traumatic memories. The process we use is one of retelling or "revisiting" the past trauma. It is based on the principles of exposure therapy, particularly as developed by Edna Foa and her colleagues (see Rothbaum & Foa, 1999). Some therapists immediately recoil when they hear the words "exposure therapy" used in treatments for survivors of trauma. Therapists fear inflicting pain on their clients, or even feel themselves to be sadistic in encouraging the practice. In actuality, clients can experience palpable relief at having an opportunity to discuss and describe their trauma in a safe environment and in a structured and contained way. The reality is also that clients with PTSD relive their memories every day in some form or other—reenactments, flashbacks, nightmares, intrusive thoughts, and images that are far more painful than the trauma-focused session work any of us has implemented. In addition, the clients' past traumatic experiences often profoundly dictate much of their present behavior. In reaction to the intrusion of the past into the present, clients avoid reminders of the past. They may keep relentlessly busy, misuse substances, and spurn romantic attachments. The failure of one set of avoidance strategies often begets additional avoidance strategies. The clients' experiential worlds get smaller and smaller.

Consequently, the clients' memories of the past control their lives. The intrusive, uncontrollable, and unpredictable symptoms reinforce the helplessness generated by the original trauma. At one time, the clients were subject to an ongoing reality of threat that they had no power to end or avoid. Now they are subject to the capricious and random intrusion of the memories of these events. But the reality is that the trauma is in the past, and the fear that persists is of the memories. The only exception to this situation occurs when a person is currently in a traumatic environment; in this case, the interventions should be supporting the client in protecting themselves, removing themselves from a dangerous situation, and building skills to help them do so. In cases of past trauma in a currently safe environment, the situation is different. Here, they can contextualize the traumatic memories. For example, although clients with childhood trauma could not control the original traumatic events, they can have full authority over the impact of their memories in the present. In the process of examining and exploring their memories, clients confront them, own them, and ultimately determine their value and meaning. The process of confronting the traumatic memories reverses the relationship between the clients and their trauma. In confronting and telling about their past, the clients gain mastery over it. They move from being passive recipients of a burdensome history to becoming active agents in determining its place in their lives.

A BRIEF HISTORY OF EXPOSURE THERAPY FOR PTSD

The Evolution of Exposure Therapy for Memories

The first documented efforts in resolving PTSD through the direct emotional exposure and processing of traumatic memories were made by behavioral psychologists working with combat veterans in the late 1970s and 1980s. The PTSD symptoms of fear and avoidance of situations reminiscent of the trauma were often behaviorally quite evident. The sound of a car backfiring, evoking a memory of gunfire, could elicit a startle response from a veteran. For veterans of the Vietnam War, the sound of rain and feel of humidity, reminiscent of the combat zone, could induce increased heart rate, sweating, and muscle tension. Later work with survivors of rape revealed similar physiological and behavioral responses. A woman raped in an elevator, garage, or park might suffer intense hyperarousal in these settings or avoid them altogether, leading to significant restrictions in movement and travel. Effective interventions for these problems were derived from understanding this pattern of behavior as an example of a conditioned response: The sights, sounds, smells, and sensations that occurred during a traumatic event, while not necessarily intrinsically frightening, are associated so strongly with the event that their recurrence months or even years after the trauma can elicit a fear response in the absence of any real threat.

This phenomenon has been reliably observed in a series of studies where veterans with combat-related PTSD were exposed to sounds, pictures, or film clips of combat experiences. These veterans responded with strong fear reactions, as measured by affective response, blood pressure, and increased flow of epinephrine in their bloodstreams, particularly as compared to similarly exposed veterans who had not developed PTSD (e.g., McFall, Marburg, Ko, & Veith, 1990). Accordingly, treatment to resolve these maladaptive reactions involved the "decoupling" of the fear response from the stimuli in a traditional behavioral manner. Via repeated exposure to the stimuli in the absence of any real threat, the clients would experience decline in the fear reaction. The stimuli, once paired rather capriciously with a real and powerful threat, now lost their potency. They became ordinary objects in the world, neutral features of the environment.

A remarkable evolution in this research occurred when it was noted that fear reactions of equivalent strength could be elicited simply through the evocation of these stimuli in memory. The physical presence of trauma-related stimuli was not necessary to elicit a fear response; the memory of these stimuli was sufficient. Increased heart rate, blood pressure, and muscle tension, all measurable aspects of a fear reaction, were induced simply by the thought of the trauma (e.g., Pitman, Orr, Forgue, de Jong, & Claiborn, 1987). PTSD became reformulated as more of a disorder of memory: The feared "object," so to speak, was a memory. The process of habituation previously applied to external stimuli was adapted to mental stimuli. The rationale for the treatment was that if a therapist could induce a client to bring up the image of the trauma in sufficient detail and for a sufficiently long time in the context of a safe environment, the client's fearful reactions to the memory would diminish, and PTSD symptoms would resolve (see Shalev, 1997). A series of randomized, well-controlled treatment studies with veterans in the late 1980s and early 1990s, however, indicated that the intervention was only partially successful: PTSD symptoms improved but did not entirely resolve (Cooper & Clum, 1989), or veterans reported little change in subjective distress despite reduction in physiological arousal (Keane, Fairbank, Caddell, & Zimmering, 1989). In one study PTSD symptoms were not reduced, even though veterans were rated as better adjusted (Boudewyns & Hyer, 1990).

The Strength of Fear Memories

Independent of these efforts to characterize and treat PTSD, a line of research exploring the neurobiological basis of fear responses was being conducted in animal laboratories. Joseph LeDoux and his team were among the leading scientists who determined that a relatively primitive brain structure, the amygdala, was the center of learning and unlearning of fear reactions. They were particularly interested in determining the parameters of this process. Early research tracked electroencephalographic (EEG) patterns in the amygdala during extinction of a conditioned fear response, with the expectation that the firing of the neurons related to the fear response would diminish with repeated exposure to the stimulus. In a critical study of this design, the investigators found that while there was an overall reduction in neuronal activity, the activity in cells that had been identified as specifically related to the learned fear did not diminish. The fear reaction as represented in the neuronal activity of the amygdala did not go away (see LeDoux, 1998).

LeDoux (1998) originally described this phenomenon as the "indelibility" of emotional memories. It was proposed that certain aspects of fear memories were indelibly etched into memory. The implications of these findings, translated into human functioning, suggested that traumatic memories could never be entirely freed of the overwhelming fear with which they had been encoded. This notion was supported in a substantial number of empirical studies among both animals and humans (e.g., Bouton & Swartzentruber, 1991; Jacobs & Nadel, 1985).

The idea that there are indelible aspects to traumatic memories provided an explanation for diverse observations about traumatic memories among those who suffered from PTSD. If the emotional quality of traumatic memories could never be entirely extinguished, then the memories could be activated or reactivated with sufficient cueing or under circumstances of sufficient emotional power. This proposition is consistent with the observed relapse of PTSD symptoms on anniversaries of the trauma ("anniversary reactions"); delayed onset of PTSD when a survivor is presented with emotional or physical environments similar to the circumstances of the trauma; "recovered" memories that have lain dormant for years or decades; and the emergence of PTSD among elderly persons confronting chronic illness or mortality, such as World War II veterans and Holocaust survivors (see Shalev, 1997).

Updating of Fear Memories

Shortly after the identification of the work that fear memories were so strong that they appeared to be indelible, a second line of research by the same investigators found that while fear memories were powerful, they were not necessarily "indelible." LeDoux and colleagues found that when a memory is first called up, it enters into an activated or labile state, where it can be revised and the fear associated may be eliminated or reduced (e.g., Nader, Schafe, & LeDoux, 2000). As a practical matter applicable to psychotherapy, the revision of the memory occurs through the introduction of new information. For example, a person who is recalling a rape event and feeling to blame for it can introduce the idea that the attacker, with whom the person was on a date, actually exploited the client's trust and committed a crime, and the perpetrator is to blame. Alternatively, the person recalling the rape can introduce the fact that the event is in the past and they are safe now.

During this period of activation, the new information is integrated, resulting in a revision of the memory—a process called "memory reconsolidation." It is not that aspects of the memory are "erased" (as it is sometimes described in the popular media), but rather that new information is introduced, so that old information becomes less important and the emotional valence of the memory changes. Scientists have described memory reconsolidation as a process that allows the updating of memories in order to maintain their relevance as circumstances change (Lee, Nader, & Schiller, 2017). This research provides one way to frame the process that occurs during narrative work, and it offers a potential explanation for the resolution of symptoms. During the narrative work, the client calls up an old memory, adds new information, and reevaluates its meaning. The new information results in a revised or updated memory of the event that takes into account new insights and new feelings. In the narrative work, the client also integrates the traumatic memory within the context of previous and subsequent experiences. The old memory is "updated" in two ways: as a specific event, and in the context of a life that is being lived.

The disruption of old memories and their updating via introduction of new and alternative information is a core principle of many cognitive therapies (e.g., Ehlers & Clark, 2000; see Ehlers & Wild, 2015). This principle is applied in STAIR Narrative Therapy as well.

THE TRAUMA NARRATIVE

The review and elaboration of trauma memories in STAIR Narrative Therapy involves both an appraisal of the event and well as the elaboration of the event in the context of the person's life. The therapeutic power and necessity of both of these aspects of the process was demonstrated to us in the case of a man suffering from PTSD symptoms and burdensome grief that literally left him gasping for breath. The man, in his 70s, came into treatment after losing his son in the September 11, 2001, terrorist attack on the World Trade Center. He could not stop imagining his son's final moments and the particulars of his death. So frequent and extreme were these intrusive thoughts and images that when he was asked to describe his relationship with his son, he could recall nothing. It was as if the horrendous images of his son's death obscured access to any other memory about him. The situation was devastating to behold. The man had lost his son twice over: once in the World Trade Center, and now again, in his imaginal world. It was clear that a review of the traumatic event, in and of itself, was insufficient to resolve the PTSD.

The therapist shifted the work to include a discussion of the son's death in the larger context of the life he had lived. The therapist began by asking the man to tell about his son as a young child, and then about his son's middle school years, his performance as a high school athlete, and his marriage to a neighborhood girl. Over time, several stories were told, and the death of his son became one of several belonging to the narrative that was his son's life. The last story was a terrible story, to be sure. But the formation of the narrative had placed the death in the context of a life lived; it was no longer simply the story of a death. When the man thought of his son, he had a narrative of how his son had lived joyfully, or another narrative about the relationship with his son and its various ups and downs. In either case, the narrative did not end with the son's death, but was continued by the creation of positive memories of the son to be handed down to his grandson.

THE TASKS OF NARRATIVE THERAPY

Telling the Story

As the description provided above indicates, the primary function of narrative work for the survivor of trauma is to create the story of an unfolding life, in which the trauma is only one of many events have occurred and that are possible for the survivor moving forward. A particular traumatic event is described several times. It is expected that through repeated tellings, the associated fear reactions will diminish and the memory will become organized and internally coherent, so that questions about the facts of the matter (what happened and when) can be answered as clearly as possible.

Identifying Themes

After the trauma narrative is shared, however, the client and therapist continue the work by listening to the narrative and identifying interpersonal relationship models within it. These models identify the client's core beliefs about the self in the world, and are typically driven by feelings of fear, shame, and loss. Examples of such beliefs include (1) "The world is a dangerous place, and I am not able to live in it without being hurt again and again" (a theme of fear); (2) "I did something to provoke this and did not stop it, so I am to blame" (a theme of shame); and (3) "I never had what so many take as 'given' in a normal childhood, and I cannot ever have it" (a theme of loss and grief). The treatment sessions described in Chapters 23–25 of this book provide specific guidance about how to work effectively with the commonly occurring themes of fear, shame, and loss, respectively.

SUMMARY AND IMPLICATIONS FOR TREATMENT

This chapter has highlighted the importance of and rationale for addressing the traumatic past, as well as the strategies we use to make this process engaging, relevant, and therapeutic. The overall goal of the Narrative Therapy work is to create an integrated sense of self—one that incorporates the traumatic past in a respectful way, and that allows the person to live in the present and have hope for the future. This is accomplished via the identification of old trauma-generated relationship models embedded in the trauma narrative. These models are validated as adaptive or inevitable, given the conditions of trauma from which they emerged. In addition, the old trauma-generated models and the new emerging relationship models are directly compared side by side. The therapist guides the client in identifying ways in which the old model may no longer be applicable, given changing circumstances (e.g., the client is out of the traumatizing circumstances, is no longer a child, or is no longer in a war zone), and the new model may offer opportunities for better relationships. Each model is validated as appropriate for a particular context. Both sets of beliefs are validated by placing them in the context of time and place, and by acknowledging the value and possibility of change.

The distinction between the past and the present is reiterated in all sessions. A symptom of PTSD (and a mental characteristic of many survivors of trauma) is that time has collapsed. The traumatic events define reality as it was in the past and will be in the future. Traditional narration, with its underlying chronological structure, helps clients to anchor these events to moments in time and to assign them meaning in the context of the passing of time.

CHAPTER 7

Extending the Narrative
Transforming Shame and Loss

The dark does not destroy the light; it defines it. It's our
fear of the dark that casts our joy into the shadows.
—BRENE BROWN (2010, p. 82)

The Narrative Therapy phase of the treatment gives clients the opportunity to develop a coherent life history with various themes that follow the thread of critical, emotionally charged experiences. In addition to fear, central emotional burdens for those who have experienced sustained interpersonal trauma (particularly abuse by caregivers) are shame and loss. There are, however, very few established trauma-focused treatments that intentionally and specifically address these often debilitating consequences. Narrative work is assumed to be therapeutic in the resolution of fear through repeated exposure to the traumatic memories and the consequent habituation/extinction of the fear-laden responses. As discussed in Chapter 6, given what is known about emotions, there is no reason to think that feelings of shame and loss would be resolved through repeated exposure to or systematic reexperiencing of shaming or grief-eliciting memories. Still, it became clear in our own narrative work that feelings of shame and of grief were almost inevitably brought forth at some point in the telling of traumatic memories—and, furthermore, that the telling was therapeutic. We suspect that the aspects of narrative work making the process therapeutic are the act of constructing the narrative and the task of imbuing it with meaning. Narrative work contributes to the resolution of shame and grief not through habituation, but through their transformation via the meaning the client attributes to the trauma and through the call to action that these feelings often prompt.

Narrative Therapy—which includes both the telling of the story and the particular meaning analysis that follows—is organized so that clients' understanding of who they are, because of where they have been or what they have experienced, is no longer a source of shame or irremediable loss. Rather, it now supports the evolution of a sense of dignity, purpose, and self-compassion. The reparative actions that transform shame and loss can begin with the simple act of telling about the event. Narration as an act, through both its process and its content, is an "antidote" to shame and loss.

Shame, which often arises from a perception of the self as being ineffectual and weak, is countered by the experience of agency in the creation of the story. Through telling the brutal facts of their traumatization, clients clearly see, often for the first time, the difficulties of their early lives and can appreciate and even marvel at their success in having survived these difficulties. The telling of their trauma stories in therapy can also liberate the clients from the dark weight of secrecy that often paralyzes the capacity for self-expression. If clients can tell about the trauma, they can tell about myriad other thoughts and feelings; stories begin spilling out; connections are made; multiple past events that have seemed to follow separate tracks come together; and important patterns are identified.

The act of narration has a similar transformative potential with experiences of loss. Narration provides a means by which a ritual for grieving and remembrance can take place. Telling about and putting words to the loss affirm that the experience has importance. Its meaning, though, is often discovered only through the process of telling the story. The loss, often initially understood rather abstractly as an "absence" of something in the life history (e.g., a loving parent, a secure home), is transformed into something with presence. This comes in the form of awareness, wisdom, or insight, and ultimately in a conscious and purposeful decision about what to make of the losses and their assigned role for life in the future.

This chapter focuses in depth on shame and loss, which, despite their importance, have historically received relatively little attention in empirically based trauma-focused treatments. Studies implementing treatments that focus on reevaluating the meaning of events associated with shame and grief have reported reduction in these feelings (e.g., Gilbert, 2010; Kubany et al., 2004; Shear, Frank, Houck, & Reynolds, 2005). From our combined decades of clinical experience, we characterize shame and loss as we have observed them in treatment and identify different thematic aspects expressed by clients in the narrative phase of the work. We present this information to provide some guidance in the exploration and recovery from feelings of shame and loss. Examples of Narrative Therapy sessions with these themes are provided in Chapters 24 and 25, respectively.

SHAME

Therapists and survivors alike have been acutely aware that shame is a pervasive emotional state associated with interpersonal trauma, with far-reaching detrimental consequences. As Judith Herman (2007) has described, humiliation, degradation, and shame are so central to a survivor's experience that the resulting posttraumatic stress can be viewed as both an anxiety and a shame disorder. Only recently, however, have changes been made to diagnostic systems to reflect these lived experiences of survivors. Specifically, in DSM-5 (American Psychological Association, 2013), PTSD has been moved out of the anxiety disorders category and into its own category of trauma- and stressor-related disorders. PTSD criteria have been expanded to include the cluster of negative alterations in cognitions or mood

(Criterion D), and for the first time shame is incorporated as a PTSD symptom (persistent negative trauma-related emotions, such as fear, horror, anger, guilt, or shame). There have been similar shifts in ICD-11, which now includes CPTSD as a separate diagnosis (Cloitre, Garvert, Brewin, Bryant, & Maercker, 2013; Maercker et al., 2013), as mentioned in Chapter 1 and discussed further in Chapter 9. In addition to core PTSD symptoms, CPTSD includes disturbances in self-organization that typically result from repeated or chronic exposure to traumatic stressors from which one cannot escape. Here too shame has been specifically added; it is included within the category of negative self-concept (persistent beliefs about oneself as diminished, defeated, or worthless, accompanied by deep and pervasive feelings of shame, guilt, or failure related to the traumatic event).

Empirical research on shame is still in its infancy, but continues to expand with increased recognition of how shame can contribute to difficulties in adaptation across the age spectrum (Andrews, Brewin, Rose, & Kirk, 2000; Bennett, Sullivan, & Lewis, 2005; Orth, Robins, & Soto, 2010; Stuewig et al., 2015; Tilghman-Osborne, Cole, Felton, & Ciesla, 2008). Studies have shown a significant association between shame and PTSD symptoms (Feiring, Taska, & Chen, 2002; Leskela, Dieperink, & Thuras, 2002). In the first comprehensive review of this literature, Saraiya and Lopez-Castro (2016) synthesized results from 47 experimental studies on shame and PTSD. Taken as a whole, this research to date provides evidence for the following:

1. The detrimental impact of shame is most pronounced in the aftermath of relational and repeated traumas characterized by social subordination, powerlessness, and lack of control.
2. Shame is strongly associated with both psychological and physiological symptoms of PTSD; has a functional role in the development of PTSD; and is a significant predictor of PTSD, independent of fear.
3. For a subset of individuals with PTSD, shame is *the* primary response to traumatic experiences, suggesting the existence of a shame-based variant of PTSD.
4. Trauma-related shame has an impact on PTSD treatment outcomes. Addressing shame during intervention may not only expressly diminish shame, but may also affect overall posttraumatic symptom changes, whereas not effectively ameliorating shame may impede recovery.

Many of the findings listed above provide corroboration for our view of shame as inextricably linked to fear, the "core" emotion resulting from trauma. Fear is a biologically hard-wired and evolutionarily ancient emotion; it alerts people to potential life threat and functions to maximize survival behaviors. Shame includes a sense of threat to survival or well-being as it relates to how individuals are perceived by others or within a community or social context. Shame arises in a threatening situation when persons feel that they have failed, that others perceive the failure as a sign of weakness, and that it places them at risk for ejection or rejection from the community. Most often the failure is a defeat that is interpersonal in nature, such as a rape, a robbery, or ongoing sexual abuse (see Andrews et al., 2000; Brewin, 2003). Those so intimately injured feel that they have failed in the essential task of self-preservation, as compared to what others might have done or as compared to what is socially expected.

The beliefs associated with feelings of shame include thoughts that the persons are marked as inferior, are viewed as blameable for their defeat, and that ultimately they will be rejected by others. A cycle of shame gets perpetuated as individuals whom experience being harmed by, rejected, and alienated from their communities are likely to respond by further isolating and withdrawing, which may lead to a further sense of rejection or reinforce that sense of rejection. Isolation deprives a person from a social network or relationships that could counter the person's negative beliefs about the self and could provide respect and admiration for the person—a form of nurturing that can contribute to recovery from shame. Based on our clinical experience, we have identified four different shame themes that emerge in narrative work and that are often reflected in the day-to-day functioning of survivors: "self as inferior," "self as bad," "self as annihilated," and "self as identified with the perpetrator."

Self as Inferior

As discussed above, shame commonly emerges following interpersonal traumas when the traumatized persons carry a sense of defeat or failure. Reactions of helplessness and powerlessness are part of the definitional landscape of a traumatic experience. In contrast, shame results from the survivors' belief that they should have done better—that they should have been able to protect themselves and did not do so. This belief gives rise to a sense of inferiority: "Others would not have reacted the way I did," "Others would have escaped this circumstance," or "Others would have fought back, and I did not." The judgment about self is in relation to others and relative to the perceived capacities of others for self-preservation. Shame is especially intense when a survivor responded to traumatic circumstances by "freezing." Although freezing is an involuntary response, and one that may be most adaptive in cases where fighting or fleeing is not possible or is dangerous, survivors often interpret the freeze response as evidence of cowardice or deficiency.

In addition, shame is tied to people's capacities for self-protection as members of a social group. Individuals who have been victimized by members of their own social network feel shamed and inferior. They believe that in the social hierarchy, they are "less than" others who have not experienced this form of interpersonal defeat. Social recognition or observation of defeat by others is threatening, as it carries the identification of the defeated persons as victims, and therefore as demonstrably vulnerable and at risk for further victimization. For this reason, many victims of crime feel greater shame when their victimization has been witnessed by others (e.g., gang rape), and often witnesses themselves feel shame for the victims. Shame results from experiences of being "acted upon" and having no recourse or resources to avoid the victimization, escape from it, or emerge victorious.

Thus, for example, children victimized by sexual or physical abuse feel shame and inferiority because they not only *did not*, but *could not* help themselves. Feelings of shame and inferiority are further exacerbated in this as in other sexual or physical crimes, because the defeat in these events has a specific intimacy—the defeat of one's body, which leads to feelings of profound vulnerability and self-disgust. This is the focal point of the inferiority and shame felt by victims of physical and sexual abuse.

Victims of crime often ruminate about whether they could have done anything differently to alter the outcome of the event. One purpose of replaying traumatic scenes is to determine the critical elements in the victimization. If the trauma can be attributed to unfortunate and unforeseeable circumstances, then the victims may feel that anyone would have reacted the way they did, and that the outcome does not reflect any intrinsic inferiority. They are "victims of circumstances," not victims of their own inherent weakness or vulnerability.

Survivors of childhood abuse or neglect also often ruminate about the transgressions they have experienced. The fact that they were small children with limited resources, and thus were inherently vulnerable, is of little comfort. In fact, it brings their analyses of the events to the larger social environment: If they could not be expected to rely on their own resources for protection, then who should have been providing the protection? The closest members of their social world—namely, their caregivers. Yet the caregivers were also often the victimizers, and in any case they provided no protection. Still, these survivors ask, "Why me?" During the years of maltreatment, the children often construct an answer that includes and reinforces their own sense of shame: They must have deserved it.

Self as Bad

Children who are maltreated often believe that these events are expressions of their own intrinsic "badness." This occurs for several reasons. First, explicit statements of the children's inherent badness, inferiority, and worthlessness are frequently made by those who are inflicting the maltreatment. The children are identified as the cause of these events (e.g., "Look what you made me do"). This is self-evident in many cases of physical abuse, where the pain that is inflicted is often called "punishment" for the children's "bad behavior." In cases of sexual abuse where there is little or no pain, or perhaps even pleasure, the children still understand that these activities are "bad," "dirty," or "wrong," because such activities deviate from typical, day-to-day touching experiences and because they are inevitably carried out in secrecy.

In addition, the perpetrators are aided by children's cognitive predisposition to interpret experience in a self-referential way. When bad things happen, children tend to view themselves as the sources of the problems. Beatings, other physical assaults, and sexual abuse convince children that they themselves are inferior or bad. Both moral and social justice are filtered through the developmentally immature, self-referential forms of cognitive processes that define childhood. A negative assessment is not circumscribed to an event (e.g., "A bad thing happened with Daddy") or designated to another actor ("Daddy did a bad thing"), but is absorbed by a child as part of their identity: The child *is* bad for being involved in something bad. In contrast, adult victims of crime have the cognitive abilities to differentiate between internal and external causes of events, and can engage in a cognitive reevaluation that delineates the difference between events that made them feel inadequate and being inadequate persons. This type of analysis is not typical of children, and may not even be possible for younger children. Notably, even when children do recognize that the adult perpetrators are to blame, they do not necessarily excuse themselves from blame (Fei-ring et al., 2002; Kolko, Brown, & Berliner, 2002).

Labels of self-blame and "self as bad" stick through the years of adolescence, young adulthood, and maturity. Looking back on their childhoods, adult survivors can usually see past the treachery of the self-referential logic of childhood and recognize the vulnerability of their childish minds to self-blame. This often does not help them to give up, resolve, or reorganize beliefs of self-blame, however. The resistance to relinquishing these beliefs has many sources.

Self as Annihilated

Shame is associated with feeling oneself to be inferior to others and of less worth. Beyond the feeling of being "less than others" is that of being "nonexistent." One survivor described it as "being erased." These are experiences where victims feel that their very lives are of no value or regard. Brewin (2003) reports that victims of crime sometimes describe hav-ing felt that their survival was of no consequence. Prostrate bystanders at a bank robbery describe being stepped over as impediments to the goal of a successful robbery, or perhaps even being used as "human shields" to enable the robbers to escape. Brewin describes such circumstances as "encompass[ing] a total surrender of oneself and one's rights and expecta-tions as a human being" (2003, p. 80).

This intensely disturbing state is often a chronic condition for children who have been abused or neglected. A sense of self develops in the context of a caregiver who responds to a child's needs; soothes the child's distress; laughs when the child is funny; and engages in play, teaching, and learning. Through all of these interactions, the caregiver reflects back or "mirrors" the presence of the child, provides recognition of the child as a particular person, and acknowledges the child's agency. Physical and sexual abuse, and neglect, undermine these experiences. Like the victims of robbery described above, children who have been maltreated become objects of another's will. Parents who beat their children in fits of rage often report that their anger overwhelms them and they lose all ability to see (sometimes lit-erally), to reason, and to control their actions. Empathy for and connection to their children have vanished, and so have the children.

Although little is known about pedophiles in general or about parents who sexually abuse their children, some research indicates that such adults do not actually see the chil-dren as persons, but rather as objects of desire—objects without any volition or emotional experience. In an unusual study of convicted pedophiles (Chaplin, Rice, & Harris, 1995), a series of pictures were developed to look like children in erotic poses and shown to the men, during which time measures of sexual arousal (i.e., erection, heart rate) were taken. The emotional states of the children were varied: One set of photos showed distressed children (crying); in the second set, children looked happy; and in the third, they had neutral expres-sions. The study results revealed that the levels of sexual arousal exhibited by the pedo-philes were the same, regardless of the children's emotional state. These findings suggest that pedophiles experience children as sources of erotic stimulation—literally as "sexual objects"—and have little empathic connection to the children as persons in distress.

Annihilation through self-betrayal

If children do not exist in the eyes of their caregivers, they have difficulty existing for themselves and within themselves. Even if a child's growing identity incorporates experiences, values, and opinions obtained from outside the family, it is hard to hold on to these self-constructions while still participating in the family system. Because the sense of self is anchored in the recognition that parents or other caregivers give to their children, children are likely to compromise their moral codes to protect the family system.

As a result, children who have been maltreated are agents of their own annihilation through these routine acts of self-betrayal. Although they wish to tell the truth, they often find themselves lying about the conditions of their home lives; they hide their bruises and maintain the secret of abuse or neglect. Adult survivors of maltreatment often feel shame in recollecting their childhood behaviors. They feel shame in having become accomplices in something wrong, being held captive by their circumstances, and being ineffective in escape from these circumstances. And, perhaps most damaging, they experience shame in betraying themselves and their own dignity.

Children may also preserve important relationships by attributing negative emotions they are experiencing to their own perceived flaws and deficiencies, rather than recognizing that the harm is being caused by trusted adults (Platt & Freyd, 2012). There are some findings consistent with this theory, indicating that shame may function in survivors of trauma by reducing awareness of betrayal in a relationship, especially when it is a needed relationship (Platt, Luoma, & Freyd, 2017). Although in the short term shame may serve as a mechanism to maintain necessary bonds with attachment figures, in the long term it greatly impairs a survivor's ability to develop new and healthier relationships.

Self as Identified with the Perpetrator

Rather than have no sense of self (i.e., in order to avoid annihilation), children who have been abused will sometimes actively or purposefully participate in abusive behaviors. Some survivors report instances in which they provoked their own abuse by triggering the perpetrators' tempers and getting (although sometimes escaping) a beating, or actively participating in or even initiating sexual activities. In much the same way that having any caregiver is better than having no caregiver, it seems to be the case that having any self, even a terribly abased self, is better than having no self. Identifying with a perpetrator's attitudes and behaviors provides self-coherence. It means that the victim can move from helplessness and passivity to active agency. The victim takes on an action plan, so that there is a capacity to act; takes on victim–perpetrator relational patterns, so that a relationship exists; and takes on the perpetrator's beliefs, in order to have a system of meaning.

The relationship of the victim and perpetrator is likely to have special meaning, although not necessarily in any positive sense. It has been reported that relationships among individuals who have survived the same traumatic event have a special quality. It is forged from the mutual recognition that they have experienced something beyond typical experience and beyond the power of words to describe in normal conversation or day-to-day life that sets them apart from others (e.g., Gurewitsch, 1998). A relationship of a similar nature can occur between a survivor of childhood victimization and a perpetrator. These experiences have potent meaning to the victims; the events have formed their view of themselves and contributed to their self-definition. In the case of sexual abuse and sometimes in physical abuse, there is often no one else who knows about the experience, no one who was witness to the events, and no one with whom a victim has shared what happened. Recognition of a large part of the victim's identity is bound up with only one person—the perpetrator of the victimization.

A critical aspect of recovery from trauma is the disclosing and sharing of the event with a sympathetic person outside the experience. If a traumatized person is able to share and convey the reality of the experience in this way, it becomes known to a social world beyond the perpetrator. The bond between the victim and perpetrator, sustained by secrecy, is loosened and ultimately dissolves. The victim can become known in full to others, and then can have relationships with others in which the person's whole history and whole self are known, understood, and accepted. This work is described further in Chapter 24 (on narratives of shame).

Shame, Social Functioning, and Interpersonal Relationships

Shame burdens survivors of interpersonal trauma with a pervasive sense of alienation from others and diminished confidence in social interactions. Avoidance, often employed as a strategy for managing toxic shame, furthers isolation and strengthens negative beliefs such as "If you knew I was abused as a child, you would not connect with me." The survivors have internalized a view of themselves as "bad," "weak," "ineffective," "damaged," or "defeated." These beliefs are reflected in reports of their interpersonal problems, as described earlier, with problems such as assuming blame for events they are not responsible for ("If something is wrong, it must be my fault") and being too controlling ("I am not going to let anything bad happen again"). In addition, when survivors do confront difficulties, they often exhibit a "blind spot" about calling on social support to help resolve a problem. This disinclination may be based on a general sense of being "outsiders" or not part of a particular social network or community. It may also be a result of what they have experienced and learned from their traumatizing situations: "Help" was not forthcoming then, and is now no longer expected. Some may believe that asking for help would expose them as the "weak" persons they fear themselves to be. In circumstances where help from others is necessary to complete a task or reach a goal, this attitude leads to failure and defeat, reinforcing the view of themselves as weak, ineffective, and critically regarded.

Survivors' negative and critical views of themselves also affect their evaluation of others. The trauma has led survivors to view certain characteristics as unacceptable—not only in themselves, but in others as well. For instance, survivors who internalize the views that vulnerability is weakness, and that weakness is bad, not only view themselves with contempt but judge others in the same fashion. These survivors may prize self-confidence and self-sufficiency in others, and derogate those who show confusion, emotionality, vulnerability, or limited competence. The familiar mode of critical regard that is applied to the self is applied to others. The limited compassion that the survivors have for their own past experiences is now applied to others' experiences. These attitudes diminish opportunities for positive social experiences and the development of sustained interpersonal relationships.

The development of a sense of self-compassion allows such clients to live much more easily with themselves, and perhaps even with some pride and enthusiasm for themselves. In addition, a positive and more generous process of self-evaluation may lead to more generous appraisal of others. Positive changes in self-regard go hand in hand with positive changes in regard for others. The clients benefit in their relationships with others, as well as their relationships to themselves.

LOSS AND GRIEF

Childhood maltreatment is inevitably an experience of loss. This includes loss of protective and supportive caregivers, of a healthy sense of entitlement, and of unencumbered connectedness to others; of a child's innocent pride and easy comfort within their own skin; and of what the child "could have been" and the life they "could have had" in the absence of the maltreatment. Identification of losses can be, at bottom, the most difficult and painful aspect of recovery. It requires clients to acknowledge that they have received less than they humanly deserved in their childhood. This can reinforce feelings of shame, because the survivors may view these losses as a reflection of their personal worthlessness. In addition, recognition of these losses can ignite feelings of grief and anger.

These losses, while very real and painful, have not been addressed in any systematic way in established trauma-focused treatments. The incorporation of themes of loss in the Narrative Therapy component of our treatment is intended to alleviate this gap. Indeed, the use of narrative to address and resolve loss borrows directly from established rituals for mourning, which almost always include storytelling as a means of shared remembrance. This process acknowledges and confers reality on the loss. Stories about the person who has died elaborate and clarify the importance of that person to the survivors and often formulate ways of continuing to remember the person. In addition, rituals of mourning are almost always social processes that bring members of a community together. In this gathering, a network of social support is formed, reflecting the understanding that grief can be all-consuming and can paralyze the ability to function and the will to live in the present. The community cares for and protects those who grieve, and keeps them emotionally and socially engaged in the present by sharing recognition of the loss and understanding of the consequent pain.

When addressing the client's losses, Narrative Therapy shares many functions with those observed in socially sanctioned rituals of mourning. As a witness or listener to the story, the therapist confers a social reality on the client's losses, even though they are far in the past. The elaboration of the aspects of loss intrinsic to trauma, especially childhood maltreatment, is an important step to understanding the past, its impact on the client's present life, and its role in the client's future. In the community of two that is the treatment, the therapist provides care, emotional support and validation of the client as they recognize and mourn these losses together.

In addition, however, the therapist facilitates the transformation of grief into the purposeful selection of changes in loss-related attitudes and behaviors that have restricted the client's ability to function and live well. There is a certain paradox in the experience of grief, in which recognition of loss can ignite energy to repair the damage and even bring forth greater effort, imagination, and determination to create meaning and value to life than would have otherwise have been the case.

Below, we have identified some common and specific loss themes that surface in client narratives. These themes are "loss of protective parental figure," "loss of childhood innocence and pleasures," "loss in interpersonal relationships," and "loss of time."

Loss of Protective Parental Figure

Children tend to accept their lot in life, for the simple reasons that they know no better and have few other choices. Their reference points for evaluating their relative degrees of life hardship are their immediate environments, particularly their families. Only through the exploration of the larger social world, via school and peer relationships in the middle school, preteen, and early teen years, do children who have been maltreated actually begin to realize that their home lives deviate from those of other youth. By the adolescent years, youth who have experienced abuse or neglect recognize that the goings-on in their lives differ from those of other teenagers. They recognize that their peers are *not* having the kind of experiences with which they are familiar. It may take many more years for the adult survivors to recognize that they differ from their peers not only in the *presence* of maltreatment, but also in the *absence* of loving care, good regard, and benign adult guidance in the world.

Exploring the reality of abuse or neglect and the context in which it was allowed to occur through the narrative work often leads survivors to painful clarity about the limited capacities and caregiving behaviors of their parents and/or parent figures. Identifying relationship models from childhood and comparing these to the ones they are forming in the present may also highlight survivors' awareness that the warmth and comfort they can now experience, or see others experience and wish for themselves, were not theirs in childhood. The persons whom they relied on for a sense of worth did not value them. Many survivors have never known "unconditional positive regard" and have never experienced a parental figure as a consistent or soothing presence. As awareness of these truths sets in, clients begin to understand on a more profound level how their most basic human rights—to be regarded with value, and with respect for their autonomy and agency—were denied them.

Loss of Childhood Innocence and Pleasures

The experience of not being protected and/or of being maltreated by caregivers stands in stark contrast to the innocence, safety, simplicity, and carefree ways that we, as a society, usually equate with the childhood years. Even if a child who is abused or neglected is given the opportunity to participate in positive childhood rituals, such as playing with friends, going on first dates, or receiving honors for graduations or sports activities, the effects of trauma often pervade and overshadow the pleasure and satisfaction of these experiences. In particular, abuse and neglect by parental figures significantly decreases children's engagement with their environment and openness to others, diminishing the typical pleasures of childhood and positive memories. Such children have experiences beyond or quite different from those of their peer group. For instance, sexually abused children are prematurely forced into the world of adult sexual knowledge.

At the time of the maltreatment, the survivors may simply feel confused, angry, or alienated from their peers. As adults looking back on the experience, clients often feel aggrieved: They begin to see themselves as having their innocence—an attitude to life that belongs to the domain of childhood—stolen from them.

Loss in Interpersonal Relationships

The actual truth—essentially, their betrayal by their parents or other trusted adults—often takes years for survivors to recognize and to accept. Teens who have been intrafamilially maltreated often still cling to their attachment for and love of their parents or other caregivers, even when these adults have been egregiously abusive or have repeatedly failed in parenting tasks. This connection, however, serves to maintain a template of relatedness. The affection and attachment that a child or adolescent shows to a caregiver, however unresponsive, undeserving, or implausible the caregiver may be, has an important function: It maintains the young person's capacity for human connection. The template of relationship models remains intact.

Nevertheless, specific relationship models developed in this context lead to several problems in adulthood relationships. For example, survivors of abuse or neglect are more likely to choose relationships with individuals who are unreliable and unavailable—even to the point of being abusive and/or neglectful—since this is expected and accepted. Even in relationships where there is potential for support and caring, the clients may not be able to see or cultivate these aspects of the relationship. Clients sometimes report that while they can identify the presence of support or help from others, they reject these overtures, because such giving cannot possibly match what they didn't get and still long for from parental figures. In line with this understanding, our treatment in such a case does not necessarily involve the revision or dissolution of a client's connection to the caregiver. Rather, the treatment supports the growth of the client's persistent capacity for attachment. As such, it sets the goal of helping the client establish alternative relationship models and behaviors in the service of developing new and different relationships. The treatment helps the client to identify old working models of relating that were established in the context of maltreatment; to understand that they no longer need to live by the old models in new relationships; and to invite them to develop new, alternative, more positive relationship models that include mutual respect and support.

Loss of Time

Once clients begin experiencing fewer symptoms and improved functioning, review of their past leaves them aghast at the many years that they have not had the capacity to function well and engage in their lives. Clients sometimes feel resentful that they will never recapture the time they have lost. They consider, for example, their teen years when they could have been studying rather than abusing drugs, or their 20s when they were too angry and hostile to establish themselves in the work world or to experiment with relationships. Coming to recognize the extent to which their development has been derailed by trauma often leaves survivors feeling that they were "left behind" and that they will never be able to "catch up" to their contemporaries.

The developing awareness of the profound and pervasive negative impact the trauma and related PTSD symptoms have had on a client's life trajectory can elicit anger and dismay. This loss, like many others related to early maltreatment, is irreversible. However, the client does have the opportunity of the present, which, if spent in anger, will only add to the mountain of lost hours accumulated through the years. Feelings of anger, resentment, and sadness are natural parts of understanding loss. But the client and therapist need to titrate this experience so that it does not exclude the possibility of pleasure and satisfaction. Ideally, awareness of loss can contribute to an understanding of its value and effective use by the client.

A client brought this insight to her session. She reported:

> "On my 30th birthday, I thought about myself as I was 10 years ago at the age of 20. I made a list of all the things that I did not have then (no education, no career training, no money, no partner) and do not have now. As I made the list, though, I realized that when I turned 40 I could be doing the same thing: making a list of all the things I did not have when I was 30. I realized that it was up to me not to waste my time now—that I was free to choose what to do and how to do it. When I am 40, I want to be able to turn back and be pleased by what I did in my 30s. I put my pencil down and felt really free."

This insight is the gist of the work with all of the losses described above. In recognizing the losses and their consequences, the client has the opportunity to choose to live differently. Doing so gives meaning to the past, makes it "count for something," and so honors it.

Traumatic Loss and Bereavement

As discussed above, interpersonal trauma is always associated with loss. Loss, however, is not always associated with trauma. It is important to acknowledge the group of survivors who have experienced traumatic loss, although this type of loss is not the focus of this treatment. According to Barlé, Wortman, and Latack (2017), "a death is considered traumatic if it occurs without warning; if it is untimely; if it involves violence; if there is damage to the loved one's body; if it was caused by a perpetrator with the intent to harm; if the survivor regards the death as preventable; if the survivor believes that the loved one suffered; or if the survivor regards the death, or manner of death, as unfair and unjust" (p. 127).

Children and adolescents who lose a family member or significant other through traumatic means face unique challenges, which can interfere with their daily functioning and development. They often exhibit significant PTSD symptoms, which in turn complicate the ability to process grief and may make it impossible for them to remember the person who has died without being emotionally and physically triggered. In the past, there has been little overlap between the study of the adaptation to trauma and the study of adaptation to chronic bereavement. More recently, however, the complex interactions between posttraumatic stress and traumatic grief are being examined more systematically (Layne, Kaplow, Oosterhoff, Hill, & Pynoos, 2018), and treatment integrating evidence-based strategies from both fields is available (Pearlman, Wortman, Feuer, Farber, & Rando, 2014).

In work with clients who have had multiple traumatic experiences, it is not unusual for a traumatic loss to be among these experiences. In fact, traumatic loss in childhood can be a risk factor for subsequent victimization. For example, we have worked with clients who have lost a significant caregiver through murder or suicide. As a result, they were placed in living situations (such as foster care or with other relatives) that were ultimately not safe and led them to be exposed to additional trauma. In such a case, the traumatic death can be integrated into the therapy as one of the client's several traumatic events and can be included as part of the client's narrative work in the course of treatment.

SUMMARY AND IMPLICATIONS FOR TREATMENT

The guiding principle and central purpose of creating a life narrative is to transform a life viewed with fear, shame, anger, and loss into one that gives the client a sense of purpose, meaning, and dignity. It is unlikely that deeply entrenched feelings of shame and loss, and associated patterns of thoughts and behaviors, will be entirely transformed during the course of a single treatment. Given the layers of life experience that shame and loss have infiltrated, this task is more likely to be a long-term process. However, the narrative work can establish one or more templates for an improved and alternative sense of self and relationship to others, and demonstrates a process that the client learns and can use after treatment ends.

CHAPTER 8

Guidelines for Implementing Treatment

The paradox of structure is that it demands flexibility to be stable.

—ANONYMOUS

Treating survivors of trauma poses particular challenges and rewards, over and above those encountered in standard outpatient psychotherapy. Survivors of trauma have many and varied difficulties in different domains of their lives. It can be hard for a therapist—and a client—to decide exactly where to begin. Our treatment program is organized into two relatively self-contained modules, STAIR and Narrative Therapy, each with distinct goals. This modular approach provides flexibility in selection of treatment goals and processes. In addition, the rationale for each treatment module is clearly described in Chapters 5 and 6, and these descriptions can facilitate the process of deciding where to start and what to do. In this chapter, we address and provide guidance on potential concerns related to using a manualized treatment, deciding which clients may benefit from STAIR Narrative Therapy, developing a strong therapeutic alliance, and addressing issues specific to working with clients who have experienced early interpersonal trauma. The specific issues we address include concerns related to trauma memories (seeking corroboration, confronting the perpetrator); client self-harming behaviors; a client's sharing the trauma history with others; the role of a couple in individual therapy; and concurrent therapy. We conclude by discussing therapist self-care.

USING A MANUALIZED TREATMENT

Therapists interested in using STAIR Narrative Therapy come from a variety of clinical backgrounds and training experiences. When we talk to therapists in the community, many express concerns about using a manualized treatment in practice with their clients. As authors of this manualized treatment, we understand these concerns, because all of us have had extensive training in nonmanualized, nondirective forms of psychotherapy as well as manualized treatment. For this reason, we would like to address doubts some therapists have about using a manual for treatment—even one intended to be used flexibly, such as this one—right up front. Commonly heard concerns are as follows:

"I am a therapist, not a technician."

"If I use a manual, I will lose myself as a therapist."

"Manualized treatments are scripted and will feel forced, not allowing for spontaneity or creativity."

"I will not be able to give my full attention to my client if I am trying to follow a manual."

"Therapy is an art, not something you can learn from a rulebook."

"My client is a unique human being, not a piece of equipment to be 'fixed.'"

"If I use a manual, I'll be controlling the sessions and won't be able to work collaboratively or follow my client's lead."

"Manuals just don't provide the flexibility needed to manage complex situations."

STAIR Narrative Therapy: A Guide, Not a Technical Manual

We know that STAIR Narrative Therapy works in the format described in this book. However, the treatment has been used by all five of us authors in both lengthened and abbreviated forms, and it has an intentional structure and logic that allows flexibility in its implementation. Indeed, the treatment has been used in New York City for survivors of the September 11, 2001, terrorist attacks with substantial success (see Cloitre, Levitt, Davis, & Miranda, 2003). Flexibility in use of treatment modules, types of interventions, and number of sessions, as well as in application to a variety of clients, has led to uniformly beneficial outcomes—often equal to those obtained in the more restricted conditions and client selection characteristic of an RCT (see Chapter 4).

Flexibility in Use of Modules

Again, this treatment contains two distinct components. The first module is focused on developing emotion regulation and interpersonal skills. The second is focused on processing the client's trauma history. In our research, we complete the modules sequentially, with Module II immediately following the completion of Module I. Nevertheless, a therapist can choose to use either module alone or to reverse the order of modules if it suits a client's needs and preferences. This flexible multimodular approach is consistent with recommended approaches for individuals with complex trauma (Cloitre, 2015; Karatzias et al., 2019).

The STAIR module can be flexibly applied in a variety of ways, including repeating sessions, providing an abbreviated review of other sessions, or even skipping some sessions if the material is already familiar and the client has mastered it. Some clients, for example, may be relatively skilled in emotion regulation, but have more challenges in managing relationships. In this scenario, we recommend a condensed review of emotion regulation skills in one or more sessions, followed by several sessions focusing on the identification of interpersonal difficulties and development of skills to help manage them. STAIR alone is also useful for clients who do not feel ready to address their trauma memories, or whose life situations are unfavorable for their engaging in trauma processing. For example, adjustments to the treatment structure were needed in a case where the client was diagnosed with cancer during Module I. In order to focus attention on the crisis that the client was now facing, the Module I component of the treatment was extended with skills training interventions directed to issues relevant to the client's current stressors and challenges.

Alternatively, there may be some clients who are prepared for directly addressing their trauma memories and need only be provided with a few preparatory sessions before entering the Narrative Therapy component of treatment. These may be clients who have successfully completed a skills-based treatment previously and want to address remaining trauma memories.

Lastly, there are some clients who are curious about their traumatic past and start treatment with Narrative Therapy, and then realize they still have some issues they want to address in day-to-day living. In this situation, the clients might begin with Narrative Therapy and then add STAIR to resolve any remaining daily problems.

Regardless of the starting point, it is critical that a client and therapist spend some time getting to know each other before engaging in the narrative work. Our research has informed us that a key factor in good outcome of trauma memory processing in particular is a strong therapeutic alliance. The alliance is generally established relatively quickly (usually in three to five sessions) and tends to remain stable thereafter. This early phase of treatment is useful for showing the therapist's ability to listen empathically, understanding the client's goals in treatment, identifying the client's coping strategies and current life stressors, assessing the impact of the trauma history on current functioning, and mapping out and agreeing upon a treatment plan.

Flexibility in Use of STAIR Sessions

Although the development of social skills and the development of emotional skills overlap and evolve dynamically in relationship to one another, the topics and skills addressed in STAIR are sequenced in a way that reflects the basic logic of skills development. For example, identifying feelings is a prerequisite for effectively communicating them to others, and establishing basic skills in communication is useful before attempting to resolve conflict-ridden or highly charged interpersonal problems.

The therapist can begin treatment with a session and topic that make sense for the client. For example, some clients are very aware of their feelings and have no difficulty in naming them or describing situations in which these feelings emerge and are difficult to manage. In these cases, identifying relationship models and interpersonal patterns or specific problems in issues of assertiveness may be a reasonable place to begin. Our experience, however, has been that it is useful to do a quick review of feelings identification and other assumed skills before going forward. This review may take only one or two sessions, but it establishes a reference point for the client's level of competence and comfort with skills that will soon be called upon. In a few cases, this review can take as little as one session and a week of practice exercises.

Flexibility in Use of Narrative Therapy Sessions

The skills and planning involved in successful use of Narrative Therapy are less variable, given that these sessions share one central task. It will still be necessary to complete the basic preparatory work for conducting narrative processing (in the first two sessions of Narrative Therapy, described in Chapters 21 and 22). This preparatory work is as important as taking a good life history and identifying the client's presenting problems before initiating treatment. These sessions involve explaining the overall approach and rationale for the narrative work and identifying memories from which the narrative work will be drawn. They are the nuts and bolts of the procedure, and the client must be comfortable and familiar with them in order to proceed with confidence and a sense of being able to master the task ahead. The actual material about which the client chooses to create a narrative, however, is unique to the client and selected collaboratively by therapist and client. In Chapters 6 and 7, we have identified three emotion-driven themes that are inevitably all part of interpersonal trauma in childhood: narratives of fear, shame, and loss. The client's particular history, symptoms, stage of recovery, and life circumstances will determine which theme is of most importance to them.

If clients are experiencing PTSD symptoms such as intrusive images and flashbacks, narration of fear-laden trauma memories is a good place to begin. However, some clients enter treatment with PTSD symptoms but feel more burdened by shame or loss. Often such feelings come to the surface as a result of recent life stressors. For example, in our work with survivors of 9/11, 60% also had a history of childhood trauma; of those, many experienced powerful depression, with the PTSD symptoms being of secondary importance. The loss of so many lives had reawakened unresolved feelings of loss, such as loss of a belief in goodness or in the possibility of a happy future. Treatment included STAIR to support symptom management, while Narrative Therapy focused on the telling about the losses, clarifying their meaning, and formulating activities or ways of living that honored the losses intrinsic to both the clients' childhoods and to 9/11.

Flexibility in Number of Sessions

This treatment was originally organized into 16 sessions, but now consists of approximately 18–24 sessions. It has been completed successfully in 16 weeks with 8 STAIR and 8 Narrative Therapy sessions conducted weekly (Cloitre et al., 2010), as well as in 12 weeks with 8 STAIR sessions completed weekly and the 8 Narrative Therapy sessions conducted in a more condensed fashion, twice per week (Cloitre et al., 2002b; Levitt et al., 2007). We encourage therapists in practice to use as many sessions as needed to address the problems that are the focus of the interventions. This kind of flexibility can mean either extending the number of sessions to cover material at a pace appropriate for a particular client, or skipping material that is not relevant.

In our study of STAIR Narrative Therapy applied to 9/11 survivors (Cloitre et al., 2003), treatment was flexibly applied so that emotion regulation, interpersonal problems, and trauma memory processing all were expected to be addressed to some degree, but the number of sessions selected for each problem cluster was matched to each client's problems and preferences. The number of protocol sessions implemented averaged 18 across all clients and ranged from 12 to 24. Data suggested that application of the treatment in this way produced benefits equal to those achieved in the standardized approach. For example, the effect size for PTSD symptoms in the standard 16-session trial was 1.76 (Cohen's d); the same effect size was obtained in the flexible application.

Another adaptation of STAIR we have developed is a trimmed-down 5-session version for clients in primary care settings. STAIR for Primary Care (STAIR-PC; Cloitre, Ortigo, & Gupta, 2018c) focuses on the development of emotion regulations skills in a way that can be individualized to clients' specific needs. Initial findings on STAIR-PC are encouraging. (See Chapter 27 for more discussion.)

Though these data are preliminary, they give us confidence in the benefits of adjusting the session number and content to the needs of each client and the specific treatment setting. We recommend that therapists in practice determine how best to structure the treatment on a case-by-case basis.

FORMAL TRAINING AND CONTINUING EDUCATION

In this book, we provide theory, diagnosis, treatment principles, session-by-session instruction, and numerous clinical examples to guide a therapist in a real-world application of the treatment. Still, a book, no matter how good it is, cannot replace excellent clinical training, experience, and supervision. We strongly recommend that therapists working with survivors of childhood interpersonal trauma receive specialized workshop education to become informed about issues specific to working with these survivors and about implementation of cognitive-behavioral strategies. We recommend that therapists interested in working with this population complete at least one multiday training workshop provided by experts in PTSD related to interpersonal trauma and/or in the treatment of survivors of childhood maltreatment. This type of training experience sets a general framework for thinking about childhood maltreatment, often provides hands-on experience in intervention demonstration and practice, provides a forum for asking questions relevant to a particular client or caseload, and often builds therapists' skills and confidence to work even more effectively with clients who have experienced such maltreatment. If trauma treatment is new to a therapist, then ongoing supervision and consultation are required to implement the treatment effectively.

THE THERAPEUTIC ALLIANCE

The two-module format of this treatment aids in building a strong therapeutic alliance. The alliance is important, because the therapy requires active participation and collaboration from both the therapist and the client. In STAIR, the therapist is working with the client to develop emotion regulation and interpersonal skills to reach real-life goals that the client values, This work is collaborative, with the goal of improvements in the client's day-to-day functioning. As such improvements begin to occur, the client's trust in the therapist grows, building a strong foundation for the trauma-processing work of Narrative Therapy. During the Narrative Therapy component, the therapist bears witness to the trauma the client has suffered. Thus the client is leading the treatment within certain guidelines offered by the therapist.

DECIDING WHICH CLIENTS MAY BENEFIT FROM THE TREATMENT

Survivors of Physical Abuse

When we present this treatment to therapists in the community, they often raise the question about who is appropriate for this treatment. The treatment was initially developed specifically for women with PTSD related to childhood sexual abuse. It quickly became apparent that most of these clients had also experienced physical abuse. About 70% of women seeking treatment for sexual abuse also have a history of physical abuse—sometimes by the same person, but often by one or more additional persons (see Cloitre, 1998; Cloitre et al., 2002a). Over time, we provided treatment to women who had experienced only physical abuse, and found that they did not differ in symptom profile or clinical needs and did just as well in the treatment (Cloitre et al., 2002b).

Clients with Significant Traumas in Adulthood but Not Childhood

As noted earlier, we provided STAIR Narrative Therapy to adults exposed in some way to the 9/11 collapse of the World Trade Center. About 60% of our clients also had a history of childhood abuse. Evaluation of the treatment indicated that these clients showed significant improvement both in their PTSD symptoms and in their coping strategies—including gains in emotion regulation and in obtaining and seeking out social support, and decreases in using alcohol and other substances to cope (see Cloitre et al., 2003). The improvements in social support were especially striking, because these 9/11 survivors experienced substantial deterioration of social networks (through death, building destruction, and/or job-related moves), which required them to apply coping strategies that had not been of particular importance or necessity before 9/11. The use of STAIR Narrative Therapy may be relevant with clients who have recently been traumatized and are faced with the need to adapt to new environmental or social realities. We know that among these clients, the treatment provided moderate to large benefit, and that those with and without childhood abuse histories had equally good outcomes.

Clients across the Gender Spectrum

This treatment was originally developed for women, because the index trauma was sexual abuse—a form of trauma experienced approximately five times more frequently by women than by men. Through our work with 9/11 survivors, however, we found that men did just as well in the treatment as women did (see Cloitre et al., 2003). Indeed, the benefits for men were greater in certain areas, particularly in reduction of aggressive behaviors and of alcohol use as a coping strategy. In reduction of PTSD, depression, and other trauma-related symptoms, men showed benefits equal to women's. Men with a history of childhood interpersonal trauma tended to have more severe symptoms than men without early life trauma, but showed changes equal to or greater than those of men without histories of early trauma. These preliminary findings suggest that the treatment is applicable to men. From a clinical standpoint, we have observed that the interventions and narrative process are just as relevant to men as to women, and that men accept and tolerate them just as well. It remains to be seen whether additional sessions or more refined interventions for certain symptom areas, such as aggressive behaviors or use of alcohol, would provide even greater benefits than those we observed.

Despite the fact that much of this research has focused on cis-gender women and men, individuals across the gender spectrum can likely benefit just as much, as long as the therapist carefully considers that transgender and "questioning" individuals confront additional barriers to treatment, experience greater trauma exposure rates, and require culturally competent and sensitive client-centered care. Therapists who do not have experience in working with these issues will benefit from consultation, but the overall nature of the interventions and theoretical framework still broadly apply. As a reflection of the field's growing awareness of gender diversity, we have carefully replaced gendered third-person singular pronouns in this edition of the book with the gender-neutral "they," "them," and "their." We hope that this concrete change provides one example of how to consider the impact of language when creating a sense of safety for diverse clients, no matter how they personally identify. As with any work in the area of diversity, open, collaborative conversations with clients will go a very long way in ensuring that these issues can be part of the work in treatment.

Clients with Subthreshold PTSD

Our research with people who have "subsyndromal" or "subthreshold" PTSD indicates that such clients find both the STAIR and Narrative Therapy components of treatment useful. It seems impractical and nonsensical to exclude individuals from treatment just because they have less than a full diagnosis. For clients who have minimal PTSD symptoms, the application of STAIR alone may be sufficient. In some cases, Narrative Therapy can still be implemented as a method of exploring shame- and loss-related emotions or other important parts of the meaning-making process after trauma.

Clients with Borderline and Other Personality Disorders

Therapists working with clients who were abused as children often note that these clients have many features of borderline personality disorder (BPD), even if they do not meet full criteria for the disorder. BPD is the most common but not the only personality disorder characterized by significant disturbances in areas of emotion regulation, sense of self, and relationships with others. These difficulties are precisely the sorts of problems that several of the STAIR interventions were designed to address. Indeed, we have used this treatment successfully with clients who had several features of BPD, or even met full diagnostic criteria for BPD and other personality disorders, by mindfully adapting the treatment as appropriate. Thus, the presence of a personality disorder diagnosis alone does not warrant automatically referring a potential client to another treatment. However, certain characteristics of personality disorder symptoms may indicate that another treatment, such as Transference-Focused Psychotherapy (TFP; Yeomans, Clarkin, & Kernberg, 2015) or DBT (Linehan, 1993, 2015), would be a better treatment match. For example, individuals with chronic, severe suicidal ideation and attempts may be appropriate for DBT, as the treatment has been developed specifically for these types of difficulties and has a successful track record in managing them (Linehan et al., 2015). Individuals with a severe sense of abandonment and emptiness may benefit more from TFP, a long-term therapy that can help build a strong and stable sense of self and reassurance about the enduring presence of others.

Clients with Motivation for Skills Development

Our experience suggests two important prerequisites for determining the potential for successful treatment. These are a client's identified goals for therapy and the client's perception of the therapeutic relationship. These two issues are related. Specifically, the client's motivation and goals for the therapy must be *skills-based* rather than *relationship-based*. We have found that treatment is not effective or appropriate for clients whose treatment focus is on the relationship with the therapist, rather than on learning skills with the therapist's guidance. In these cases, the clients' needs drift toward analysis and feelings about the relationship, and away from self-reflection, self-transformation, and skill acquisition as guided by the therapist. For example, one client who we soon realized was inappropriate for this treatment felt that the between-session exercises were the therapist's way of punishing her and trying to control her outside of sessions. The treatment quickly became primarily about the therapist–client relationship, rather than about how the client could develop skills to help her improve her life. The therapeutic relationship is critical to the success of the treatment (as we discuss below), but this relationship supports change rather than being the primary tool or medium for it.

ASSESSING READINESS FOR TREATMENT

Review of Treatment History

Clients who experience strong feelings of emptiness and, in conjunction, report volatile relationships may be driven by such problems to the extent that they preclude the clients' ability to set and follow through on skills-based treatment goals. One way to identify risk of a poor client–treatment match is to review each client's history of prior treatment. Indicators of poor fit would include reports of difficulty in making and keeping commitments to therapy in the past; having started and terminated many treatment relationships; and stormy relationships with several previous therapists. Also of note are clients who don't seem able to view previous therapists as having both strengths and weaknesses, but only idealize or denigrate them.

Alternatively, a good record of effort in previous treatments might indicate an appropriate match, despite the presence of a full diagnosis of BPD. For example, an assessment of a

30-year-old lawyer who had been sexually abused by her grandfather yielded a diagnosis of PTSD and BPD, as well as a history of disordered eating behavior (bingeing and purging). Normally, such a client might not seem appropriate for this or any short-term treatment. However, the client had engaged in long-term psychodynamic psychotherapy for several years. She was seeking this treatment in combination with her other therapy, and her other therapist was supportive. It was clear from this woman's treatment history that she would be able to form a collaborative relationship with a therapist.

Engagement during Initial Sessions

In some cases, it is not possible to determine that a client is appropriate for STAIR Narrative Therapy until the treatment has started. If a therapist starts this treatment with a client that the therapist is unsure about, it is wise to pay close attention to the client's participation in the early treatment sessions. Does this client participate actively in sessions? Can they identify specific areas of their life they would like to work on? When they do between-session exercises, are they less focused on learning about themselves and more focused on what the treatment work says about the therapeutic relationship? Clients may raise objections to some skills work or may not complete skills exercises for all kinds of reasons. However, it is notable if a client's reasoning about these behaviors concerns their reactions to the therapist rather than to the intervention.

THE THERAPEUTIC ALLIANCE

In the introductory chapters of this book, we have reviewed how caregiving environments characterized by sustained maltreatment (sexual, physical, or psychological abuse, or neglect) disturb the development of healthy attachment, emotion regulation skills, and relationship models (e.g., Malatesta & Haviland, 1982; Shields & Cicchetti, 1998; Shipman & Zeman, 2001). Clients bring their attachment difficulties, emotion regulation deficits, and interpersonal problems into the therapeutic relationship. The success of this treatment, and indeed of any psychotherapy, depends on the therapist's ability to build a strong alliance with the client in spite of these problems.

What Is the Therapeutic Alliance?

The foundation of a strong therapeutic alliance is unconditional positive regard (Rogers, 1951). We believe first and foremost that therapists should, in general, enjoy working with their clients. It is difficult for a therapist to enjoy the work and to maintain such regard for a client they do not like. Authentic positive feelings for a client go a long way toward building an alliance.

Second, the therapists must believe that they can help clients improve their lives. Using a treatment that has empirical data supporting its efficacy, such as this one, contributes to holding and conveying that attitude.

Due both to the complex nature of this work and to the range of interpersonal and attachment difficulties with which clients present, therapists will inevitably encounter situations in which experiencing and/or maintaining positive feelings for clients is challenging. In these instances, it is essential that therapists practice self-awareness, take time to reflect on their own reactions, and increase efforts to understand and accept their clients' perspectives and struggles. In most cases, a therapist who has a sincere desire and determination to connect can usually find something positive about working with any client. If, for whatever reason, the therapist cannot find a way to experience or communicate positive regard for a client, given the degree to which the therapeutic relationship determines treatment outcome (as detailed below), it is the therapist's responsibility to facilitate a referral to another qualified therapist. Seeking consultation or supervision from another professional, in order to manage this situation and process in the most ethical and sensitive way possible, is recommended.

The Importance of the Therapeutic Alliance

Through our research, we have demonstrated the importance of the therapeutic alliance to the success of this treatment (Cloitre et al., 2002b). In particular, the strength of the therapeutic alliance established during the first component of treatment predicted successful reduction of PTSD symptoms during the treatment's second component (Cloitre et al., 2002b). Furthermore, this relationship was mediated by participants' improved capacity to regulate negative emotions during the Narrative Therapy module of the treatment. These data suggest that a strong therapeutic alliance facilitates a client's ability to manage negative emotions during trauma processing (Cloitre et al., 2004). Other investigators treating clients with PTSD have reported similar results. In one study, Chemtob, Novaco, Hamada, and Gross (1997) found that PTSD-related anger symptoms caused ruptures in the therapeutic relationship that directly compromised treatment outcome, including premature termination. Similarly, Tarrier et al. (1999) found that clients' feelings regarding the credibility of treatment—a contributor to the therapeutic alliance—predicted dropout from treatment.

The strength of the client–therapist relationship appears to be a critical common factor across treatment modalities, including short-term CBT, interpersonal therapy, psychodynamic therapy, and gestalt therapy. Notably, the relationship between the therapeutic alliance and good outcome for clients with childhood abuse histories in STAIR Narrative Therapy was twice as large as that usually observed in other treatment modalities and populations (Cloitre et al., 2004). This finding suggests that the role of the therapeutic alliance in the treatment of survivors of childhood abuse is particularly important, which makes sense, given the interpersonal context in which their trauma occurred. Specifically, a positive alliance may serve to reverse or repair some of the interpersonal disturbances that so often undermine success in a variety of life tasks.

Threats to the Therapeutic Alliance

When managed well by the therapist and worked through, threats to the therapeutic alliance can actually improve the client–therapist relationship and model effective interpersonal communication skills—all of which increase the efficacy of the treatment. This successful resolution of ruptures can be achieved by framing threats to the therapeutic alliance as communications from the client to the therapist. Often a client's apparent difficulties with the therapist or treatment are ways of conveying fear, conflict, or a host of other problems that the client may be unable to express in other ways. If the therapist attends to alliance problems in this way, it is more likely that issues affecting the treatment relationship can be recognized and directly addressed.

Below, we identify four common problems in the therapeutic alliance that occur with survivors of interpersonal trauma. Therapists may benefit from reminding themselves about these patterns from time to time and asking themselves if these patterns are operating in any of their relationships with clients. If this is the case, or if a therapist feels vague discomfort or confusion about the nature of the therapeutic relationship, consultation with a trusted colleague can help to determine and resolve these difficulties.

Breaks in understanding

It is inevitable that there will be occasional lapses of understanding between a therapist and client. To minimize the impact of such lapses, the therapist can at the beginning of treatment predict their occurrence and provide the client with guidelines about how to respond. The therapist may say something like this:

> "At some point, I'm going to say or do something that upsets you, makes you angry, or makes you feel misunderstood. Although I'll try my best to help you, at some point I'll probably make a mistake. You may not even recognize my mistake at first. You may not be aware of it until you go home and think about it. When this happens, it's important that we have an opportunity to address the issue. If you're angry with me or feel hurt by me, please come back to the next session and tell me. I want to hear about it and then make corrections to how we proceed! This is your treatment, so it's my job to help it work for you and to help you feel cared for."

By letting the client know that ruptures in the relationship will occur, the therapist has taken away some of the ruptures' power and made it more likely that the client will stay in the therapy and repair them. The therapist is also showing that they are not unduly afraid of ruptures in relationships, that these are to be expected in the course of a relationship, and that they can be overcome. This approach has the added benefit of being an opportunity to model good interpersonal skills to the client.

We have also found it helpful for the therapist to make extra efforts to reach out to the client when breaks in the relationship do occur. These may include calling, rescheduling sessions, and sending letters. As we have discussed in the opening chapters, clients who were maltreated as children did not develop the skills to address conflict or ruptures in relationships. They tend to be easily hurt but avoidant of conflicts, and as a result, they may simply break off relationships when difficulties occur. The extra efforts the therapist makes reassure the client that the therapist values the relationship and believes in the client's ability to complete the treatment successfully.

Lapses in perceived empathy

A second issue related to the therapeutic alliance is a client's uncertainty about the therapist's ability to understand what they have been through. For some clients, this uncertainty is manifested in a question about whether the therapist is also a survivor of trauma. It is important for the therapist to avoid taking such a question too literally. Often what the client really wants to know is whether or not the therapist can help them, not the details of the therapist's trauma history. Even if the therapist is a survivor of trauma, this personal experience does not necessarily make them better able to understand the client's unique experience. In some cases, rather than facilitating understanding, the therapist's own experience may cloud their ability to see the client clearly. Addressing the concern behind the question, the therapist might respond with a statement like this:

> "No one can really understand someone else without standing in that person's shoes. And no one's experience is exactly the same. My goal is to understand your experience as you have experienced it. I will listen carefully to you. In addition, I have worked with many people who have experienced childhood trauma, and I can share with you things that I have learned from them, if you think that would be helpful."

Sexualization

Sexualizing the therapeutic relationship happens often—perhaps particularly often—with clients who were sexually abused in childhood. Indeed, behaving sexually with therapists may be almost automatic for some clients. A client may wear provocative clothing to session, flirt openly with the therapist, and ask the therapist questions about their personal life. The therapist may react with discomfort or even with horror at finding themselves attracted to the client and reacting unconsciously or emotionally to sexual advances or flirting in response.

Many clients who act in very sexualized ways are not conscious that they are doing so; even if they recognize their behavior as such, they do not know how else to act. It is important that a therapist take care to address such behavior without embarrassing or shaming such a client. A therapist may feel inclined to reprimand the client or tell them directly that their behavior is inappropriate. In actuality, the client is often merely trying to find some way to communicate or forge some connection with the therapist. The underlying relationship model at work may reflect the client's belief, based on their abuse history, that "to be attached means to be sexual." The therapist's task is to recognize how this relationship model has shaped the client's expectations, and to provide an alternative way of relating. The therapist can demonstrate in words or actions that the client is important to the therapist for reasons not having to do with their sexuality, and that a sustained connection to another person need not be expressed in sexual terms.

If the client is looking for a way to connect with the therapist or to experience positive regard from the therapist, strategic comments will help move the client away from sexualized behavior and toward the exploration of other important and positive aspects of themselves. For example, the therapist can explicitly note and express interest in the client's skills at their job or ability to compliment others. The therapist can also remark on the courage the client has shown in coming to therapy and engaging in the treatment tasks.

As a more direct alternative, the therapist may wish to express how they experience the client's sexualized behavior, but this approach requires great sensitivity. Observations such as "When you said that, I felt like you were flirting with me," or "Sometimes I feel like you are behaving toward me like you might if you wanted to date me, rather than as your therapist," or "Sometimes I feel like you ask me questions about my personal life to distract us from focusing on you" can be experienced as reprimanding or belittling; the client may feel "caught being bad." Rather, reactions to sexualized behavior need to be conveyed with empathy, kindness, and even humor, and always in a spirit of collaboration.

Ideally, this direct approach is taken only when the therapist feels confident that the therapeutic relationship is stable and that the client feels respected and well regarded by the therapist. Under these circumstances, any sense of guilt or blame that the client experiences for the appearance of sexual expression can be quickly dissipated. The therapeutic goal is to have the client understand that sexualized modes of relating are not inherently "bad," but also are not necessary in creating strong and effective relationships. This perspective contributes to the evolution in the client's sense of self and to the development of more varied relationship models that free them from the narrow constraints of relating to others in a predominantly sexualized way. The therapist conveys to the client that they are free to be more than a sexual object or being, and that in the therapeutic relationship, the strength of the bond comes from growth in areas other than the appearance of sexual value and attraction. In some cases, explicitly stating, in a compassionate but clear way, that a sexual relationship will not and must not develop may be necessary. In situations that require it, unambiguously setting such a boundary can actually be a very comforting and healing experience for a client.

Conflicts

The therapeutic relationship is also fertile ground for replaying the power and control conflicts that are so frequently part of victim–perpetrator relationship dynamics. For example, the client may feel victimized by the goal-directed nature of the therapy. The client may say, "You're forcing me to do these exercises—what gives you the right?" Or "You're hurting me by having me think about my trauma." Alternatively, the therapist may feel placed in the victim role and maltreated by the client. This dynamic may be expressed in the client's anger, criticisms, and rejection of the therapist's attempts to provide help ("There's nothing you can do for me," "I tried it, and it didn't work"). The client may begin missing sessions but calling for help on weekends, may come to sessions late, or may not pay fees as agreed upon. The therapist may feel overwhelmed, incompetent, and helpless to do anything to aid the client, or may feel exploited and disrespected. If the therapist's reactions go unchecked and unexamined, they will ultimately lead to countertherapeutic behaviors that may be expressed directly to the client through verbal attacks, or indirectly in ways that are equally rejecting. It is important that a therapist in this situation closely monitor their feelings and behavior toward the client and work to regain empathy for the client's difficulties.

One goal of the treatment is to address and reframe power/control conflicts in the therapeutic relationship. A guiding principle of treatment implementation is that the client takes the lead in setting both the pace and the goals. This philosophy of treatment, and the particular goals and pace of treatment, are articulated in the process of the assessment and initial session work (see Chapters 9 and 10). Ideally, this structure will not so much prevent as extinguish future conflicts around power and control that could arise. The therapist may choose to reassert the agreement and remind the client that the client is in charge of the process. More importantly, it may be useful to ask the client, "What do you really want?" Often the appearance of resistance to treatment or criticism of the therapist's technique reflects clients' anxiety about going forward in the treatment and resentment about their predicament. As one client put it, clients often have this simple human desire: "I wish I did not have to do this. I wish I could be magically better." This type of question and response can break the stalemate in the conflicts of power/control and can unify the therapist and client in working toward the same goals, with adjustments as needed in the pace, process, and goals of the treatment.

SPECIAL CHALLENGES IN TREATING SURVIVORS OF CHILDHOOD ABUSE

This section focuses on the special challenges we have encountered in working with survivors of childhood abuse while implementing this treatment. These challenges include issues involving a client's seeking to validate the truth of their trauma memories (including seeking corroboration of memories and/or confronting the abuser); client self-harming behaviors; a client's sharing their abuse history with others; the role of a couple in individual therapy; and concurrent therapy. We review each in turn.

Seeking to Validate the Truth of Trauma Memories

In our clinical experience, most individuals reporting childhood abuse have always remembered something about what they experienced. At the same time, even those who have always remembered their abuse have had doubts or questions about some aspect of what really happened. Many of these clients find themselves wondering whether specific memories or specific details about the abuse are true.

Clients' concerns about the veridicality of their abuse memories have several sources. Many clients find that they experience an increase in memories of abuse and heightened distress when they begin trauma-focused treatment. Often such memories are not really "new" ones; they are memories that a client has always had, but that are now more accessible and present because the client is focusing on those memories. Additionally, clients sometimes report that they now remember more details of their abuse experiences. They may wonder if these details are accurate. Lastly, some clients find that in the process of therapy, they come to a different understanding of their histories and may reframe certain experiences they had previously thought were "normal" as abusive. For example, a client reported in the initial assessment that her trauma history consisted solely of being sexually abused by her stepfather. While reviewing her history in therapy, she also reported that her mother engaged in very severe corporal punishment. In fact, the corporal punishment was so severe that the client often wore long-sleeved shirts to school in warm weather, to cover the bruises on her arms. The client had not initially considered those experiences as physical abuse, but over time she came to label them as such and to view them as an important part of her abuse history that she addressed in treatment.

Many individuals who were abused as children and have come to treatment in adulthood have disclosed the abuse at some point, only to have their experience denied completely or invalidated. At the worst extreme, clients report having disclosed to a trusted adult when the abuse was happening, and being told that they were lying and punished for making up stories. Clients also commonly report experiences of being invalidated when sharing their abuse experiences. Clients often first try to share their abuse stories with friends in adolescence. Such friends, in their immaturity, are unprepared for these disclosures and may have responded by denying the abuse, minimizing it, or just not wanting to hear about it. For example, when she was 15, one client told a friend about being sexually abused by her uncle. Her friend at first responded by wanting all the lurid details, and then stopped her from talking about it further by saying, "That is really gross. You shouldn't say those things." Another client tried to talk to her 17-year-old boyfriend about her experience of sexual abuse by her older brother. He responded by getting angry and calling her a "whore." He then tried to pressure her to have sexual intercourse with him, saying that it should be "no big deal" for her, as she had "done it all before."

Clients who have disclosed their abuse and received these types of responses may come to doubt the reality or meaning of their own experiences. Clients may find themselves wondering at times if the abuse really happened or if they did make it up—or, even if they are sure it did happen, whether they are making "too big a deal" about it. This is especially true of clients who disclosed their abuse in childhood, found its reality denied, and then continued to be abused. Such clients had to live with two realities: one of their personal reality in which they were being abused, and one of their social reality in which the abuse was denied. Minimizing or denying their experience becomes a way of coping with it in such cases. As a result, even when clients come to understand and accept the abuse they endured later in life, they still often feel the need for "objective" verification and acknowledgment.

Seeking corroboration of the abuse

By beginning trauma-focused therapy, clients are making a statement that at least some part of them believes that the abuse happened and is worthy of serious consideration. Some clients may begin seeking external corroboration of their abuse experiences from family members or childhood friends. Or they may pore over childhood documents, pictures, letters, and school records, to see if they can find inconvertible evidence that they were abused and can thus silence any possible doubt. Clients may wish to confront their abusers and, in some cases, to pursue legal action against them.

What is a therapist's role in such a client's search for "the truth"? There is no one accepted answer to this question, so we give our opinion, based on our clinical and research experience with survivors. First, the therapist's job is to help the client explore what they hope to gain from external corroboration of the abuse. Second, the therapist can help the client ponder how they might go about getting external corroboration. Third, the therapist can help the client think through the consequences of getting or not getting the corroboration they so desire.

Clients' reasons for seeking corroboration are as varied as their experiences. What many clients want is understanding from family members or friends. Clients want those individuals most important to them to recognize that these terrible experiences really happened, that they have caused the clients much pain and anguish, and that they have had long-term adverse effects on them. Often they have tried to talk with friends or family members about the abuse, but have not felt understood. These clients hope that presenting some type of corroboration will be more convincing than mere words.

One woman we treated was physically abused in childhood by her mother, who had her own mental health problems. Her father was caring but usually physically absent: He dealt with his wife's illness by working long hours and traveling a great deal. The client and her siblings were therefore often left alone to cope with their mother's abusive behavior. When the client reached adulthood, after her mother's death, her father and siblings talked about their mother's problems; however, they greatly minimized how abusive and chaotic the household had been. They also minimized the relationship between the abuse and our client's and her siblings' difficulties in functioning in their adult lives. This client remembered receiving medical care related to her mother's physical abuse—in particular, being taken to the emergency room for a broken arm caused by her mother's throwing her down some stairs. She wanted her medical records to show her father and siblings, so they would admit how bad her childhood was.

Her therapist asked her, "And if you get these records and show them to your father, what do you hope will happen?" The client answered, "Daddy will finally admit that my mother was a terrible mother. That she abused me and my siblings. That he never should have left us with her. That he should have protected us. He'll say he is sorry and hug me. We'll be a family again without this barrier—this ghost of my mother—between us." The therapist did not argue or debate with the client about whether or not to get the medical records or, if she got them, to show them to her family. Rather, the therapist focused on helping the client explore how else her father and siblings might react to the medical records (e.g., with more denial), and how that might affect their future relationship.

Exploring what clients hope to achieve with corroboration is important, because often the type of corroboration clients can realistically obtain is unlikely to achieve their goals. Family members, friends, and partners who deny or minimize the clients' experiences are likely to maintain this stance even in the face of external evidence. This response can reflect some level of motivated reasoning or denial, but is often possible because most corroboration, such as the medical records sought by the client described above, can be explained in other ways (e.g., childhood accidents). However, obtaining corroboration can be helpful to clients for other reasons. For example, one client we saw remembered having done very well in school until she started being sexually abused by her new stepfather when she was 11 years old. She obtained her school records, and they confirmed her memory: Her grades started dropping when she was 11, and her teachers noted her being more distracted in class and withdrawn, commenting on her drop in performance. Reading these report cards was very validating for the client, but they were not helpful in convincing her mother, who always denied that the abuse occurred.

Confronting the abuser

Many clients, at some point during treatment, consider confronting their abusers. This idea is particularly common if an abuser is a family member with whom a client still has some contact. Almost all clients wish for a confession from their abusers—the ultimate form of corroboration and validation. Many clients imagine the day when they will confront their abusers, who, in the clients' imagined view of the confrontation, will break down, confess their wrongdoing, and apologize.

The therapist's approach to the idea of confronting the abuser is similar to the approach used with other forms of corroboration. That is, the therapist focuses on helping the client identify what they hope to accomplish through a confrontation. Many clients are seeking the ultimate confirmation to themselves that their experiences are real and true. Other clients want to prove their abuse to those who denied their experiences. Clients may also be driven by the desire for revenge: to make their abusers pay emotionally, legally, and/or financially for the pain they caused. Occasionally clients may want to have adult relationships with their abusers, but feel that this option is not possible until the abusers have acknowledged the abuse. We find that once clients explore what they hope to get from confronting their abusers, they often realize that the confrontation is too risky or will not achieve what they hope. After realizing this likelihood, they decide to move forward in a different way.

For a client who wishes to pursue confronting the abuser, a therapist can help the client think through and plan the confrontation, so that the client has the best chance of achieving their goals and has a plan in place for self-care, regardless of the outcome. The therapist can help the client decide when, where, and how they wish to conduct the confrontation. The therapist can also explore potentially negative outcomes (e.g., denial by the perpetrator) and ways the client can cope with them. In rare cases, the abuser may be willing to meet with the therapist and client together. This situation sometimes occurs when the abuser has been in therapy. In such cases, the abuser's and survivor's therapists may decide that a joint meeting is most appropriate.

Mandated reporting and other legal issues

Clients also seek confrontations with their abusers for reasons other than corroboration. For example, some clients are driven by the desire to protect children from potential abuse if they believe that a perpetrator still has the opportunity to exploit other children (e.g., a priest or other spiritual leader, or a relative who may be abusing other children in a family). Situations where clients are reporting abuse by individuals who are at risk of continuing to abuse others place special ethical and legal demands on therapists. Mandated reporting statutes differ by state, but in general therapists are required to report an individual if they believe that the person is at risk of currently physically or sexually abusing children.

Clients who pursue restitution from their abusers through the legal system also pose special challenges to their therapists. If a therapist has a client pursuing legal action, we strongly recommend seeking legal advice from attorneys who have dealt with such cases. Many professional organizations, such as the American Psychological Association, have contracts with attorneys who deal with these and other mental health issues. The therapist may have to address issues relating to the confidentiality of therapy records, or may face a subpoena to testify in the case. Pursuing legal action can also have direct consequences for clients' motivation to recover from the abuse. In order to receive financial compensation for the abuse, clients may have to show that the abuse was mentally damaging in an ongoing way. This situation may result in clients' needing to remain symptomatic to obtain a financial settlement. During the period when a legal process is ongoing, a therapist and client may choose to focus therapy on supporting the client through the process, rather than doing trauma-focused work. The legal process in itself can be very time-consuming and stressful, and often leaves clients with few resources to focus on other areas in treatment.

Acceptance of ambiguity

For most clients, part of the therapeutic process involves accepting that they will likely never receive external corroboration of their abuse or achieve certainty. They may never know for sure whether specific details of the abuse happened, or be able to fill in lapses in their memories of traumatic experiences. The evidence for their abuse may never reach the standard of proof demanded by the legal system. Some clients will continue to have family members, partners, and friends who minimize or deny what they experienced. Ultimately, the therapeutic process is different from the legal process: The aim of therapy is not to determine truth, but to help a client understand their subjective experience, the impact of that experience, and the process for moving away from the past and more fully into the present and future.

Client Self-Injurious Behaviors

Some clients who have completed STAIR Narrative Therapy have had a history of self-injurious behaviors such as cutting or burning. Self-injurious behaviors are common aspects of the symptom profile of survivors of childhood interpersonal trauma, and clients with mild to moderate self-injurious behaviors are appropriate for and can benefit from STAIR Narrative Therapy. A self-injurious behavior often functions as an attempt to cope with emotion dysregulation—either to reduce or organize a "flooding" experience, or to elicit a focused feeling when acutely distressed by either numbing, dissociation, or fear of lapsing into a dissociative state (Brodsky et al., 1995). In STAIR, these behaviors can often be resolved and replaced with more effective coping skills. Developing a more positive view about the self and the capacity to share urges for self-injury with an empathic, nonjudgmental therapist can contribute to recovery from these maladaptive coping behaviors. Moderate to very severe self-injurious behaviors (e.g., head banging, deep cutting) need to be addressed immediately, however, as they create significant and long-term health risks. Such clients may need to be referred to other providers who specialize in the reduction and prevention of self-injury.

Sharing the Abuse History and Treatment with Others

When clients begin a trauma-focused treatment, they may also have the desire to share their trauma history and their treatment with members of their social network. This desire may be more or less appropriate, depending on the type of relationship a client has with a particular person. Clients who are survivors of childhood abuse sometimes have not yet developed good judgment about whom they can trust or who would benefit from hearing their trauma history. A client may be inclined to tell nothing to their intimate partner, but to relay a detailed history to a passing acquaintance. Part of the therapy is to help clients learn with whom they can and cannot safely share their trauma histories, and what exactly about their experience is helpful to share.

For example, one client who came to treatment was socially withdrawn and had no close relationships. Her closest "friend" was the elderly woman who worked at the bakery where she bought her coffee and bagel every morning on the way to work. Each morning, the client and this woman engaged in small talk about what each was doing that day. On the day she started treatment, the client told this woman that she was going to therapy because her father had sexually abused her as a child. The elderly woman responded by saying, "In my day, one didn't talk about such things!" and walked away. Naturally this encounter was distressing to the client, who only realized over time that her disclosure in that situation was inappropriate to the context and relationship, regardless of how hurtful and lacking in compassion the woman's response was.

Couples Issues

A client who has an intimate partner may wish to have the partner included in the treatment. Although this treatment program was not designed to be used with couples, we routinely meet with a client and their partner if the client requests such a meeting. For those clients who desire couples therapy, such treatments have been developed for partners of veterans with combat-related PTSD (Monson & Fredman, 2012) and may be adapted for working with couples where one member has experienced childhood trauma.

In STAIR Narrative Therapy, we use the meeting to educate the client's partner about the relationship between the client's history of interpersonal trauma on the one hand, and their current PTSD symptoms and difficulties in functioning on the other. We find that this type of meeting can be helpful for a partner who may not understand the source of the client's problems, or feels hurt by or to blame for them. For example, a partner may interpret a client's avoidance of sexual intimacy as personal rejection, rather than as avoidance that may be related to a history of sexual abuse. Understanding the nature of the client's difficulties helps the partner be more supportive during the treatment. This meeting is also an opportunity to let the client's partner know that some of the client's difficulties may temporarily get worse during the treatment before improving, and that this temporary worsening is to be expected as part of the long-term recovery.

During this session, the therapist can also convey empathy for the partner, who may themselves be traumatized by the client's difficulties. Partners of survivors of abuse and neglect often experience anger and sadness on behalf of the survivors, as well as anxiety about the impact of the maltreatment histories on their relationships. Some partners vicariously experience intrusive thoughts and other PTSD-like symptoms as a result of hearing about the survivors' histories. As a parallel, the mental health field has understood that therapists sometimes feel overwhelmed by their clients' experiences and can find themselves ruminating about them at unexpected times. Intimate partners of clients can experience such vicarious traumatization to an even greater degree: They share the clients' lives to a much greater extent and are not professionally trained to protect themselves. Partners may also bear the brunt of the clients' difficulties in functioning and PTSD symptoms. For example, a partner is exposed to recurring difficulties when a client has nightmares and cannot sleep, bursts out in rage, or loses their job because they cannot get out of bed and go to work. Well-functioning partners may find themselves overcompensating for such clients' deficits in functioning.

In turn, partners can also contribute to the clients' difficulties and impede successful use of the therapy. Partners who are intrusive, insecure, or controlling may be threatened by the therapy, and particularly about what the clients may say about them in therapy. Although how much to share is something that always lies within a client's discretion, we encourage the client to think through what would be in their best interests. For example, in the case of a client whose partner wished to listen to recordings of their sessions, we encouraged the client to describe their experiences in therapy to their partner directly, rather than indirectly sharing these through recordings. This approach allowed the client to preserve the confidentiality of the therapy sessions, and also ensured that the client did not censor themselves in therapy.

A therapist often does not have significant knowledge about a client's relationship until well into the treatment. It is often impossible at the beginning of treatment to judge the extent of a partner's supportiveness about the client's treatment, the partner's reaction to the client's history, and the partner's own difficulties that they bring to the relationship. Some clients have compassionate partners, whereas others have maltreating partners with whom they are repeating their trauma histories. Meeting with the partner can help inform the therapist about these issues. A meeting also gives the therapist the opportunity to refer the partner or couple to therapy if indicated.

Concurrent Treatment

Although evidence supports this therapy's effectiveness in addressing the central problems faced by survivors of child abuse, it alone may not always be enough to address a client's needs. Some may need, or may come to STAIR Narrative Therapy already using, other forms of treatment (e.g., medication, couple therapy, or supportive therapy), particularly if they have been experiencing chronically stressful life circumstances. Consequently, we have routinely worked with clients simultaneously engaged in other forms of treatment. For research purposes, we have asked that clients not make changes in their other treatments (e.g., medication dosage or frequency of therapy sessions) during the length of the research protocol (3 months). The rationale has been to ensure the validity of the research protocol. This requirement is obviously not necessary in routine clinical practice where there can be much more flexibility.

Our clinical experience suggests that, given certain prerequisites (such as the agreement of all involved), STAIR Narrative Therapy can be successfully conducted concurrently with other forms of individual or group therapy or with medication management. In fact, providing STAIR Narrative Therapy to a client who is already in a long-term treatment arrangement can be very helpful. For example, we have had clients in long-term psychodynamic psychotherapies with trusted providers seek out STAIR Narrative Therapy because they also wanted to do some more directed, skills-based, and trauma-focused work. Some therapists who have been trained psychodynamically and who work in a nondirective way can see the value in such work, but may not be comfortable with or interested in a shared treatment. Other therapists, however, encourage their clients to pursue adjunctive care while they continue their long-term therapy.

Concurrent therapy can only be successful if the client's present therapist is supportive of it and feels they can collaborate well with another therapist. Occasionally a client appears to be seeking concurrent treatment, but is actually unhappy with their present therapy and is exploring other options. If that is the case, it is advisable not to begin STAIR Narrative Therapy with this client until the client has decided whether or not to continue with their present therapist. When the present therapist is supportive and the client pursues concurrent treatment, it is essential to maintain open communication among all of the client's mental health providers. Such communication ensures that all providers have the information they need to treat the client most effectively, and it prevents the client from creating conflicts between providers.

THERAPIST SELF-CARE

> The effects of trauma are catching, and the listener is always in danger of
> empathically resonating with the victim and thus converging emotionally
> within the same traumatic envelope. . . . As Euripides said several thousand
> years ago, "Where there are two, one cannot be wretched and one not."
> —SANDRA L. BLOOM AND MICHAEL REICHERT (1998, p. 145)

Psychotherapy involves "complex demands, human costs, constant risk, and often limited resources" (Pope & Vasquez, 1998, p. 1). Treating clients who were traumatized, especially as children, is particularly challenging for two reasons. First, the clients bring their difficulties in attachment, emotion regulation, and interpersonal relating into the therapeutic relationship. Second, the therapist is consistently confronted with hearing about some of the most vile behaviors human beings can inflict on one another. These circumstances are ones that most people choose to avoid or distance themselves from, but the therapist who treats clients with trauma cannot engage in such straightforward forms of avoidance. Thus cultivating self-care is essential for the trauma therapist.

Working with traumatized individuals can leave a therapist feeling disillusioned, alone, or frightened. Several authors have explained these types of reactions as an effect of "secondary exposure" or "vicarious traumatization" (Baird & Kracen, 2006; Figley & Ludick, 2017). Such traumatization is evident when therapists caring for survivors of crime, abuse, natural disaster, or combat develop a posttraumatic-like reaction from hearing about the traumatic incidents and seeing its effect on their clients. Many therapists who work with survivors talk about being surprised by the intensity of their reactions after vicarious exposure to traumatic material. It is not uncommon to hear descriptions of becoming hypervigilant and anxious, or of experiencing sleep difficulties, nightmares, and feelings of anger about the injustices clients have described. Some therapists may develop functional difficulties, such as withdrawing socially from their peers or partners. Some therapists have noted that people on whom they typically depend for support are sometimes unable to understand the difficulties involved in working with clients who have been traumatized. We do not review all the principles of good self-care here; rather, we refer our readers to other authors who have written extensively on the subject (i.e., Mathieu, 2012; Rothschild, 2006; Van Dernoot Lipsky, 2009). However, we would like to put forward a few principles we espouse in relation to self-care.

The first is the importance of seeking consultation with other trauma therapists. Throughout our work on this treatment, we have sought out other professionals' advice and wisdom about the challenges of working with survivors of trauma, and these requests for feedback have led to simple but effective revisions in our interventions. First, we have learned to be attentive to our appointment schedules. It is good practice to avoid clustering multiple appointments together, and to give ourselves time to relax, debrief with others, or take a walk in between client meetings. We have also learned to balance our caseloads. A full-time practice requires diversity; not all clients should be survivors of trauma. In any given caseload, it is advisable to avoid the intensive processing of trauma memories with several clients in the same time period. Although a therapist may feel intellectually prepared for the work, it is almost impossible to remain emotionally engaged and effective with trauma processing when the therapist is confronting multiple traumas from multiple clients while attending to their own self-care.

Through our continued work, we have also come to value maintaining a healthy lifestyle through diet, exercise, and enjoyable activities. One of the most important self-care practices is to monitor and appreciate our limitations. Our limitations make us human, and being human is a key ingredient in being an effective healer. As therapists, we all have many demands on our time. If we begin to feel overwhelmed while treating our clients, it is time to make some adjustments so that we can be more emotionally available to our clients. Self-care is not some abstract goal we achieve and then from which we can move on; it is a dynamic variable of which we all must remain mindful. Finally, we have come to realize that the social support we receive from other professionals in the field is essential. Many excellent books and websites provide further information on this subject, and we recommend that every therapist who does this type of work consider these as important resources (e.g., Baker, 2003; Pope & Vasquez, 2005).

SUMMARY AND IMPLICATIONS FOR TREATMENT

This chapter has provided guidelines that highlight *how* to deliver STAIR Narrative Therapy, how to make decisions about which clients may benefit from the treatment, and how to adapt or tailor the treatment to individuals' specific needs and contexts. The chapter has addressed the needs of the individual client, the needs of the therapist, and their relationship with each other. This chapter differs from several others in that it focuses less on the nuts and bolts of the treatment than on the real-world issues that confront the application of a protocol-based therapy (or, indeed any therapy). We expect that this chapter may be one to which therapists will frequently return.

CHAPTER 9

Assessment of Client and Match for Treatment

> Not all responses to a traumatic event fall within the orbit of PTSD, and
> many factors besides PTSD are relevant to establishing a treatment plan . . .
> and must be adequately assessed if treatment is to show maximum benefit.
> —JOHN MARCH (1999, p. 200)

The primary goal of this chapter is to provide guidelines for assessing clients with trauma histories and determining whether their needs match what STAIR Narrative Therapy has to offer. We begin with basic reminders for trauma assessment, as well as suggestions for beginning an assessment session. Next, we provide suggestions for assessing the trauma history itself, including particular types of abuse and other traumatic experiences. We then provide an overview of diagnostic profiles of ICD-11 PTSD and CPTSD, as well as DSM-5 PTSD. We also supply detailed information on these specific assessment domains: classic or core PTSD symptoms, emotion regulation problems, negative self-concept, interpersonal difficulties, harmful or risky behaviors, and resilience or coping strategies. We discuss how to assess each domain, give examples of how these problems may be described by clients, and recommend measures that therapists interested in performing a more structured evaluation can use. Finally, we talk about giving feedback and treatment recommendations to a client after the assessment has been completed.

BASIC REMINDERS FOR TRAUMA ASSESSMENT

Actively Support the Client

Some therapists, depending on their theoretical orientation, might generally assume a neutral stance with their clients. Although this approach may be appropriate in certain situations, many trauma clients who have been traumatized react negatively if therapists respond neutrally to their histories. These clients have often avoided sharing their histories because of shame or fears of rejection. For such clients, the assessment session may be the first time they have acknowledged their histories. Others may have shared their histories previously but have had them denied or refuted. These clients are especially sensitive to a therapist's reactions and will quickly interpret neutrality as denial, condemnation, or rejection. Openly supportive statements that acknowledge such a client's difficulties can go a long way in building an alliance with the client. For example, a therapist might say, "Thank you for trusting me enough to share that experience with me," "That must have been very frightening/upsetting," or "I appreciate your difficulty in telling about these events."

Seek Behavioral Descriptions, Not Value Judgments

The cardinal principle of trauma assessment is to ask questions that describe traumatizing behaviors, rather than asking a client to evaluate whether or not they have been traumatized. For example, a therapist assessing for physical abuse might ask the client, "When you were a child or adolescent, did a parent or someone who took care of you ever do something on purpose to you that gave your bruises or scratches, broke bones or teeth, or made you bleed?" rather than "When you were a child, were you ever physically abused?" The second question requires the client to make a value judgment about their experience and to define it as abuse.

Although clients may have experienced what trauma research typically defines as abuse, they may not view it in those terms. For example, Marta, a 37-year-old Puerto Rican woman, at first reported being sexually abused by her father, but denied experiencing physical abuse. However, in response to the first question above, she answered affirmatively and went on to describe how her mother regularly punished her by making her kneel with bare knees on gravel for hours at a time. After Marta had done this for a while, her knees would start bleeding. She would not be allowed to get up to go to the bathroom and would sometimes wet herself. Marta had not previously viewed this as physical abuse, as her initial definition only entailed physical beatings, which her parents did not engage in.

Contain the Client's Narrative

Some clients come to treatment overwhelmed by memories of interpersonal trauma. These memories intrude on their work, their sleep, and their relationships. The therapist may find that such clients can't seem to stop talking about their trauma histories once they begin. Rather than avoiding the therapist's questions, they will talk about their experiences in great detail. The therapist needs to help such clients contain their trauma narratives during the assessment. Letting them go into too much detail in the first assessment session may lead them to feel overly or unexpectedly vulnerable, and make them less likely to return to treatment. Alternatively, after the assessment, a therapist may determine that a client is not appropriate for their practice or program. If the client has disclosed a great deal of personal information, they are more likely to feel rejected and take the therapist's decision personally.

An effective way to contain a client is to describe explicitly the task at hand. The therapist can say something like this:

> "Now I am going to ask you some questions about some difficult experiences you may have had in childhood. I am not going to ask you to go into detail at this time, but just collect some general information about things you have been through."

If the client's narrative becomes overly detailed or extended, the therapist may say,

> "I am going to stop you from going into more detail here. I appreciate the difficulties of telling your history. But there are still many aspects of this consultation remaining, and I am hoping to help pace us through it all. Telling all of your history is an important part of treatment, but not necessary right now, and can be very tiring and painful. Is this all right with you?"

Keeping an opening for the client to respond is key, as the client may have been working toward disclosing a critical part of their history.

Model Nonavoidance

Traumatic events such as child abuse are difficult to talk about. Even therapists find it difficult to ask clients questions about their traumatic experiences, for fear of upsetting them or even upsetting themselves. One of the principles of trauma-focused therapy is that clients' avoidance of memories, feelings, and thoughts related to their traumatic experiences has played a role in maintaining their symptoms. Therapists must therefore be careful not to avoid asking about traumatic experiences, and not to subtly redirect clients who are talking about such experiences.

This advice may seem contradictory to our preceding recommendation about containing a client. A therapist must perform a delicate balancing act in terms of containing a client without promoting avoidance. Given that clients are often very sensitive to therapists' reactions to their disclosures, they may take redirection from a therapist as a message that the therapist can't manage hearing about their trauma. Countering this expectation is another reason why we recommend being openly supportive of a client's disclosure, rather than maintaining a neutral stance. When containing a client, we use direct language and explain why we are not going into more details about the trauma at this time. We also state explicitly that we will go into more detail later.

Expect More

Whatever a client reveals in this session, a therapist can be fairly confident that they have held back some experiences. Usually clients seem to hold back their "worst" experiences. For some clients, these will concern their most brutal abuse episodes; for others, these will be their most shaming or grief-provoking experiences. Clients will reveal more about themselves as they come to know and trust their therapists more.

Below are guidelines for a therapist to keep in mind from the first contact with a client and throughout the assessment process.

INITIAL CONTACT

The first contact between a therapist and a potential client will often take place on the telephone. For some therapists, this contact may merely involve getting the client's name and contact information and setting up the initial assessment session. Others may also choose to obtain information about why the client is seeking treatment. If a therapist's practice is primarily trauma-focused, questions concerning current problems and trauma history will help determine the appropriateness of this type of treatment. Through assessment, it may become evident that the primary focus of treatment will not be on trauma. For example, if there are current significant life-threatening behaviors or other disturbances, such as sustained substance misuse, eating disorders, self-injury, or initial reactions/working through of recovered memories (see Chapter 8 for discussions of the last two issues), the primary focus will be on these. If the therapist does not specialize in these problems or have consultation available for these types of treatment, a referral, kindly and reassuringly provided, will save the client time and frustration.

BEGINNING THE ASSESSMENT SESSION

The assessment session will generally be the first time a client and therapist have met in person. It is a time to gather systematic information about whether or not the client is appropriate for the treatment. It is also the first opportunity to start building the therapeutic alliance.

"What brings you to treatment now?" is the most important question to be asked and answered in the assessment session. This question begins the process of building the therapeutic relationship by demonstrating that the therapist cares about the client's concerns and reasons for being there. The client's answer to this question will provide preliminary information about their goals and hopes in coming to treatment. The client's response to this question will also give the therapist information about the client's level of insight into the relationship between their trauma history and current difficulties. The answers we have heard to this question are varied. In response to the question "What brings you to treatment now?", clients have said the following:

> "I have never been able to get past a first date with a man. If anything remotely sexual happens—like he tries to kiss me or even just hold my hand—I freeze. Last weekend, at my friend's wedding, I met a man I like. He has asked me out, and I don't want to blow this chance. I need to find out what is wrong with me."—Susan, a single, heterosexual, 35-year-old Jamaican woman and successful architect

> "I visited my parents at Passover for the first time in years. Since getting back to New York, I have been completely blocked in doing my art. I can't concentrate, get frustrated, and lash out at my studio-mates. I thought it would pass, but it hasn't."—Rachel, a single, lesbian, 50-year-old unemployed Jewish artist

> "I find myself losing my temper with James [her 3-month-old son] all the time. It's all I can do to stop myself from hitting him, so I end up screaming at him instead. If he

starts crying and doesn't stop right away, I feel overwhelmed and helpless and like a terrible mother. I know what I am supposed to do, but my feelings just get in the way."— Jane, a 30-year-old European American married woman

"I used to be able to keep going no matter what. I just kept busy all the time, worked hard, went to the gym, went out with friends, took active vacations, traveled. I just can't do it any more. I can't keep going. I don't know what to do."—Selena, a 40-year-old Latina advertising executive

"I am here because my husband says he can't take it any more. If I don't change, he will leave. He is tired of my irritability, my yelling, my distance, and my lack of interest in sex. I don't want to lose him!"—Kashana, a 35-year-old African American married woman

As indicated in the examples above, clients will not always state their trauma histories as the reason they are coming into treatment, even though they may be aware that the service or therapist they are calling specializes in trauma-focused treatment. Rather, clients tend to focus on the problems that are currently causing them difficulty. Although they recognize that they have been abused, they don't necessarily connect their history with present problems. Clients typically do not come into a consultation and state, for example, "I am coming for treatment because I have PTSD symptoms related to being sexually abused as a child." Rather, clinicians need to obtain information on clients' trauma histories through careful assessment.

Many therapists working in nonresearch settings find it helpful to use standardized assessment measures. Such instruments can help assure the therapists that they are covering all the relevant domains thoroughly. We have found this especially important with regard to a client's trauma history, as often a therapist will remember to ask about certain types of traumatic experiences (e.g., abuse) and forget others (e.g., sudden, unexpected death of a close friend or relative). Conducting a complete assessment is essential for treatment planning, as the more information the therapist has in the beginning, the more effective they can be in connecting the interventions to the client's specific difficulties. Below, we cover the seven domains we believe are important to assess. As we describe the assessment process, we also mention and provide references for some specific self-report and therapist-administered instruments that we have used in our assessments.

TRAUMA HISTORY

Before obtaining the client's trauma history, the therapist can say something like this:

"Now that I know why you are coming to treatment at this time, I would like to go back and ask you some questions about your childhood. In order to make sure I gather all the information I need to help you, I have a list of questions I ask everyone who comes to see me. Some of these questions may not apply to you, and other questions may seem very personal or difficult to answer. You don't have to answer anything you don't want to. Please also feel free to stop me at any time if you want to ask me something or need a break. OK?"

The therapist can begin eliciting the client's history in a nonthreatening way by asking for some basic background information, including where the client grew up, with whom they lived, whether they had siblings, and so forth. The therapist can then move to asking the client about abuse and other specific trauma experiences. How the clinician introduces this topic will depend on whether they are using a specific assessment instrument or conducting an entirely open-ended interview. In either case, the therapist reminds the client that they should feel free to decline answering any questions about areas the client does not wish to discuss at this time.

Therapists who do not have experience in assessing trauma histories will need training and supervision in how to conduct a trauma assessment. Using structured interviews designed to assess histories of child abuse can be very helpful, particularly for therapists with less experience in this area. Such interviews have been designed to give specific wording on how to ask about different forms of abuse. As we have stated previously, questions about abuse experiences should be worded behaviorally. We give some examples of such wording below, following descriptions of the specific types of abuse (most of these descriptions are adapted from those provided by John Briere, 1992).

Sexual Abuse

Sexual abuse includes activities by a parent or caregiver, such as fondling a child's genitals, penetration, incest, rape, sodomy, indecent exposure, and exploitation through prostitution or the production of pornographic materials. Sexual abuse can also occur between peers or siblings, if a substantial age difference exists between the victim and perpetrator or if the sexual activity is performed without the victim's consent.

Sample question: "When you were a child, did a parent, family member, or someone else in charge of your care ever touch or fondle you in a sexual way?"

Physical Abuse

Physical abuse can range from minor bruises to severe fractures or death as a result of punching, beating, kicking, biting, shaking, throwing, stabbing, choking, hitting (with a hand, stick, strap, or other object), burning, or otherwise harming a child. Such injury is considered abuse, regardless of whether the caregiver intended to hurt the child.

Sample question: "When you were a child or adolescent, did a parent or other caregiver—such as a grandparent, other adult relative, or babysitter—ever do something on purpose to you (for example, hit or punch or cut you or push you down) that gave your bruises or scratches, broke bones or teeth, or made you bleed?"

Emotional Abuse

Both sexual and physical abuse of children often co-occur with emotional abuse. Emotional abuse is a pattern of behavior that impairs a child's emotional development or sense of self-worth.

> *Sample question:* "When you were a child, did a parent or other caregiver say things repeatedly to you like 'You will never amount to anything'?"

Emotional abuse may also include constant criticism, threats, or rejection, as well as withholding love, support, or guidance.

> *Sample question:* "When you were a child, did a parent or other caregiver ever threaten to hurt or kill either you or someone (a friend) or something (a pet) you cared about?"

Physical Neglect

Physical neglect involves the failure of a child's caregiver to meet the child's basic physical or medical needs.

> *Sample question:* "When you were a child, were you ever not properly fed or clothed by your parent or other caregiver?"

Emotional Neglect

Emotional or psychological neglect is the failure of a child's caregiver to provide adequate nurturing and affection to a child, or a refusal to ensure or delay in ensuring that a child receives needed attention to emotional or behavioral problems.

> *Sample question:* "When you were a child, did your caregivers show you affection and make you feel special (for example, celebrate or acknowledge your birthday)?"

> *Sample question:* "When you were a child, did your caregivers comfort you when you were hurt or distressed?"

When the therapist has completed the assessment of the client's childhood trauma history, we recommend taking a few moments to check in with the client and ask how they feel having shared what they did before moving on to assess other traumatic experiences.

Revictimization History and Other Traumatic Experiences

One of the most profound consequences of childhood victimization is subsequent, repeated victimization in the form of rape, physical assault, and domestic violence (Jaffe, DiLillo, Gratz, & Messman-Moore, 2019; Messman-Moore & Long, 2000). Women with childhood sexual abuse are acutely aware of these problems, which are often among their most pressing reasons for seeking treatment. Trauma assessment therefore includes reviewing clients' adulthood as well as childhood trauma histories. We have found using a measure designed to screen for a wide range of traumatic experiences to be helpful in assessing clients' victimization histories and other traumatic experiences. Many of these screening measures, such as the revised version of the Life Stressor Checklist (LSC-R; Wolfe & Kimerling, 1997), have been designed for clients to fill out themselves, but they can also be used to guide a clinical interview.

Challenges in Reviewing Trauma History for Diagnostic Purposes

It should be noted that in order to receive a diagnosis of CPTSD or PTSD, a person must have experienced a traumatic event, and often the person is asked to identify their "worst trauma" as a point of reference for reporting symptoms. Since survivors of chronic trauma have often experienced multiple traumatic events, is most helpful for the therapist to talk about childhood abuse, domestic violence, or even combat as a set of *experiences* rather than as discrete events. During the evaluation, the therapist can ask the client to identify and focus on the experience that they consider the worst or most impactful. The trauma experience that the client chooses is not necessarily the event that the *therapist* views as most severe or distressing, but the one that troubles the client the most at the time of assessment. Diagnostic instruments such as those described below often include or identify life events measures by which to assess all potentially traumatic life events and determine which is currently the "worst" event for the client.

DIAGNOSIS OF ICD-11 PTSD AND CPTSD

Since the first edition of this book appeared in 2006, CPTSD has been formally recognized as a diagnosis in ICD-11 (WHO, 2018), as noted in Chapter 1. ICD is the diagnostic system that all insurers in the United States use, as do all hospitals, many clinics, and many therapists in private practice. It is a diagnostic system that includes both mental health and physical health disorders and is used by all disciplines (psychiatry, cardiology, immunology, gynecology) in hospital and clinic settings. In contrast, DSM, now in its fifth edition (DSM-5; American Psychiatric Association, 2013) is a diagnostic system that is specific to psychiatry and no other type of health problems. Clinicians have a choice of whether to use ICD or DSM in making diagnoses and submitting insurance claims. We devote some space to ICD-11 CPTSD here, because it is a new diagnosis but likely to be relevant to clients with chronic or prolonged traumas. For those interested in more detailed discussion of the similarities and differences between ICD and DSM diagnosis, we recommend Bisson, Brewin, Cloitre, and Maercker (2020).

Symptom Profiles

ICD-11 has been innovative in formalizing a conceptual distinction that has long been proposed—namely, that between PTSD and CPTSD (Herman, 1992). The latter refers to symptoms that are typically associated with prolonged trauma such as childhood abuse, intimate partner violence (IPV), or being a prisoner of war (see Brewin et al., 2017, for a review). ICD-11 PTSD includes the classic posttraumatic reactions of fear and horror, as well as three symptom clusters: (1) reexperiencing symptoms (constant replaying of images and thoughts about the event); (2) avoidance of thoughts, places, and feelings that are reminders of the trauma; and (3) a sense of threat that is manifested by excessive hypervigilance and or excessive startle response.

CPTSD comprises all three sets of PTSD symptoms, but also what are called "disturbances in self-organization," which include three problem domains: affect dysregulation, negative self-concept, and interpersonal difficulties (Maercker et al., 2013). CPTSD symptoms thus represent a broader spectrum of problems than PTSD symptoms. The CPTSD diagnosis acknowledges not only the role of traumatic stressors in generating horror and fear, but also the consequences that exposure to sustained, repeated, or multiple types of traumatic stressors have on self-organization, particularly when they occur during childhood. The affect dysregulation is evidenced by heightened emotional reactivity, violent outbursts, reckless or self-destructive behaviour, or a tendency toward experiencing prolonged dissociative states when under stress. In addition, there may be emotional numbing and a lack of ability to experience pleasure or positive emotions. Negative self-concept includes persistent beliefs about oneself as diminished, defeated, or worthless. These can be accompanied by deep and pervasive feelings of shame or guilt related to, for example, not having overcome adverse circumstances, or not having been able to prevent the suffering of others.

Interpersonal disturbances are defined by persistent difficulties in sustaining relationships. These difficulties may present in a variety of ways, but are exemplified by difficulties in feeling close to others. Some individuals will avoid relationships or feel incapable of getting and staying close to others, often because managing conflict and engaging in authentic communication is fear- or anxiety-producing. Others may actually deride or belittle relationships due to past disappointments. In sum, starting relationships is challenging and anxiety-producing, and maintaining them requires emotion regulation, psychological tolerance, and interpersonal skills the person may not have or cannot use when in a distressed state.

A substantial literature is accumulating indicating that individuals with CPTSD are more likely to have experienced prolonged trauma than those with PTSD, supporting the conceptual basis for this distinction (see Brewin et al., 2017). The practical clinical benefits of this distinction are that it can facilitate more refined characterization of symptom profiles for subgroups of survivors of trauma, and, most importantly, can help shape more personalized, effective, and efficient treatment plans (see ISTSS, 2019b).

Measures

There are at least two measures developed for the assessment of ICD-11 PTSD and CPTSD, both of which have validity and reliability data. The International Trauma Questionnaire (ITQ; Cloitre et al., 2018d) contains 12 symptom items that assess the three domains of PTSD (reexperiencing, avoidance, and chronic threat), as well as the three domains related to self-organization difficulties (affect dysregulation, negative self-concept, and interpersonal difficulties). It is intended to be brief and easily implemented, allowing for a designation of a probable diagnosis of ICD-11 PTSD or CPTSD. There is also a clinician-administered interview, the International Trauma Interview (ITI; Roberts, Cloitre, Bisson, & Brewin, 2018), which includes questions covering all of the symptoms described in the ITQ but in a more detailed way. This measure allows for the client to elaborate on the specific nature of the symptoms, age of onset of symptoms, and degree to which the client feels that symptoms are related to their trauma. The ITI is still under development and is not currently available for distribution. The ITQ has been translated into several languages and can be downloaded for free (*www.traumameasuresglobal.com*). The ITI will be posted on the same site when it becomes available.

DIAGNOSIS OF DSM-5 PTSD

Symptom Profile

DSM-5 covers many of the symptoms and perhaps even more than those presented in ICD-11 PTSD and CPTSD combined, and for that reason it has sometimes been called the "big tent" approach to diagnosis. DSM-5 is likely to capture a large number of people but without specific reference to type of trauma or salience of symptoms, which may be a benefit of the ICD-11 system. DSM-5 PTSD shares with ICD-11 PTSD what are considered the "core" or "classic" symptoms of PTSD—namely, symptoms of reexperiencing, avoidance, and what is called "hypervigilance."

DSM-5 also includes symptoms described as "negative alterations in cognitions and mood," which include symptoms such as negative emotional states (shame, guilt), social withdrawal (a type of interpersonal problem), and inability to experience positive emotions (a version of numbing). In addition, DSM-5 includes "alterations in arousal and reactivity," which include the symptoms of chronic threat in ICD-11 (irritable behavior, angry outbursts, poor concentration, and sleep difficulties). Lastly, DSM-5 includes a dissociative subtype, which is represented by symptoms of derealization and depersonalization. To date, there has been no research investigating whether different therapies may be valuable for individuals who experience or are concerned about particular symptoms associated with DSM-5 PTSD, although this situation may evolve over time.

Measures

Two validated and reliable instruments are most commonly used to assess DSM-5 PTSD. The PTSD Checklist for DSM-5 (PCL-5; Weathers et al., 2013b) is a self-report questionnaire with 20 items. The Clinician-Administered PTSD Scale for DSM-5 (CAPS-5; Weathers et al., 2013a) is administered as an interview. Both measures (English-language versions) are available on request from the U.S. National Center for PTSD.

It will be important to conduct research examining the degree of overlap between individuals who receive a diagnosis of DSM-5 PTSD and those who receive a diagnosis of either ICD-11 PTSD or CPTSD. ICD-11 PTSD and CPTSD may together represent a similar population but provide a more refined description of the range of clients' concerns. Further details about these diagnoses, their development, and their similarities and differences are available in other publications (e.g., Bisson et al., 2020).

SPECIFIC SYMPTOM DOMAINS

Regardless of which diagnostic system a therapist or client prefers, assessment of specific problems and strengths is part of good clinical evaluation. Below, we describe important symptom domains associated with trauma, their presentations in the clinical setting, and measures for assessing them. The descriptions of assessment measures are by no means exhaustive, but rather are intended to provide some suggestions for interested therapists. These measures can be given directly to clients to complete or simply to review. Alternatively, a therapist can use them as a basis for further queries. Often, when clients complete or review the items on these measures, they are surprised but also comforted that the difficulties they experience are identified. Some clients have commented that they are relieved that their experiences are known and understood, and that other survivors share the same problems.

Classic or Core PTSD Symptoms

The symptoms discussed below are those that have been consistently identified as symptoms of PTSD across diagnostic systems (DSM or ICD) and across changes within a diagnostic system.

Reexperiencing symptoms

Clients may express that thoughts or images of the trauma come into their minds without warning. They may describe having nightmares about the trauma (or nightmares that evoke emotions similar to those they experienced when the traumatic events were occurring). At the extreme, clients may have flashbacks, in which they actually feel as if they are experiencing the feelings, sensations, and thoughts associated with the trauma in a "here-and-now" way. Such flashbacks are sometimes so real that they can be misdiagnosed by clinicians unfamiliar with PTSD as psychotic symptoms. For example, one of our clients, who had been severely physically and emotionally abused by her mother, reported to her psychiatrist that she was "hearing voices" that insulted her and told her to punish herself. During our assessment of this client, we discovered that the "voices" were actually flashbacks of her mother yelling at her. The client knew that such voices were not real, but when these flashbacks occurred, she felt as if she was a child and the abuse was happening again.

Avoidance symptoms

Avoidance symptoms consist of clients' avoiding thoughts, feelings, places, or persons that remind them of their traumatic experiences. Such symptoms are particularly challenging to assess in clients who experienced childhood abuse, because often avoidance began early in life and has become such a part of the clients' ways of being in the world that they are not even conscious of it. For example, a 47-year-old client who was sexually abused was very socially withdrawn. She had never had an intimate relationship, had few friends, and supported herself financially by editing scientific publications (which she could do from home). Her social withdrawal started in adolescence as a way of avoiding sexual attention from males, because such attention reminded her of the abuse and made her extremely anxious. At 47 years old, this client had been socially withdrawn for over 30 years. She had structured her entire professional and personal life to avoid being around people, particularly men. She did not even fully recognize how her avoidance had shaped her life.

Chronic sense of threat

Hypervigilance and exaggerated startle responses are typical expressions of perceived threat. In a survivor of childhood abuse, chronic hypervigilance may be manifested by general unease around men or discomfort when in close physical proximity to men if the perpetrator was a man. Individuals without trauma histories may also experience exaggerated startle responses when in an anxious state. Among those with trauma exposure, however, the startle responses are consistently present, and the clients tend to notice and report them.

The classic or core PTSD symptoms can be assessed via interviews such as those described above, but it is likely quicker and just as useful for nonresearch purposes to use self-report measures such as the ITQ (Cloitre et al., 2018d) or the PCL-5 (Weathers et al., 2013b).

Emotion Regulation Problems

Emotion regulation is the ability to modulate powerful affective states. As noted above, clients with histories of child maltreatment find themselves fluctuating between two emotional extremes: either being overwhelmed by their feelings or alternatively feeling nothing or "numb." Clients report that these extreme states often occur unpredictably. They also may find that they get highly distressed unexpectedly over minor things, have trouble letting go of upsetting things, and have difficulty calming themselves down. At other times they feel numb, particularly in circumstances that would typically elicit emotion (including positive emotion, such as at a wedding or birthday celebration).

"Numbing" refers to the tendency to experience restrictions in emotional experiences. Some researchers argue that individuals who report numbing are hyperreactive to negative triggers (particularly those related to the traumatic events), which deplete their capacity for emotional response and therefore need more intense positive stimulation to experience positive emotions (Litz & Gray, 2002). Survivors of childhood trauma may describe feeling at times "numb" or "dead inside" or "nothing" or "like a zombie." They may report difficulty feeling love or joy, as well as anger or sadness. They often describe being confused because things that produce emotion in other people often have no impact on them. Thus numbing is a component of the emotion dysregulation characteristic of individuals with trauma histories, who tend to cycle between feeling overwhelmed by emotion and feeling "nothing."

The therapist may begin the assessment of emotion regulation by saying something like this:

"Some people who experience trauma have difficulty managing their feelings. Sometimes they may feel nothing, numb, or empty. At other times, for seemingly no reason, they may be overwhelmed by feeling too much. At these points, they may not even know what they feel—only that they are 'upset.' Does this sound familiar to you?"

For emotion regulation problems, the 16-item Difficulties in Emotion Regulation Scale (DERS-16; Bjureberg et al., 2016) can be used. The DERS-16 identifies five types of emotion regulation problems, including difficulties in clarifying feelings, difficulties with impulse control, difficulties in maintaining focus on goals when emotionally distressed, limitations in skills or strategies to manage emotions and lastly, ability to accept emotional distress. All five types of emotion regulation problems are relevant to individuals who have experienced early interpersonal trauma.

Negative Self-Concept

Negative self-concept relates to beliefs about oneself as being worthless or a failure. It can also be associated with feelings of shame and guilt. Survivors of childhood maltreatment often feel worthless because they have been told this directly (i.e., verbal abuse) by caregivers, who say this to justify their actions. In particular, although sexual abuse is sometimes framed as a "special" experience for a prized child, the secrecy required suggests that there is something bad or shameful about it. Often as the child grows up, they become aware that in fact they have engaged in something inappropriate, but blame themselves rather than the perpetrator. Assessing feelings of low self-worth is a delicate task that needs to be approached with support and psychoeducation. For example, clients often have firmly rooted beliefs of their inferiority and can assume that the therapist is asking about this problem because their inferiority is so evident. The therapist can introduce the inquiry by saying something that references the trauma as the cause of the problem, not the person. For example, the therapist can ask, "One of the consequences of being subjected to abuse is a sense of worthlessness. Do you have any of those kinds of feelings?" Repeated reassurance that the client is not alone in these feelings (normalization) will help reduce the client's shame, guilt, and other negative beliefs they hold about themselves.

A brief and well-established measure to assess self-esteem and sense of worth is the Rosenberg Self-Esteem Scale (RSES; Rosenberg, 1965), a basic 10-item scale that has been translated into several languages and used in several countries.

Interpersonal Difficulties

As mentioned throughout this book, many clients cite interpersonal problems as their primary reasons for seeking treatment. Therapists can get a sense of clients' interpersonal difficulties by asking about their social support networks; whether they have close friends;

and whether they are in or have ever been in an intimate relationship, and, if so, what those relationships have been like.

Problems with emotion regulation and mood often lead to interpersonal problems among those with histories of childhood abuse. Several studies have found that depression and anger, rather than PTSD symptoms, are the predominant correlates of the interpersonal difficulties reported by individuals with abuse histories (e.g., Beckham et al., 1996). A therapist can query whether a client has noticed that they get depressed or angry, and whether these feelings seem to interfere with relationships at home, at work, or in social life. The therapist may ask (in regard to depression), "Do you cancel social events or call in sick because you are feeling too down to go out?", or (in regard to anger), "Do you ever find that when you are angry, you do or say things that you later regret?"

A study of the types of interpersonal problems experienced by survivors of abuse revealed that, compared to those who had never been abused, those with abuse histories reported significantly more problems in being both too submissive and too controlling, greater difficulty in being assertive, and more problems in taking on too much responsibility in situations for which they might not be responsible (Cloitre & Koenen, 2001). These data suggest that survivors of childhood abuse often have significant difficulties centering around issues of power and control in relationships. A therapist can gently inquire whether a client experiences these sorts of difficulties, with questions such as "Do you find yourself having difficulties standing up for yourself or afraid of conflict?" or "Do your friends ever say that you are argumentative or need to have your own way?"

For problems in relationships, the 32-item version of the Inventory of Interpersonal Problems (IIP-32; Barkham, Hardy, & Startup, 1996) is useful, as it inquires about a range of interpersonal difficulties we have commonly found among survivors of chronic trauma. These include difficulties with being either too submissive or too assertive; difficulties with being too caring for others at the expense of oneself, or, alternatively, difficulties with being supportive of others; and difficulties with being sociable, including in romantic and intimate relationships.

Harmful/Risky Behaviors and Comorbidity

The assessment of harmful or risky behaviors has been addressed in detail by other authors (e.g., Linehan, 1993, 2015). The present discussion is limited to the task of identifying whether STAIR Narrative Therapy is a good match for individual clients presenting with PTSD or CPTSD. Clients whose difficulties demand immediate attention—such as imminent suicidality, alcohol or other substance use disorders, severely disordered eating behaviors (such as regular bingeing and purging), or severe dissociation that meets criteria for a dissociative disorder diagnosis—are most likely to need more intensive interventions and should be directed to a higher level of care or a setting in which these behaviors can be directly addressed.

Self-harming or risky behaviors are strongly associated with a history of child abuse, and therefore should be assessed in clients presenting with a history of trauma. Clients who have these difficulties may be appropriate candidates for STAIR Narrative Therapy at a later time, when they are stabilized and are no longer a threat to themselves or others. We have had several clients who engaged in STAIR Narrative Therapy after successfully completing an inpatient or residential treatment program for one of the above-mentioned problems.

Resilience and Coping Strategies

The topics of resilience and coping among survivors of childhood maltreatment are receiving growing attention (e.g., Harvey, Liang, Harney, & Koenen, 2003). We view clients who were abused as children and are now seeking treatment as showing resilience. Such clients must have had some coping strategies that were effective for their environments and have enabled them to survive. Our interest in resilience is reflected in our assessments, which attempt to gather information about the clients' resilient domains of functioning and successful coping strategies. Such information can help therapists tailor interventions to best utilize clients' resources and strengths.

A therapist may begin to engage a client in talking about strengths by asking how the client coped when the maltreatment was going on: "How did you manage to function?" The therapist can then guide the client toward evaluating those strategies and whether they continue to work in the present. Another way of talking about the client's strengths is to ask them what they think they are. However, many clients have trouble identifying anything positive about themselves. If this is the case, the therapist might have the client talk about what their boss, best friend, neighbor, or significant other might say are their best qualities. The therapist might gain information on the client's strengths by talking about their intellectual or social interests or activities, such as drawing, reading, church/temple work, or volunteer work.

A well-established and well-known measure to assess coping capacity is the Coping Orientation to Problems Experienced (COPE; Scheier & Carver, 1985). It is a 60-item inventory that measures five problem-focused coping styles, including active coping, planning, suppression of competing activities, restraint coping, and seeking instrumental social support.

ASSESSMENT FEEDBACK
AND TREATMENT RECOMMENDATIONS

Match for Treatment

If a therapist is considering using this treatment with a particular client, a simple rule of thumb is to ask whether the client's primary presenting problems involve difficulties in emotion regulation or interpersonal problems that appear to be connected to a history of trauma, particularly child abuse or neglect. If the answer is yes, and if the client is not at imminent risk from self-harming behaviors, then it is appropriate to consider using this treatment with the client. Therapists may wish to use only the STAIR module (Module I) to address these difficulties, and to use the module or particular sessions as often as needed. If the client also has significant PTSD symptoms, then the addition of the Narrative Therapy module (Module II) is indicated.

Readiness for Treatment

If the client's presenting problems indicate that the treatment is appropriate, the therapist will want to consider whether the client is motivated and has the time and other practical resources to participate. STAIR Narrative Therapy requires a commitment of 18 weeks and additional time to complete between-session exercises. The trauma-processing work during the Narrative Therapy module in particular requires a sustained and consistent effort for a minimum of 4 weeks (if sessions can be scheduled twice per week). The treatment as a whole requires not only a time commitment, but a commitment to use all available emotional and social resources to complete the work. During STAIR Narrative Therapy, clients are asked to confront not only their trauma histories, but also parts of themselves and their lives that they have avoided for years. Clients who enter into this treatment must therefore be motivated to make changes in their lives and to commit the practical and emotional resources it demands.

Clients who cannot attend treatment regularly—say, because of personal or professional demands, or generally chaotic lives—are likely to obtain less benefit from this treatment. For instance, clients who travel a great deal on business and will miss sessions for weeks will not obtain maximum benefit. Such clients can be provided with supportive or other forms of therapy until they are able to attend treatment regularly.

It is also common for clients to come to treatment in the middle of a personal or family crisis, such as when a parent is terminally ill. Such crises seem to trigger unresolved trauma histories or exacerbate PTSD and other trauma-related symptoms. However, some clients in such situations may not be able to commit to an intensive, trauma-focused treatment. They may benefit from a less directive, more supportive form of therapy until the crisis resolves.

It is difficult to predict ahead of time which clients will be able to commit to the treatment. Therapists will have to think through these situations on a case-by-case basis. Some clients are able to overcome great odds to participate fully in the treatment. One client we treated was an impoverished single mother, who worked full-time while raising four children. She was also in recovery from alcoholism and regularly attended Alcoholics Anonymous (AA). Despite these barriers to treatment, she never missed a session and regularly completed between-session exercises. This success was partly the result of good planning. Early in treatment, the client and therapist thought very practically about how to arrange her schedule to maximize her ability to complete the therapy. The client made backup arrangements for child care with friends, and got up 30 minutes earlier in the morning to complete her skills practice. She was also fortunate enough to have a supportive supervisor at work, who allowed her to attend her AA meetings during the day. Thus this client was able to activate her social supports in order to commit to treatment, in spite of having few financial resources and large family responsibilities. We encourage therapists to work with clients to help them identify barriers to treatment and address those barriers before they become insurmountable obstacles.

Feedback

After completing the assessment, the therapist is in a position to give feedback to the client. This includes summarizing the therapist's understanding of the issues the client has presented, describing the connection between the client's trauma history and current symptoms, and discussing how these are addressed in STAIR Narrative Therapy. This process can be therapeutic in and of itself. It can provide an experience in which the client feels listened to and understood, and can offer the opportunity for the client to clarify the therapist's understanding if needed.

We have found that that most clients, including those who have already been in therapy, have never received this kind of direct feedback. Many have never been assessed for or diagnosed with trauma-related disorders; have never discussed with a therapist how their trauma histories continue to affect them; and/or have never been given a rationale for the treatment being offered and how it will address the difficulties that led them to seek help.

CASE EXAMPLE

Annie was a 35-year-old divorced woman with three school-age children. She worked as an administrative assistant for an official in a local government agency. Her husband had left her when her children were very young, and she had since been preoccupied with supporting her family and raising her children. She reported a history of sexual abuse by her father from ages 7 to 10, and verbal and physical abuse by her mother throughout childhood (*trauma history*). She called our clinic after she saw an advertisement for our treatment in a local newspaper. She came to treatment when she reached her 35th birthday.

In Annie's initial session, she described herself as "an alcoholic," but noted that she had been sober for the last year. She was actively involved in AA (*history of harmful behavior [substance use] but not current*). She reported that since she stopped drinking, she had become increasingly anxious and irritable, and had difficulty not snapping at people in response to what she knew was minor provocations (*emotion regulation problems*). Nightmares of the abuse had become more frequent (*PTSD symptoms: nightmares*). She also reported that when she felt particularly down on herself at work for failing to do a task correctly, she would occasionally have images of the abuse come into her head, hear her mother's voice deriding her, and have the urge to crawl under her desk for safety but restrain herself from doing so (*PTSD symptoms: flashbacks*). She also noted that she tended to be on guard all the time, even when doing simple tasks like grocery shopping, and was easily startled (*PTSD symptoms: chronic sense of threat*).

Annie reported that she had coped with her symptoms by keeping very busy. She had been at her current job for 7 years and had a good record (*resilience and coping strategies*). Her work experience revealed a consistent pattern of good employment. She appeared to have a record as an excellent employee, but had never built on that to request any sort of advancement for herself, such as asking for a raise or new duties (*interpersonal problems: lack of assertiveness*). She stated that her agency was currently offering a training program for employees who wished to move from administration to management. Her supervisor at work wanted to nominate her as a candidate for the program, but Annie was convinced she would never be selected. She did not believe she "had what it takes" to make it in management, and generally considered herself to be worthless (*negative self-concept*).

Annie reported several close friendships with members of AA (*resilience: good social support*). However, she felt that she would never get into another intimate relationship again (*interpersonal difficulties: problems with getting close*). Her husband's leaving her had reinforced her feelings of failure as a wife and mother (*negative self-concept*), and she was terrified to allow herself to be vulnerable again. She struggled to be a good parent to her children, but frequently found herself caught between being overly indulgent because she felt guilty about not being more available to them, and being overly controlling and strict (*interpersonal problems*). She reported that sometimes she lost her temper and found herself screaming at them, which left her feeling like a terrible mother and bad person. She reported impulses to hit her children, but had never done so (*emotion regulation problems*). If she found herself particularly enraged, she would lock herself in the bathroom until she calmed down. She reported suicidal thoughts, but had never attempted suicide and reported no plans or intention to make such an attempt. She reported a tendency to overeat when she was anxious or depressed, but denied bingeing or purging (*risky behaviors not a priority*).

Interpreting the Assessment Findings

If Annie was imminently suicidal, actively self-injurious, or currently misusing substances, she would have been inappropriate for this treatment. If this had been the case, the therapist would have given Annie the reasons for needing to be provided with an alternative treatment and would have referred her to a treatment program focusing on her suicidality, self-harm, and/or substance misuse. Often we encourage clients to return to us for treatment after they have addressed problems such as substance use disorders.

Annie was a client who was clearly appropriate for STAIR Narrative Therapy. She presented with PTSD symptoms (flashbacks, nightmares, chronic sense of threat) related to her history of childhood abuse. She also reported emotion regulation difficulties that were affecting her interpersonal relationships (snapping at others, difficulty managing her children). Annie's alcoholism was under control, and she did not report any other self-injurious behaviors that would have taken priority at this time.

Therapist Feedback

After completing and evaluating the assessment information, the therapist informed Annie that her problems were appropriate for STAIR Narrative Therapy. In speaking about how STAIR Narrative Therapy would help Annie, the therapist focused on three specific issues: her nightmares and flashbacks of the abuse; her difficulty with managing her emotions in a range of situations and relationships; and her challenges with pursuing advancement at work. The therapist spoke with Annie about how part of the treatment would focus on how to manage her feelings in interpersonal situations to achieve goals she had identified. As an initial goal to focus on, the therapist suggested that Annie might choose speaking with her boss about being nominated as a candidate for the training program. She could ask questions and get more information about the program and possible position, so that she could make a decision based upon her goals rather than based upon fear.

The therapist noted that Annie's self-esteem seemed to be low, despite such accomplishments as holding a steady job and being a single parent. The therapist also noted that developing mastery in managing her feelings and developing more skills both at work and at home might help boost her self-esteem. This might give her sufficient confidence and security to begin exploring the deeper sources of her negative views of herself, which might have been rooted in her abuse experiences. The therapist also spoke about how the trauma-focused work in the second part of the treatment would help reduce Annie's nightmares and flashbacks. It would also allow her to reappraise the abuse experience and consider whether the abuse and insults she had experienced as a child might have had more to do with her parents' own difficulties than with who she really was. Through this discussion, the therapist was able to tie the specific problems Annie was currently experiencing to the interventions used in STAIR Narrative Therapy.

SUMMARY AND IMPLICATIONS FOR TREATMENT

This chapter has focused on orienting therapists to the process of assessing clients and considering the match between clients' needs and STAIR Narrative Therapy. We have discussed how to talk to clients about their trauma histories. We have provided information about the ICD-11 diagnoses of PTSD and CPTSD, as well as the DSM-5 diagnosis of PTSD. We have provided detailed information on specific symptoms and strengths and on how they may present in the assessment. Finally, we have offered some suggestions for determining whether a client is appropriate for this treatment and for giving feedback to the client after the assessment has been completed.

PART III

STAIR Narrative Therapy, Session by Session

Skills Training in Affective and Interpersonal Regulation (STAIR)

Building Resources

CHAPTER 10

The Resource of Hope
Introducing the Client to Treatment

> The very making of an appointment with a total stranger
> to deal with the greatest intimacies and vulnerabilities
> of one's life is an act of profound faith.
> —DIANA FOSHA (2000, p. 5)

By the time a client with trauma comes to therapy, they have often reached the limits of their capacity to function adequately on their own. They are likely to be feeling substantially demoralized and defeated. Visiting a professional is often an act of desperation. Still, by coming to therapy, the client is holding on to some vestige of hope. The therapist's primary task is to sustain and strengthen this hope. Hope emerges from both a sense of being understood and cared for, and a belief in the possibility of change. Thus the therapist's first task is to listen carefully to the client and reflect back an accurate and empathic understanding of the client's symptoms and life circumstances. In addition, the therapist must then propose a treatment plan that addresses these problems, and, in a collaborative process with the client, must come to a shared understanding about the goals of the therapy and the means by which these goals will be reached.

WELCOME CLIENT TO TREATMENT AND IDENTIFY FOCUS OF THE SESSION

The therapist begins the session with a warm welcome and polite check-in on how the client is doing the day of the meeting. The check-in is brief, but if content comes up related to the client's symptoms or experiences, the therapist provides genuine empathy while containing any affect and reassuring the client that they are here today to start (or continue) their journey of recovery. The therapist can also let them know the broader goals of this first session, which are to review the client's symptoms and goals, orient them to the intervention plan, and learn their first skill. Box 10.1 outlines the session contents and major tasks.

Theme and Curriculum for Session 1
The Resource of Hope: Introducing the Client to Treatment

By the time a client with a history of trauma comes to therapy, they have often reached the limits of their capacity to function. Still, by coming to therapy, the client is holding on to some vestige of hope. The therapist's primary task is to sustain and strengthen this hope. Hope emerges from both a sense of being understood and a belief in the possibility of change. Thus the first of the therapist's tasks is to listen carefully to the client and reflect back an accurate and empathic understanding of the client's symptoms and life circumstances. In addition, the therapist must then propose a treatment plan that addresses these problems, and, in collaboration with the client, must come to an agreement about the goals of the therapy and the means by which these goals will be reached. The therapist will also give the client "something to go home with" by beginning skills training in a mind–body exercise (Focused Breathing).

PLANNING AND PREPARATION

Review client's evaluation materials, particularly trauma history, symptoms, and coping skills. Bring handouts on treatment rationale and Focused Breathing (Handouts 10.1 and 10.2). The work in the session is estimated to take about 60 minutes; a flexible application is assumed (i.e., not every client will need all interventions).

AGENDA

- Welcome client to treatment and identify focus of the session.
- Review client's evaluation experience, trauma history, and symptoms.
- Establish the therapeutic contract.
- Provide overview of treatment plan.
- Explain goals of Module I: STAIR (emotion regulation and interpersonal skills development).
- Explain goals of Module II: Narrative Therapy (PTSD symptom reduction and creation of life narrative, if relevant to client's treatment plan).
- Review rationale for and benefits of a two-module treatment (if relevant to client's treatment plan).
- Provide a coping skill: Focused Breathing.
- Provide rationale for between-session skills practice.
- Summarize the goals of the session.
- Plan skills practice:
  - Practice Focused Breathing twice a day.

(continued)

REVIEW CLIENT'S EVALUATION EXPERIENCE, TRAUMA HISTORY, AND SYMPTOMS

The therapist begins by inquiring about the client's experience of the evaluation process, which established the client's baseline symptoms and appropriateness for the treatment. This discussion will provide an understanding of the client's emotional state and potential concerns about the treatment. If someone other than the therapist completed the evaluation, it will be important to make clear that the therapist has become acquainted with the evaluation materials and presenting problems. If the therapist completed the evaluation, it is still useful to summarize the material from the evaluation, including trauma history, symptoms, and presenting problems. Doing so serves multiple purposes, including verifying that the information is correct and providing the client an opportunity to add anything further that feels important for the therapist to know.

The therapist is actively working here, conveying that they have made an effort to know the client, and also that the therapist is not overwhelmed by the client's history or symptoms. At the same time, the therapist is careful not to overwhelm the client by confronting them with too stark a summary of their trauma experiences. Thus the therapist may often pause to make room for the client to confirm, clarify, or add information, conveying an expectation of collaboration. This task may take 10–30 minutes, depending on the complexity of the client's trauma history and/or inclination to elaborate.

Many clients can be emotionally reactive to hearing their trauma histories summarized. In fact, a key symptom of PTSD is often a client's experience of being upset upon confronting memory triggers of what has happened to them. The therapist needs to be alert to this possibility, and addressing it with the client is often necessary. In some cases, previewing this possible reaction before conducting the review can help prepare the client and reassure them that their feelings are normal, that these reactions are not signs of weakness, and that the therapist is sensitive and caring about the client's experience. All of these messages help bolster the therapeutic alliance at this early stage of therapy. Furthermore, reassuring the client that this treatment will help them better manage these reactions over time can be very important and motivating. Although reviewing assessments and trauma history may trigger symptoms in the moment, this reaction will become manageable as the therapy proceeds. In fact, this phenomenon is a core aspect of many posttraumatic reactions and a key treatment target.

ESTABLISH THE THERAPEUTIC CONTRACT

The initial and perhaps unarticulated agreement when the client walks through the door is that the client has come to therapy for help and the therapist has agreed to help them.

How this will take place is the next question, and the answer to it needs to be discussed and negotiated in a collaborative, respectful way. Alongside the spoken words of this contract are process-oriented components; both are crucial in establishing an effective contract.

The Initial Treatment Description

Certain parameters guide this process when a therapist plans to implement an empirically based treatment like STAIR Narrative Therapy. In this situation, the therapist begins with the proposal that the results of the assessment—particularly the client's identified PTSD symptoms, problems with emotion management, and difficulties with relationships—indicate that STAIR is a good match to their needs. The therapist can express confidence in this approach by saying something like this:

> "This treatment was developed specifically for people with problems similar to yours. The therapists who created it relied heavily on input and feedback from survivors of trauma who came to treatment and had the same kinds of problems and issues as you. Because of this history, we know that this treatment works. It's been systematically evaluated with several hundreds of people similar to you over the last 20 years, and the results have shown it's effective. People who've completed STAIR Narrative Therapy have also shared that the treatment process itself was, although sometimes difficult, a positive experience and worth the effort. Because of all of this history and evidence, I'm looking forward to our work together, and to helping you find your way toward recovery and living the life you deserve."

If the client is concerned that the treatment may be too rigid or structured and will not take into account their individual needs, the therapist can reassure them. As described in Chapter 8, the treatment has built-in flexibility. The therapist can say something like this:

> "STAIR Narrative Therapy has become flexible enough over time to be tailored to each person's needs without compromising its effectiveness. For example, increasing or decreasing the number of sessions—as well as the emphasis on some types of skills training over others, depending on your needs—in no way decreases the effectiveness of the treatment. In fact, applying the treatment in this way is known to provide even greater benefits. We'll work together on how to tailor this treatment so that it's most effective for you."

Cautious enthusiasm is the most common response to hearing this initial introduction to treatment. Clients are typically relieved to hear that their problems are not unusual; are well known to professionals; and (most importantly) have received considerable amounts of sensitive thought, research, and treatment development. The therapist can then proceed to a more specific review of the treatment rationale and specific interventions. As described below, the therapist engages in a dialogue with the client to make sure that each aspect described is matched to the client's specific needs in a way that is understandable and relevant to them. The number of sessions, length of treatment, and areas of concentration for skills training are discussed and planned, but the client and therapist can be assured that whatever may come up in the process of therapy, both of them will collaborate to adapt it to the client's specific needs and response.

Reminders about the Therapeutic Alliance

The therapeutic alliance is a working partnership between the therapist and the client, and it is an integral if not critical part of any effective treatment. In particular, therapy settings "pull" for power dynamics, owing to the therapist's perceived position of authority. The power balance between therapist and client can be delicate to negotiate, given the client's experiences of misused authority.

On the one hand, the therapist is placed in the position of an "expert" or an authority figure, as they have skills that are intended to help guide the client in reaching desired goals. This role has legitimate aspects and positive value for the client. The therapist's knowledge and capacity to implement the treatment provide much-needed structure and containment for the tasks at hand. It also provides the client with a sense of safety and security, which is a prerequisite for effective treatment.

On the other hand, the client's reactions to authority figures, especially in the case of childhood abuse, may include feelings of fear, hostility, and/or suspicion toward the therapist. The client may feel disregarded and controlled by the therapist, and ineffectual in managing themselves in this setting. To counteract this obviously negative interpersonal dynamic, the therapist must make clear that their role as an "expert" is in the service of the client's needs and desired recovery, and that it ideally complements—not invalidates—the client's perspective on their personal experiences. The interventions, their use, and their timing/pace follow the client's experiences and wishes. The treatment has been developed to be flexible for this very reason. Given the client's background, they are likely to have had little opportunity to be attended to, taken seriously, and truly seen and heard. The therapist's attitude of receptivity and responsiveness to the client's experience is a therapeutic intervention in its own right. For many survivors of childhood abuse, openly sharing their perspective, especially when it contrasts with another person's viewpoint, is a very challenging but important opportunity to practice appropriate levels of assertiveness—a skill more explicitly introduced in the second half of STAIR Narrative Therapy.

Ideally, agreement about the therapy goals and means will be readily established between therapist and client, and therapy will proceed. Therapist and client will remain attuned to each other as treatment goals evolve and as the means by which these goals are to be met are determined. The support of the therapist will empower the client and affirm their value and crucial role in the effort. The client in turn will appreciate the therapist's expertise as an instrument of support, rather than as a negation of their needs or experience. Any ruptures that may occur in the therapeutic alliance, as in any kind of therapy, will require immediate attention, communication, and healing to ensure that the therapeutic work is effective. Therapeutic ruptures cannot all be avoided, but if they are openly and respectfully addressed, the repair of ruptures can actually strengthen the alliance and reinforce important lessons about relationships and communication.

PROVIDE OVERVIEW OF TREATMENT PLAN

The therapist explains that this treatment has two modules, which usually (when combined) last for a total of 16–20 hour-long weekly sessions. The first module focuses on learning skills for living more effectively, with specific emphases on emotion management problems and interpersonal difficulties. In the second module, sessions focus on the emotional processing of the client's traumatic experiences, as well as continued work on enhancing life skills. Handout 10.1, Treatment Overview: What Is STAIR Narrative Therapy?, can be used to provide the client with an overview of the STAIR Narrative Therapy treatment. (Note that all client handouts are grouped together at the ends of treatment chapters, for ease of reproduction.)

EXPLAIN GOALS OF MODULE I: STAIR

Emotion Regulation Skills Development

The therapist explains that one main goal of the first module is to help the client develop emotional awareness and learn skills to modulate negative feelings and tolerate distress. The client may benefit from learning that many people who were traumatized (especially as children) have difficulty knowing what they are feeling and/or how to manage their feelings. Some people feel overwhelmed by their feelings, while others may have learned to cope by not feeling anything at all—through either numbing or dissociation. The therapist can stop and ask the client about their experience with these common patterns. It may help to give examples such as the following: "Some people are never able to feel anger, while others don't feel able to manage their anger at all, so that they 'blow up.' Does either of these patterns match your experience?"

The therapist explains that the treatment will involve learning how the client can experience their feelings without becoming overwhelmed. This will first involve the client's becoming more aware of their feelings and what triggers them. People traumatized as children may have particular difficulty experiencing and labeling feelings, because their feelings were mislabeled or disregarded by others. Again, the therapist both gives examples and elicits examples from the client.

To get an initial sense of how others responded to the client's feelings when the client was a child (this subject is pursued in more detail in Session 2), the therapist engages the client in a discussion. If the client does not spontaneously respond to what the therapist is describing, inviting them to do so may help with comments such as "Does this strike a chord anywhere for you?"

Interpersonal Skills Development

A second goal of the STAIR module is for the client to learn how to improve interpersonal skills by using interpersonal goals rather than feeling states to guide their interactions. The therapist and client will also talk about how the client can use these skills in their relationships—specifically, to manage certain emotions that can at times interfere with or overshadow their relationship goals. The therapist may ask the client about difficulties they experience in interpersonal relationships, prompting with examples and questions as necessary—for instance, saying something like: "Some people who were maltreated as children have a hard time being assertive, or they let people take advantage of them. Is this familiar to you?" or "Are there certain feelings you have problems expressing to people? What makes it difficult?" The client's answers likely will highlight elements of their interpersonal style and areas of concern. Later sessions explore these topics again in more detail.

Selection of Specific Coping Skills

Finally, the therapist tells the client that the client will have the opportunity to learn a number of emotion management and relationship skills, and will select what they think will work best for them from a "menu" of options. The therapist and client will use the results of any preliminary assessment measures to evaluate the client's relative strengths in cognitive, behavioral, and social support strategies for managing current distress. This information will inform, later in treatment, the selection of coping skills that best match the client's current problems.

EXPLAIN GOALS OF MODULE II: NARRATIVE THERAPY (IF RELEVANT)

If the treatment plan involves both modules of STAIR Narrative Therapy (or the possibility of continuing to Module II), the therapist can preview that in the second half of treatment, the client will systematically identify and explore their feelings about their traumatic experiences. One important goal of this work is for the client to be able to think about the trauma, or encounter reminders or triggers of it, without experiencing their particular symptoms at the intensity they do now at the start of treatment. A second goal of Narrative Therapy is to help the client make meaning of their traumatic experiences—to respect their history of pain, but also to put it in the past.

Review of PTSD Assessment Results

If not done earlier in this session, the therapist can provide a brief overview of the symptoms that constitute the diagnosis of PTSD or CPTSD (whichever is more appropriate), and explain how some or all of the client's symptoms fit into the diagnosis. PTSD is described as a syndrome that can develop after a person has been exposed to a traumatic event, such as childhood abuse, rape, combat, being in a plane crash, or witnessing a murder. Often PTSD develops soon after the trauma; however, it can begin at any time after the event. Using the client's self-reported PTSD symptoms (obtained from evaluation materials), the therapist and client together review the four DSM-5 PTSD symptom clusters (i.e., reexperiencing, avoidance, negative cognitions/moods, and arousal); determine which of these symptom clusters match what the client reported in the assessment; and clarify their understanding of what the symptoms are and how they fit into each category.

Another diagnosis that might be a better match for people who have experienced prolonged trauma is CPTSD, a diagnosis that is now included in ICD-11 (see Chapter 9). In addition to symptoms relating directly to the traumatic event (such as flashbacks, avoidance of trauma-related material, and hyperarousal), CPTSD identifies three additional sets of symptoms: difficulties with emotion regulation, negative self-concept, and relationship problems. The interventions in STAIR particularly help with emotion regulation and relationship difficulties. Negative views of oneself are addressed in both STAIR and Narrative Therapy.

For example, some people may have negative feelings about themselves because they feel that they are not competent to manage day-to-day difficulties, have problems in managing their emotions, or have problems managing relationships (or having any relationships at all). STAIR interventions help people develop skills and resources to address these difficulties. Ultimately, however, traumatic experiences often lead people to feel ashamed of themselves, guilty, worthless or bad. Narrative Therapy allows a client to go back to the trauma and reassess where those feelings and beliefs came from and resolve them. This task is a difficult one, but often very liberating once completed.

Narrative Work for the Purpose of Decreasing Fear and PTSD Symptoms

The client's current symptoms (nightmares, flashbacks, anxiety, etc.) indicate that there is "unfinished business" related to the past trauma. The therapist notes that some people try to cope with this by avoiding traumatic memories and triggers, which is understandable but ultimately ineffective. Avoidance can work in the short term, but in the longer view, it only maintains and exacerbates PTSD/CPTSD symptoms. Even when triggers and memories are avoided to the extent possible, many people find that they cannot completely avoid their memories and feel overwhelmed by them when they come up. The aim of the treatment is to help the client process the memories of their trauma in such a way that they attain more control *over* them, rather than being controlled *by* them. The therapist can tell the client something like this:

> "The goal will be to help you make meaningful connections between your feelings and your experiences in a safe and supportive environment. Staying with these memories rather than running away from them can be very distressing at first, but over time it will help decrease the anxiety and fear that are associated with them. This process is called 'deconditioning' or 'habituation.' It works because the body is drained by the 'fight, flight, or freeze' system. That system works to protect us from danger. When you're not in danger, your body can save its energy. That's the point of this second module of treatment. That is, your body will be learning over time that in a safe environment, remembering is not the same as experiencing the trauma. Don't worry if even

talking about this approach brings up some anxiety for you now. We'll get there when you're ready, and I'll be here all along the way to support you."

Narrative Work for the Purpose of Organizing Traumatic Memories

A second goal of the narrative work is to help the client to assimilate and integrate their experiences. The therapist can elucidate this more abstract goal with the use of the following analogy:

"The mind can be viewed as a kind of library in which a person's experiences are organized and stored, helping the person to make sense of them and put them in their right place. So, for example, children might have a section of their library for 'birthday parties,' where they store memories of particular parties, plus their growing knowledge about what one brings to a party, what to expect at a party, and so forth. But where does a child file and organize the experiences of trauma? Typically, the traumatic experiences are not labeled and discussed. So the feelings and memories continue to interfere with life in the present, frequently in the form of depression or posttraumatic stress. The symptoms often reflect the unorganized and unassimilated feelings tied to the trauma. Part of the goal of processing trauma experiences is for you to be able to organize these distressing feelings and memories and find a place for them."

Narrative Work for the Purpose of Developing a Life History

During the Narrative Therapy module of the treatment, the conclusion of each telling (or a series of tellings) will involve a review of the client's perceptions of themselves and their life circumstances during the time of the traumatic experiences, including their relationship with anyone who abused them. These past perceptions will be directly compared to the beliefs they hold about themselves now and to their perceptions of their current circumstances and relationships. Some perceptions of self and patterns of relating will be identical to those of the past. The therapist and client will review their current positive value to the client, and the client will either accept and reinforce existing perceptions or identify ones that may be due for revision. There will also be observations about the way in which the client has changed, including how they may have changed for the better. Client and therapist will identify the client's positive and more adaptive beliefs about themselves that have developed during Module I, as well as the internal and external resources for life functioning that have accumulated in response. The comparison of current self and past self often highlights the positive changes the client is making, which are easy to lose sight of during the change process. This type of contrasting activity also places a healthy emotional distance between the client's past and present. Narrative analysis organizes experience as a story with a beginning, middle, and end. The sense of time this process instills reinforces the idea that the trauma is in the past and therefore cannot hurt the client. Lastly, this analysis will yield some understanding of how the past has influenced the present but need not continue to do so. With this awareness, the client may begin to exercise choices about who they will be and what they will do.

REVIEW RATIONALE FOR AND BENEFITS OF A TWO-MODULE TREATMENT (IF RELEVANT)

For clients who are planning to complete both modules of treatment, briefly providing the rationale for dividing the therapeutic work as such may be helpful. There are several reasons for organizing treatment into two modules, each with its own specific goals. The immediate goal of the therapy is to help the client improve functioning and reduce suffering in day-to-day life as quickly as possible. The first module of treatment, STAIR, is intended to address this goal in a pragmatic and straightforward manner. These initial sessions also allow a period of time for the therapist and client to get to know each other and form a positive and productive therapeutic alliance. The client has time to become comfortable with the therapist and satisfy their valid question of whether the therapist is someone they can trust enough to engage in a process that involves experiencing painful feelings. In a complementary fashion, the therapist will develop a good working knowledge of the client's strengths and vulnerabilities, which will help the therapist guide the client in titrating the emotional intensity of the narrative work. During this time, the client will develop better skills in emotion regulation, which they can use during the more emotionally intense narrative work. The development of emotional and interpersonal resources will also build the client's self-esteem and provide them with greater awareness of their strengths, so that thinking about the past will be, if not less painful, at least less frightening and overwhelming.

Lastly, both therapist and client may review the number of times they suspect it might be useful to cycle through specific components of the STAIR module. Repeated use of skills training components can be reinforcing for some clients, particularly for those who suffer more from difficulties with daily life functioning than from PTSD-specific symptoms. This option to repeat or prolong a focus on specific skills of interest or challenge is one important way that this treatment models healthy flexibility (a theme of the emotion regulation and interpersonal work) and seeks to individualize the interventions to the needs of the client, not those of the protocol.

PROVIDE A COPING SKILL: FOCUSED BREATHING

An important and final task for the latter part of the first session is to begin instructing the client in practicing emotion regulation skills. This component of the first session gives the client "something to go home with." It is intended to boost the client's hope that the treatment will improve their functioning in day-to-day life. It also demonstrates the engagement of both body and mind that is typical of emotion regulation activities, and exemplifies the collaborative process between client and therapist that effective skills acquisition requires.

Rationale for and Overview of Focused Breathing

The therapist begins by explaining the rationale for Focused Breathing to the client:

"One way of dealing with distressing feelings involves decreasing your physiological arousal through a skill we call Focused Breathing. When people are in an aroused state, they tend to breathe from their chests and breathe more quickly. This impulse can actually increase symptoms of anxiety, including dizziness, breathlessness, and even disorientation. The aim of this exercise is to slow down your breathing and rate of oxygen intake, which will lead to a decrease in anxiety. It's like meditation in that it helps you reduce disorganized thoughts and flooding emotions by helping you focus on a single sensation and a single task—namely, breathing. Focused Breathing can be used to manage anxiety, irritation, or anger, and as a meditative tool for feeling calm and grounded. It's also an exercise that highlights the relationship between the mind and the body. By clearing the mind of all thoughts, and by directing your concentration toward regular breathing, you'll experience the influence of mind over body. In a complementary fashion, the relaxation of the body that comes from regular breathing will also reduce your flow of undirected thoughts, completing the circle so that you can experience the influence of the body over the mind. Both are intimately connected, and both can help you take charge of your reactions."

The therapist can emphasize the mind–body connection, which may be novel to some clients. Focused Breathing is an exercise that will help the client connect and integrate experiences of the body and mind in a healthful way, while not dismissing the influence of one over the other.

Instructions for Teaching Focused Breathing

By this time, because its utility is well documented in research and various therapeutic approaches, many therapists have completed at least informal training in leading mindfulness and breath-based meditations. For the purposes of this intervention, the therapist can follow these key steps of teaching Focused Breathing:

1. *Assess baseline.* Observe the client as they breathe in their usual way. Have them pay attention to their rate of breathing and whether they breathe from their chest or diaphragm.

2. *Teach technique.* Model breathing from your diaphragm, placing one hand on your chest and the other on your stomach, and have the client imitate these movements. Explain that when they are breathing from the diaphragm, only the stomach hand moves up and down, while the chest remains still. Especially if the client is a parent, it can help to invite them to think of how a baby sleeps—how only the lower abdomen moves up and down. Or they might imagine their stomach as a balloon, filling with air and expanding as they inhale, then letting out the air and shrinking as they exhale.

3. *Slow down rate of breathing.* Instruct the client to take in enough air to fill the space under the diaphragm, then gradually let it out slowly. Sometimes breathing through the nose is easier because the nostrils are smaller openings, which will help to control the rate of exhalation. Instruct the client to pause briefly after exhaling before inhaling again. Some clients will tend to hold their breath too long at first; explain that the pause is very brief and comes after exhaling. Using imagery to convey the desired movement and flow may help. For example, the ebb and flow of an ocean wave is a helpful image for some. Alternatively, consider the image of climbing up a slide (inhaling) and then sliding back down (exhaling), briefly pausing at the bottom before turning around and climbing up again.

4. *Introduce meditational component.* In order to help the client slow their thoughts and focus attention on breathing, instruct the client to count their breaths as they inhale— or, alternatively, to think of calming words like "Relax," "Just breathe," or some similar thought as they exhale. They can continue counting until they get to 10, and then go back to 1. Explain, using wording as in this example:

> "It's perfectly natural for other thoughts to come into your mind. Try not to get angry or frustrated or beat yourself up for not doing it 'right.' Just allow the thoughts to pass through your mind, without judgment for losing focus, and then gently bring your attention back to counting. Do this as often as you need. Just like any new skill, mindful breathing takes practice."

Some people find it helpful to concentrate mostly on the physical sensation of their breathing, others on the counting or use of calming words. Still others will have other ways of focusing that come most naturally to them. Encourage the client to do what works best for them. Doing so models the kinds of flexibility and pragmatism that are key to this treatment approach.

PROVIDE RATIONALE FOR BETWEEN-SESSION SKILLS PRACTICE

A core part of this treatment is independent skills practice to aid the client in newly acquiring and mastering skills. The therapist provides the client with take-home exercises, which incorporate the skills taught in sessions. There are several reasons for doing so. The first is that the practice exercises will provide the client and therapist with important data on the client's real-life experiences, which then can help inform the choice of interventions in sessions. The therapist can use examples from the client's experiences of independent practice when introducing new information or skills.

Another reason for between-session practice is that it enables the client to practice skills in the context of their real life, not just in the more theoretical space of the therapy room. Generalizing what is learned in session to real life is one of the fundamental principles of this therapy. Skills must be practical in the real world. If not, then they fail a basic test of pragmatism—doing what works! The therapist and client can share this common viewpoint, while maintaining the client's motivation to continue practicing long enough to know for sure whether a skill is effective or whether it needs some adjustments to work best. A further reason why independent skills practice is key is that because STAIR is typically a relatively brief and efficient treatment, it asks clients to learn a large number of skills in a short period of time. The only way for clients to accomplish genuine skill acquisition is to practice on their own. Some clients may benefit from comparing this kind of therapeutic skill acquisition to the skill acquisition of learning to ride a bike or play a new sport. The example used can be adjusted to match the client's experience. The therapist can adapt the following language:

> "Think about the time you learned to ride a bike. Even after seeing other people ride a bike, or hearing someone tell you how to do it, it probably wasn't easy at first, right? It likely took a lot of trial and error. But eventually you learned, and it became second nature. That's similar to what we're hoping to do with Focused Breathing and the other skills you'll be learning and practicing in this therapy. Even when it's hard, you'll learn that sticking with the practice is the best way to make it work for you when you need it most."

SUMMARIZE THE GOALS OF THE SESSION

At the end of the session (as in all future sessions), the therapist briefly summarizes the session's goals, and situates the session content within the larger framework of the client's treatment plan if helpful. The therapist can reinforce the collaborative, individualized nature of the treatment by also checking in with the client again to see how they are feeling. If the client appears in need of further encouragement, the therapist may praise the client for initiating treatment and completing their first skills practice in this session. The therapist can also assure the client that they will not be alone in their journey of recovery; the therapist will be their guide and partner throughout the process. In all cases, instilling some level of hope in the growth the client will experience as they stick with the treatment will be useful, if not critical.

PLAN SKILLS PRACTICE

At the end of this first session, the therapist gives the client Handout 10.2, Focused Breathing, for use between sessions. They can instruct the client to put aside some time each day where they will be undisturbed and comfortable, and to practice the breathing skill for at least 5 minutes twice a day. If it seems useful to revisit these points, the therapist emphasizes that the client's skill will increase with practice, and that like any practice, it takes time and patience to work. Only with regular practice will coping skills, such as Focused Breathing, be readily available and effective when the client actually becomes triggered or anxious. This emphasis on the purpose of regular between-session practice will continue to be an important point throughout this treatment.

Treatment Overview: What Is STAIR Narrative Therapy?

RATIONALE

This treatment was originally designed for adults with a history of childhood abuse who suffer from posttraumatic stress disorder (PTSD) symptoms and experience difficulties with emotion management and interpersonal relationships. Over time, it was broadened to apply to people with a range of traumatic experiences and symptoms.

The first module of treatment, Skills Training in Affective and Interpersonal Regulation (STAIR), directly addresses current relationship and emotion management problems. Module I of treatment also prepares you to work effectively in the more intense Module II, which involves discussing and analyzing painful memories of trauma.

People often try to cope with traumatic memories by avoiding them. This avoidance is understandable, but ultimately, in the long run, it does not work. The memories return in unpredictable and uncontrollable ways. The goal of Module II, Narrative Therapy, is to organize your memories of trauma and resolve your feelings about them. Doing so helps you control the memories, rather than having the memories control you.

In addition, the process of describing your past is a way for you to identify deeper beliefs about yourself and patterns of relating to others. Those patterns might have been adaptive at the time of the trauma, but no longer are adaptive and need adjustment. This process pairs nicely with the skills training from Module I, which will help you leave behind old patterns and develop new interpersonal behaviors and emotion management skills more consistent with your current life goals.

OVERVIEW

This treatment consists of two modules, as described above. You and your therapist may decide that a different number or spacing of sessions would be most appropriate to your needs. The following table provides a general overview of the treatment.

	Module I: STAIR	Module II: Narrative Therapy
Estimated session number and format	10 weekly 60-minute sessions	8–10 weekly 60-minute sessions
Focus	Learning skills to manage emotions and improve relationships	Making sense of the trauma and processing related memories and feelings
Goals	1. Develop emotional awareness. 2. Build coping skills for handling negative feelings and distress.	1. Revisit trauma memories to help emotional processing of what happened.

(continued)

	Module I: STAIR	Module II: Narrative Therapy
Goals *(continued)*	3. Review how to make decisions about whether tolerating distress makes sense to reach your goals. 4. Understand relationship patterns and create healthy alternatives to unhelpful patterns. 5. Learn interpersonal skills to pair with emotional coping skills to improve relationships.	2. Repeat tellings of the events to habituate to (get used to and decrease) the feelings of anxiety that the memories trigger. 3. Make meaningful connections between your feelings and your experiences. 4. Differentiate the traumatic past from the present, freeing your behavior and thinking from the control of the trauma. 5. Explore your life and create the story of your life, taking a long view of it, where the trauma is part of but not all of your experience and story.

Instructions for Focused Breathing

RATIONALE

One way of dealing with distressing feelings involves decreasing your physiological arousal through a skill we call Focused Breathing. The aim is to slow down your breathing to decrease anxiety, breathlessness, and disorientation. In addition, the exercise is similar to meditation, in that it helps you reduce disorganized thinking or flooding by focusing on a single sensation and single task—namely, breathing.

Focused Breathing can be used to manage states of anxiety, irritation, or anger, and as a meditative tool for feeling calm and grounded. It is also an exercise that highlights the connection between the mind and the body. By clearing the mind of all thoughts and by directing your concentration toward regular breathing, you will experience the influence of mind over body. The relaxation of the body that comes from regular breathing will also reduce the flow of undirected, distracting thoughts, which completes the circle with the influence of body over mind.

Practicing Focused Breathing will help you experience the connectedness and integrity of the body and mind in a positive, healthy way. The ability to engage in Focused Breathing in a meditational fashion is a challenge and takes practice. So do not become discouraged. Practice regularly and with patience, and your skill will develop over time.

PROCEDURE FOR FOCUSED BREATHING

Getting Started

Place one hand on your chest and the other on your stomach. Take a slow, deep breath, and pay attention to which hand moves. When you are breathing from your diaphragm, only the hand on the stomach should move up and down, with little movement coming from the chest. It may help to think of how babies sleep—how their stomachs quietly move up and down. Or you might imagine your stomach as a balloon, filling with air and expanding as you inhale, then letting out the air and shrinking as you exhale.

Slow Down Your Rate of Breathing

Take in enough air to fill the space under the diaphragm, then let it out slowly. Sometimes breathing out through the nose is easier because your nostrils are smaller openings, which will help slow the rate of exhalation. Pause briefly after exhaling before inhaling again. Some people tend to hold their breath too long at first; the pause should be brief after exhaling. Imagery can be helpful in maintaining a slow and steady rhythm. For example, seeing your breath as a wave, following it as it ebbs and flows, can be a helpful image. Alternatively, imagine climbing up a slide (inhaling) and then sliding down (exhaling), and briefly pausing at the bottom before walking around and climbing up again.

(continued)

Meditational Component

In order to help slow your thoughts and focus your attention on breathing, count your breaths as you inhale, and think "Relax," "Calm," or some similar thought as you exhale. Continue counting your breaths until you get to 10, and then start over at 1. It is perfectly natural for other thoughts to come into your mind. Try not to get angry or frustrated; just allow the thoughts to pass through your mind, and bring your attention back to counting as often as you need to. Some people find it helpful to concentrate mostly on the physical sensation of their breathing, others on the counting or "Relax" statement. Experiment with different methods, and do whatever works best for you.

Practice

Practice is essential to develop this skill, so that it becomes something you can use to decrease distress in stressful situations. It is best to practice Focused Breathing in a comfortable, quiet place where you will not be disturbed. Take a few seconds to relax, and then practice the breathing exercise for at least 5 minutes. Practicing at least twice a day is the goal. When you are beginning to learn this skill, it is best not to practice when you are already distressed. The idea is that if you practice the breathing when you are in a calm state, it will become a habit that you can then call upon more easily when you are distressed. As you become more skilled at it, you may begin practicing using it in mildly distressing situations, such as when you are feeling impatient while waiting in a line.

CHAPTER 11

The Resource of Feeling

Emotional Awareness

> Reality is when something is happening to you and you know it
> and can say it and when you say it other people understand
> what you mean and believe you.
> —ANDREA DWORKIN, quoted by CATHARINE A. MACKINNON
>   (2005, p. 13)

Identifying and labeling feelings may seem like a simple activity. But, in fact, many survivors of interpersonal trauma have not had sufficient opportunity to learn or practice this formative process. Feelings are a critical resource for living. They provide information about potential threats in our environment, guide our choices, and motivate our actions. Feelings also contribute to self-knowledge, as when they inform our preferences (likes and dislikes); subsequently, they can powerfully communicate to others our intentions and beliefs. Developmentally, awareness of feelings often grows in tandem with naming them. Naming heightens our awareness of a feeling, clarifies its meaning and potential purpose, and provides a vehicle for its expression.

Chronic trauma, especially in childhood, often leads to pervasive and long-term impairment in a survivor's ability to identify and name feelings (this impairment is called "alexithymia"). The ability to identify and name feelings facilitates emotional awareness, organizes emotional experiences, and supports effective decision making and behavior. Having difficulty with identifying and naming feelings creates disturbances in all of these experiences; perhaps most devastatingly, it undermines people's confidence in the accuracy of their feelings and perceptions, and in the authority of their actions.

In this session, a therapist helps a client find words to describe their feelings, understand their causes and value, and become aware of the physical sensations, thoughts and actions associated with them. These skills are learned through instruction and repeated practice in monitoring feelings. At the same time and of equal importance, the therapist creates a sense of safety in the client's experiencing and labeling of feelings, helps to clarify different kinds of feelings and their expressions through three channels of emotion, and furnishes support for their expression and felt reality.

Conscious awareness of feelings is a first and vital step in self-discovery. It allows clients to trust in their visceral experiences of emotions. This liberation in emotional experiencing then creates new resources for their management, gives the clients renewed energy, and contributes to their experience of a real and authentic self. Box 11.1 outlines the theme and curriculum for Session 2 of treatment.

CHECK-IN AND REVIEW OF SKILLS PRACTICE

This session and all that follow begin with an inquiry about the client's reaction to the previous session, and about any difficulties they may have had implementing the planned skills practice over the past week. Clients may have questions that need answering before they can comfortably go on with the current session. If a client reports significant difficulties with the skills work from the previous session (in this case, Focused Breathing), the therapist and client will want to plan to reserve time at the end of the session for extra practice.

In this particular session, a client may have questions or concerns about the treatment plan. Treatment goals and means to reach them must be relevant to the client and also must be adapted to the client's sensibilities, and so the therapist should address any concerns in a collaborative way. In addition, what the client has to say at the opening of the session is a demonstration of or exercise in the expression of feelings—the client's preferences, sense of collaboration, and fears about the coming weeks of work. The session thus begins with an experience of the central goal of the session: practice in identifying and expressing feelings.

IDENTIFY FOCUS OF THE SESSION

The therapist shares with the client that the focus of this session is emotional awareness, which involves helping them to enhance their ability to identify and label their feelings, and to understand the origins of their feelings (as well as of associated thoughts and actions). The therapist will also work with the client on understanding the function of feelings, clarify the different kinds of feelings the client has, and support the client in expressing feelings in a way that feels safe.

INTRODUCE CONCEPT OF EMOTION REGULATION

"Emotion regulation" encompasses the ability to identify, label, modulate, and effectively express feelings. All these aspects of emotion regulation are addressed in this and the next several sessions. The therapist conveys the meaning of the concept and explores the client's experiences with each aspect of emotion regulation. The work for this particular session focuses only on the prerequisite to all other aspects of emotion regulation: the skill of emotional awareness. Emotional awareness is learned through self-monitoring of feelings via Handout 11.3, the Feelings Monitoring Form, which gives the client practice in the specific

BOX 11.1

Theme and Curriculum for Session 2
The Resource of Feeling: Emotional Awareness

Identifying and naming feelings may seem to be a simple activity. But, in fact, many survivors of interpersonal trauma have not had sufficient opportunity to do this. In this session, the therapist helps the client enhance their ability to identify and label their feelings, their sources, and associated thoughts and actions. In addition, the therapist helps create a sense of safety in the client's experiencing and naming of feelings, helps to clarify different kinds of feelings, and furnishes support for their expression and felt reality.

PLANNING AND PREPARATION

Review client's evaluation materials related to difficulties with emotion regulation. Bring several copies of the Feelings Monitoring Form (Handout 11.3), as well as a copy of each other Session 2 handout. Prepare examples for the Feelings Monitoring Form. The work in the session is estimated to take about 60 minutes; a flexible application is assumed (i.e., not every client will need all interventions).

AGENDA

- Check-in and review of skills practice.
- Identify focus of the session.
- Introduce concept of emotion regulation.
- Explore and identify difficulties with emotion regulation.
- Introduce the Feelings Monitoring Form.
- Provide rationale for monitoring and understanding feelings.
- Use channels of emotion to help organize experience.
- Describe the functions of feelings.
- Identify and discuss client's problematic emotions.
- Discuss discrimination among different kinds of feelings.
- Practice using the Feelings Monitoring Form together.
- Summarize the goals of the session.
- Plan skills practice:
  - Practice Focused Breathing twice a day.
  - Complete Feelings Monitoring Form once a day.

(continued)

SESSION HANDOUTS

Handout 11.1. The Impact of Childhood Abuse and Neglect on Emotion Regulation

Handout 11.2. Social Influences on Your Emotional Experiences

Handout 11.3. Feelings Monitoring Form (several copies)

Handout 11.4. Examples of Emotion Regulation Coping Skills for the Three Channels of Emotion

Handout 11.5. Three Channels Skills Graphic

Handout 11.6. Negative and Positive Emotions as Messengers

Handout 11.7. Feelings List

Handout 11.8. Feelings Wheel

skills of identifying and labeling feelings and of seeing how they change based on choices before and after a triggering or impactful incident.

The therapist now introduces the notions that (1) emotional awareness and expression are skills that are learned (not innate); (2) an important aspect of childhood interpersonal trauma is that a child's feelings are often ignored or mislabeled, which itself becomes a "learning experience," albeit a negative one; and (3) negative or maladaptive habits of self-monitoring and expression can be unlearned and replaced with more adaptive functioning. The therapist can more meaningfully discuss and reinforce these ideas in the context of the client's own history and experiences. Handout 11.1, The Impact of Childhood Abuse and Neglect on Emotion Regulation, provides a summary of these ideas as they apply to these forms of trauma; the therapist can give this handout to the client at the end of the session.

EXPLORE AND IDENTIFY DIFFICULTIES WITH EMOTION REGULATION

To begin the process, the therapist can first engage the client in describing any difficulties in managing feelings they are aware of and/or would like to change. In our experiences, two simple questions yield a great deal of information and discussion: "How were feelings handled when you were growing up?" and "How have your traumatic experiences affected the way you feel?" These questions will provide specific information relevant to the client's needs.

Discuss How Feelings Were Managed When the Client Was Growing Up

Because the childhood experiences of survivors of maltreatment have a strong influence on their beliefs and management of feelings, queries into family history can be very enlightening. The client can tell about ways in which caregivers responded to their feelings in the past. For example, were their feelings considered important? Were they ignored? Were they mislabeled (e.g., the client was told, "You're fine, stop crying," when upset)? Did expression of emotion result in negative reactions from caregivers (e.g., "I'll give you something to cry about!")? In addition, the client can share how caregivers handled their own emotions. For example, did they sweep things under the rug, drink/use other substances, or express frightening, out-of-control anger?

The therapist can note where appropriate that parental guidance shapes learning via role modeling, some of which may not have been ideal or effective. Moreover, the client probably developed ways of coping in childhood—some of which are adaptive, but others of which take a toll on the client's current well-being. The client and therapist should explore and identify which emotional coping styles are problematic for the client now.

Handout 11.2, Social Influences on Your Emotional Experiences, is used in this discussion, as it offers a way to determine how emotions were managed in clients' families as well as in other important social contexts in their lives. This form is reviewed with the client in session as a way for the therapist to help the client identify their history of learning about emotions, the messages they got about emotions while growing up, and their ways of managing emotions in their current relationships and in their community or culture. For clients who have had military experience, it can be helpful to add a column to this handout about messages they got about emotions while in the service. Similarly, explicitly discussing aspects of a client's personal identity, culture, ethnicity, and other forms of community may prove very important in some cases and even highlight conflicting messages. Sometimes clients struggle to identify which emotions they were "supposed" to feel, or even share that there were no emotions they felt allowed to feel. In these cases, the therapist can shift to asking what emotions the client was most discouraged from feeling or expressing.

Discuss How Trauma Has Influenced Client's Feelings

The discussion described above often helps the client to describe how any abuse or other trauma has influenced their "habits" of emotional awareness and expression, and which of these habits the client wants to change. Below, we outline common themes in responses to the question "How have your traumatic experiences affected the way you feel?", which the therapist can use to guide this discussion.

Not all clients have the same difficulties. For example, a client may have no difficulty labeling their feelings, but may respond poorly to them or not know what to do with them. Some clients may need help primarily in being able to attenuate states of intense emotion, while others may need a lot of work to help them access any feelings at all (as we have often seen in cases of posttraumatic numbness).

Confusion

Survivors of childhood maltreatment frequently share that the most common feeling they have, even years later, is confusion. Confusion, while not exactly a core emotion, accurately represents something about these clients' state of affairs. The secrecy and denial typical in families of children who have been abused or neglected have made this particular type of trauma "the problem with no name." If the problem had no name for decades, it is unsurprising that the feelings associated with it have no names either. With few labels for their experience, these survivors often do not know what they felt as children and do not know exactly what they feel now, or how to link their childhood and adult feelings to their origins.

Chronic fear, hypervigilance, and dread

Basic needs of safety are not met and are often violated in cases of childhood interpersonal trauma. The burden of managing the trauma (which in itself is a threat to the child's physical and psychological well-being), and the frequent absence of support or intervention, often create a chronic sense of anxiety, hypervigilance in monitoring for potential danger, and a sense of dread and hopelessness about the future.

Emotions as a roller-coaster experience

It is also not unusual for clients to experience alternating acute states of overwhelming emotions and numbing—in effect, an emotional roller coaster. In response to these overwhelming emotions, some survivors learn to "shut down" altogether to protect themselves from the acute reactions of the repeated trauma, as well as the chronic fear and anxiety.

Keeping a distance from emotions

Survivors of childhood maltreatment often like to keep a distance from strong emotions. As one client who had been beaten regularly during childhood put it, "I have been on the wrong end of the stick many times, and I know the damage that anger can do to a body and soul." Survivors, by virtue of their own experience as victims, are intimately familiar with the painful and damaging consequences of intense and out-of-control emotions. Many of them shy away from experiencing intense emotions, because experience has taught them that intense emotions are linked to negative outcomes. One goal of therapy is to demonstrate to such clients that these negative outcomes are not always the case and less likely than they think.

Respect the Client and Their Experiences

Two important attitudes to convey in this discussion concern a client's feelings about themselves and about their family of origin. It is important for the therapist to acknowledge that the coping strategies of the past that create difficulty in the client's life now were almost certainly the coping strategies that were the best they could do in their given situation. Sometimes they were completely necessary and the only adaptive responses available. In addition, many clients have conflictual bonds to those who maltreated them and may feel the need to defend the perpetrators' behaviors during their childhood. For example, a client whose parents drank heavily may say, "They didn't know what they were doing. If they hadn't been drinking, they wouldn't have done any of these things." The therapist should respond in a way that respects this need, and in language that does not imply judgment—for example, "Your parents, for whatever reason, were not able to/did not help you to cope with difficult feelings."

INTRODUCE THE FEELINGS MONITORING FORM

The therapist explains that this session revolves around the introduction and use of the deceptively simple Handout 11.3, the Feelings Monitoring Form. This form provides a strategy for systematically identifying feelings, their intensity, situational triggers, and associated thoughts and behavioral responses. It is essentially a telegraphic diary of the client's emotional life and is used throughout STAIR.

The completion of this form over several weeks, and the development of the skills described above, are intended to accomplish the therapeutic goal of enhancing the client's emotional awareness. Practice in using the Feelings Monitoring Form facilitates the labeling of feelings and their links to specific events, clarifies differences between feelings, and identifies the contexts in which they happen. Lastly, the therapist can point out that the final column of the form, which asks the client to attend to their behavioral reactions to each trigger and emotion, provides information about how the client responds to difficult emotions, and so lays the groundwork for later efforts in building coping skills.

Value of Self-Monitoring for the Client

The therapist explains to the client that they will be making daily entries on the Feelings Monitoring Form between sessions. As the task is repeated over several weeks, the therapist and client can identify the range and pattern of emotions the client experiences. The therapist can provide some examples of how this form has been useful to other clients. For example, some clients discover over weeks of diary keeping that they are really almost always angry with a sister, or almost always anxious during sex. Other clients learn that feeling angry is really a cover for feeling hurt. Still others come into each session with nothing written down and report that they have no feelings. For all these clients, learning about their emotional styles is one aspect of their journey of self-discovery. It may also provide some evidence of the types of emotional reactions that clients may have during the emotionally demanding processing of trauma required during Narrative Therapy in Module II of treatment.

Therapeutic Process and the Therapist's Attitude

Beyond the immediate value of self-exploration, self-monitoring also provides a client with an experience in which someone (the therapist) is taking an active interest in the client's feelings—what they feel, how much they are feeling it, and when they feel it. This approach may be a relatively novel experience for survivors of childhood trauma, whose feelings have often been ignored, or who themselves believe that their feelings are irrelevant or too threatening, dangerous, or ugly to be given attention. The simple act and process of working together and attending to a client's emotional life ideally allows the client to have their feelings validated or feel more "real" by virtue of being named and shared.

PROVIDE RATIONALE FOR MONITORING AND UNDERSTANDING FEELINGS

Clients need a rationale for why they should take the time to monitor and understand their feelings. Discussion about feelings may elicit distress, and some clients at this point may reconsider their desire to come into contact with their feelings, their need to change, and their commitment to the therapy. It is often helpful for the therapist to provide a supportive reminder that they have chosen this therapy in order to live the life they want. Some of the reasons our clients have found monitoring feelings to be valuable are listed below:

> "My danger sensor is smashed, and I can't tell what is safe and what is threatening."
> "I never know what I'm fveeling. A friend asks, 'Are you happy?' and I don't know!"
> "I feel nothing. And then a small thing happens, and I can't get out of bed."
> "My feelings are unpredictable and seem to come out of nowhere."
> "I can't trust my feelings, so I try not to feel anything."
> "I just feel angry all the time."

Rehabilitation of the Arousal/Threat System

One of the primary reasons for clients to take the time to monitor and understand their feelings is that accurate perceptions of and reactions to emotions contribute to adaptive living. For all of us, emotions provide us with information and help guide our decisions and behaviors. The insights provided by emotions are especially pertinent for a client who requires assistance in understanding what situations to approach or avoid. One of the clients quoted above reported that she had been beaten in such an indiscriminate fashion in a series of unexpected assaults that she felt as if her "danger sensor" was smashed; in other words, she had lost all capability of distinguishing situations in which she was safe from those that might be an immediate threat to her well-being. Rather incongruously, she was chronically hypervigilant and fearful of going outdoors, but on those rare occasions when she elected to go out, she thought nothing of a stroll through a poorly lit park at night. She had been raped in broad daylight, and as a child had been assaulted for no apparent reason. The world of safety–threat cues did not apply. Her threat detection system was badly out of kilter. Persons with a history of sexual abuse are particularly prone to being victimized repeatedly and will greatly benefit from being able to interpret emotional cues accurately and then make appropriate choices to keep themselves safe. One goal of this treatment is to rehabilitate the emotional threat system that has been distorted by interpersonal trauma. Regular review of the Feelings Monitoring Form to identify feelings of threat (or their absence) is a first step in this process.

Enhanced Confidence in Using Feelings to Guide Decisions and Actions

Many survivors of childhood maltreatment have little confidence in their emotional perceptions, and thus feel stymied or suffer severe indecision because they do not trust their emotional experiences as an accurate source of information. Part of the goal in this series of interventions is to build such clients' confidence that they are having emotional experiences for good reasons, so that these experiences become a resource for the survivors in simplifying daily life. Building and strengthening emotion regulation skills are difficult tasks. Thus a therapist will want to highlight the evolution of a client's progress through treatment from developing the ability to identify and label emotions, to gaining the skills necessary to regulate them.

Enhanced Engagement in Living and the Possibility of Pleasure and Happiness

Awareness of feelings can help clients make decisions not only to live more safely, but also to live with greater engagement and satisfaction, both about themselves and about their relationships with others. Once clients feel relatively safe, they can turn their attention to experiencing positive feelings and identifying positive life goals. A survivor's increasing awareness of positive feelings, and when, where, and with whom they occur, can lead to greater clarity about the survivor's desires and wishes for their work life and personal relationships. It can lead to the pursuit of personal goals and values that are intrinsically pleasurable, satisfying, or meaningful to the client, such as sports, dance, or community engagement. Lastly, the client's ability to "follow their feelings" can ignite a sense of creativity and self-appreciation that may never have emerged or may have been lost a long time ago. It is often worthwhile for the therapist to note that approaching pleasure and positive experiences can be frightening to a survivor, for fear of disappointment or of simply being overwhelmed with sensation or arousal. One of the treatment goals will be to help such a survivor modulate their feelings and manage their distress, particularly in the pursuit of valued positive life goals.

USE CHANNELS OF EMOTION TO HELP ORGANIZE EXPERIENCE

For clients who find learning to name feelings especially daunting, labeling a sensation or physical reaction is a useful first step. Clients are usually able to identify experiences of acute sensations or rapid changes in their bodies or physical states, such as sweaty hands and racing heart. The next step is to identify the associated thoughts and behaviors and make an inference to an emotional label. For example, a racing heart and the thought "I'm going to fail my job interview tomorrow" may describe anxiety. Therapist and client can review a model of emotion that breaks down emotional experiencing into three channels or modes: body, thoughts, and behaviors. The client can learn to become more aware of bodily sensations and changes in these sensations as an entry point to connecting to feelings. Awareness of bodily sensations can be followed by questioning or observing associated thoughts and behavior. All of these combined elements ultimately contribute to the experience of an emotion.

In this part of this session, the therapist introduces the "three channels of emotion" model. The basic concepts are only briefly described here, as the model is elaborated over the following two sessions. The causal relationships among thoughts, feelings, and behaviors are multidirectional; a change in any one of these can cause or reflect a change in any other. We begin this discussion with the body channel, because many clients do not have experience with systematically linking these sensations to their thoughts and behaviors. Given that most emotions are linked to physiological changes, an effort to compose a list of commonly experienced physiological changes is worthwhile. The therapist and client can generate such a list, including such phenomena as alterations in heart rate, amount of sweating, muscle tension, and so on. This list can be followed by the names of emotions that are typically paired with specific bodily changes for the client. For example, an increase in heartbeat may reflect a myriad of emotions, such as the approach of a potential mugger or the presence of a romantic partner. Rapid breathing can be a sign of either anger or extraordinary happiness. Once these variations are noted, the client can then begin to link their own physiological changes with emotion labels, via inference and interpretation from their thoughts and behaviors.

Essentially, an emotion is a conscious or unconscious feeling associated with or triggered by behaviors or thoughts. The therapist and client should examine methods of how to recognize these changes and distinguish their meanings. The therapist can use examples, such as the one provided in Box 11.2, to illustrate how the channels interact in a dynamic process and serve to organize emotional experiences. In this scenario, the therapist and client can identify corresponding bodily sensations (i.e., muscle tension), thoughts (i.e., "Who do they think they are?"), and behaviors (i.e., yelling) as a way to arrive at labeling the specific emotional experience of anger. Using this and other examples, the therapist can then demonstrate to the client how the three channels can then be mapped onto the Feelings Monitoring Form. In turn, the channel model can also help clients in using the information recorded on the Feelings Monitoring Form to help them determine more specifically where their emotional problems lie.

Lastly, once the client understands the elements in an emotion, and knows how to identify them and how to understand their interrelationships, the therapist can then raise another important function of the three-channel model—identifying emotion regulation solutions—and indicate how this goal will be explored in future sessions. Each channel has corresponding coping strategies. Using the information in Handout 11.4, Examples of Emotion Regulation Coping Skills for the Three Channels of Emotion, the therapist can briefly preview some examples of these different strategies to be elaborated in the next two sessions. At this time the client can also be given Handout 11.5, the Three Channels Skills Graphic, with the therapist explaining that it will be used regularly from now on to help the client select some of the skills in each channel, based on their preferences and on the particular situations they are likely to encounter.

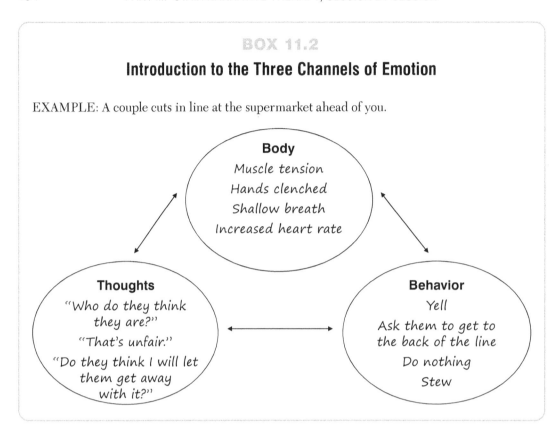

BOX 11.2

Introduction to the Three Channels of Emotion

EXAMPLE: A couple cuts in line at the supermarket ahead of you.

Body
Muscle tension
Hands clenched
Shallow breath
Increased heart rate

Thoughts
"Who do they think they are?"
"That's unfair."
"Do they think I will let them get away with it?"

Behavior
Yell
Ask them to get to the back of the line
Do nothing
Stew

DESCRIBE THE FUNCTIONS OF FEELINGS

In order to fully enlist a client in the central task of identifying feelings, the therapist needs to help the client understand why it is essential for making meaningful changes and improvements in their life. The therapist conveys to the client that emotions function in the following three critical ways: (1) They act as messengers and provide important data that help guide our decisions and actions; (2) they tell us who we are (e.g., our likes and dislikes) and help us determine our valued life goals; and (3) they help us to communicate with other people, especially concerning our needs, limits, intentions, and desires in our relationships.

The therapist shares with the client that after exposure to trauma our emotional systems are flooded, which can result in feelings' becoming overwhelmingly intense or shut down. In both responses, the ability to rely on emotions is disrupted. One goal of STAIR is to help them tap into their feelings in a safe way so they can begin to trust and use them in helpful ways. Introducing Handout 11.6, Negative and Positive Emotions as Messengers, is a way the therapist can discuss some of the specific and adaptive functions of basic emotions.

IDENTIFY AND DISCUSS CLIENT'S PROBLEMATIC EMOTIONS

This part of this session identifies the important and helpful functions of emotion and the ways in which trauma can disturb the experience and the adaptive function of emotions.

Certain emotional states can become chronic for survivors of trauma in a way that is no longer useful, but instead becomes limiting and painful. The therapist can select for discussion specific emotions discussed below with which the client may be particularly burdened. This material provides a starting point for talking about how trauma conspires to create dysregulation of these emotions, and what can be done to bring these feelings "back in line" or into synchrony with the client's goals of adaptive and healthy functioning. The aims here are to help the client understand that (1) they feel the way they do for a reason, so that they become less confused and overwhelmed by their feelings; (2) these feelings have an important and possibly beneficial presence in their life; and (3) a focused treatment goal will be to have the client learn to master and modulate their feelings. In the descriptions below, we have identified coping strategies used in this treatment that we have found to be "good matches" for modulating these particular emotions.

Anxiety

Anxiety is a state of arousal that often signals some kind of danger. It is common among survivors of trauma because it is typically generated by experiences that are unsafe, unpredictable, uncontrollable, or unfamiliar—the very characteristics of traumatic events. Anxiety has an adaptive function, which is to ensure readiness for coping with an unidentified threat. It informs us to stop what we are doing, in order to attend to and plan for response to an imminent danger. This experience of "heightened alert" often becomes chronic among survivors of trauma, however, and as a result no longer serves as a reliable indicator of threat. This reaction may persist because there are multiple, unidentified traumatic reminders in the environment that trigger anxiety, or because the trauma has caused the survivors both psychologically and biologically to adapt to and persist at an anxious set point.

A chronic state of anxious apprehension is very draining. It is often like having one's feet simultaneously on both the gas and brake pedals of a car: The individual is aroused and ready to go, but resisting the initiation of action. When the physiological arousal initiated by anxiety is used toward some action (e.g., fight or flight), the arousal may be hardly noticed; indeed, the arousal and the action can flow as one. If no action is or can be taken, however, the arousal "idles" and continues uncomfortably until it (and the individual) is exhausted. Accordingly, it is easy to see why effective modulation of anxiety involves the reduction of arousal in the body (e.g., Focused Breathing), the evaluation of thoughts ("I am safe here"), and the selection of behaviors that integrate arousal and movement. Indeed, one of the most important and long-term goals of the treatment is the perfect antidote to unfocused anxiety—that is, to replace feelings of helplessness and uncertainty with ones of competence and confidence.

Anger

Anger is a natural feeling regardless of one's exposure to trauma, and it is certainly a justified response to childhood mistreatment. Anger is adaptive when it prepares us for active coping, invigorates and sustains our actions, and fuels a healthy sense of power or agency— all part of a fight response to mistreatment. However, anger becomes problematic when it is misdirected toward people or situations *unrelated* to the trauma or other real threat, or expressed as violence toward self (e.g., self-injury) or others (e.g., physical assault). Additionally, the intensity of anger, even when it is warranted, can do harm to important relationships or interfere with valued support from others, if it is not communicated in a healthy manner. Misplaced or intense anger, particularly when it leads to destructive behaviors, can have long-term negative social and legal consequences.

To use anger effectively, a client must recognize it, modulate it, and direct it appropriately. Anger management strategies often include the combined recognition and delay of its expression (counting to 10, leaving the situation); reduction of its intensity (Focused Breathing, exercising); appraisal of the outcome of expressing the anger ("What will be the result of this action? Is it consistent with my goals?"); and appraisal of the accuracy of the source of the anger ("At whom am I angry? What in this situation has made me angry?") Skills in the ability to discriminate between feelings and goals, particularly interpersonal goals, are the topics of several later STAIR sessions (Sessions 6–10).

Sadness

Sadness is an understandable reaction to loss or change. It can serve the purpose of signaling us to slow down and give ourselves time to reflect, rest, and recover. However, when sadness becomes a more chronic and generalized state, it can turn into depression. In contrast to anxiety, which is a state of high-arousal negative emotion, depression is a state of low-arousal negative emotion. It is accompanied by a sustained absence of pleasure and excitement, and by disengagement from the world. Whereas anxiety is a state of heightened readiness to respond, depression is a state of giving up any active attempt to cope. It is associated with the view and thought that nothing can be done and no effective action can be taken. Despite their contrasting characteristics, many people experience both anxiety and depression in alternating fashion. A person may become highly anxious in anticipation of a feared or threatening event, but may then give up with a sense of severe sadness or become depressed when the outcome of the event is negative.

It is not surprising that depression is so often associated with chronic maltreatment by caregivers. Survivors of such maltreatment often reason that it happened because they deserved it—that they failed in some way, or even that they failed to protect themselves, regardless of the reason for it. In addition, sexual or physical abuse in particular is essentially a form of profound loss. Those abused by caregivers have been psychologically abandoned and have experienced losses at multiple levels, including loss of safety, security, and love. Repeated, inescapable physical or sexual abuse also contributes to a sense of helplessness and lack of control. Survivors have often experienced situations where they could not control their circumstances or create other circumstances where they could feel safe, be free from suffering, or obtain important nurturance or human warmth and connection. Thus, unlike normal experiences of sadness, the depression that results from early chronic trauma involves a lack of agency and a sense of helplessness to change one's circumstances.

Several components of this treatment serve to counter depression and similar phenomena. The client learns to recognize that their early circumstances—which more than justified their depression—no longer apply to their current situation. The client now can experience mastery of their environment, and can now actively seek safety and human connection. The reality of this proposal emerges in the treatment through the creation of new experiences of safety, mastery, and pleasure. These new experiences include the active role playing of alternative experiences later in the treatment; revision of relationship models; intentional efforts at experiencing pleasure; and the provision of energy, nurturance, and support in the therapeutic alliance. The client also experiences general mastery through growing emotional and social competence. Finally, in the second phase of this treatment, mastery of symptoms in general and of the client's trauma history in particular results from the successful completion of narrative work.

Dissociation

Dissociation is an experience in which a person feels cognitively and emotionally removed from the current environment. Dissociation is an automatic response to overwhelming emotions. It is a protective response in which the individual "escapes" from the pain or intensity of an unbearable emotion. Dissociation is most frequently a response to severe fear, anxiety, or acute nonspecific distress. It is a reaction that is fairly unique to specific types of traumatic situations—ones that are so uncontrollable, unavoidable, and threatening that physical escape is impossible.

The therapist should discuss dissociation in this session only for those clients who have experienced it. A therapist and client will be familiar with the client's tendencies to dissociate as a result of the evaluation. For clients who experience dissociation, a discussion of its nature and function can evolve as follows.

Dissociation may be seen by the therapist and experienced by the client as an emotional "shutting down," where the client shifts from a feeling state into an affectless one. In the cognitive dimension, a client may lose touch with a sense of being present in the here and now; they may perceive themselves as either "somewhere else" or "nowhere." Dissociation has a protective function, but also has a substantial cost: The individual loses touch with present reality, which can put them in greater danger or can delay a response that would be effective in the moment but will have little value later. Most important, dissociation is often reported as a distressing experience in and of itself; it can be deeply disturbing and disorienting.

The intervention for dissociation is essentially prevention, with some intervention at earlier stages of the experience when possible. Becoming skilled at modulating feelings will reduce the risk and the need for dissociation. Although dissociation may have been the only possible coping response for the client during childhood, their life circumstances have changed, and it is likely that other forms of emotion regulation will now be more effective. In addition, in the absence of the opportunity to learn other strategies, the client may have become overreliant on dissociation, so that it is now a response of habit rather than necessity. Through ongoing use of the Feelings Monitoring Form, the client can identify and track emotions that tend to trigger dissociation, as well as particular individuals and situations that tend to provoke it. The client can then act to avoid these triggers or plan for more adaptive responses accordingly. The strengthening of emotion regulation capacities, particularly in regard to triggering emotions, typically reduces dissociative responses through prevention. Nevertheless, as the client gains new mastery, they may still have moments of dissociation that need immediate intervention. For moments where the client begins to notice early signs of dissociation, the therapist can offer various options for grounding techniques that keep the client in the present moment, aware of their surroundings, and capable of more adaptive action. Skills such as Focused Breathing, other mindfulness-based exercises, Soothing the Senses, and Take a Break/Time Out are some examples the therapist can practice with the client to help them prepare.

DISCUSS DISCRIMINATION AMONG DIFFERENT KINDS OF FEELINGS

As discussed above, many people with histories of trauma become chronically anxious and frequently flooded with sensations, which interfere with their ability to differentiate feeling states. In addition, some survivors of trauma have not been encouraged to explore the wide range of feelings that can be expressed and understood. This restricted knowledge of feelings limits their self-awareness and their evaluation of and communication with others.

There are several different methods for enhancing a client's capacity for discriminating feelings and expanding an emotional vocabulary. First, we have found it helpful if the therapist provides the client with a list of feeling words (see Handout 11.7, the Feelings List). The client can savor the luxury of a rich set of feeling words and consider which are appropriate descriptors of either their current experience or their typical mood.

The Feelings Wheel (Handout 11.8) provides a visual organization of feeling states by valence, type of emotion, and intensity. It allows the client to identify a single emotion and follow the radial depiction of related emotions, or those that may result from the original emotion, given certain circumstances. Through reviewing these handouts, the client may become more aware of the wide variety of emotions and their complex relationship to one another. The therapist can point out that more than one feeling can be involved in an emotional experience. For example, sadness and anger may go together, as may demoralization and anxiety. Moreover, contrasting or opposing emotions can occur together, such as hatred and pity, or love and fear. The client can provide examples of times when they have felt such combined emotions and how they handled them in specific circumstances.

When to introduce the Feelings List and the Feelings Wheel can be determined by the therapist and client. Some therapist and clients find it easier to use these tools in an interactive way during the completion of the Feelings Monitoring Form as described below, and they are most welcome to do that.

PRACTICE USING THE FEELINGS MONITORING FORM TOGETHER

The goal of this and the next few sessions is to impart several simple and individually tailored methods for the client to be able to adequately identify and label feeling states, and to understand how such interpretations affect behavioral actions. The best way for the client to learn all this, however, is simply to work through the Feelings Monitoring Form with the therapist.

An ultimate goal of the treatment is for clients to have the freedom and ability to experience emotions with greater awareness (and less intensity, if they wish), and to engage in a broader range of behavioral reactions than those depicted in this scenario.

Typical examples of emotions that generally appear in self-monitoring exercises are feelings of sadness, anxiety, or anger. Yet there will be situations where clients will only be able to write that they felt "overwhelmed" or "upset." In these instances, the therapist can provide positive feedback regarding their ability to identify these states, and work with them to identify and label more completely the specific emotion(s) involved, often by helping a client explore the experience in all three channels of emotion. For example, the therapist can pose questions such as "Were you crying?", "What were you thinking to yourself?", "Did your muscles feel tense?", or "What other physical sensations were you aware of?" in order to tease out specific emotions and their indicators.

CASE EXAMPLE: GETTING SPECIFIC

Below, we provide a case example of how a client and therapist discussed and worked through filling out the Feelings Monitoring Form (Handout 11.3) for the first time after it was introduced. See Box 11.3 to see what the completed form might have looked like. This case demonstrates how self-monitoring provided a structure and process that helped this client develop clarity and insight about the presence and diversity of her feelings, about the way certain feelings predominated in her daily life, and about the presence of a pattern or typical mode of reaction to these feelings.

The client, Petra, had been physically and sexually abused by her father, as well as physically abused by several other caregivers throughout her childhood. Although she was able to hold a job and had achieved a relative degree of success there, she had few friends and struggled with binge eating and depression. When the therapist introduced the Feelings Monitoring Form to her, along with the Feelings Wheel, she was intrigued by the number of words she could use to describe a feeling.

Identifying Triggering Situation and Feelings

The situation Petra described when asked to identify a time when she'd had strong feelings was a conflict with her son. She said she'd felt "upset" when he would not put his phone away at the dinner table after she had asked him to repeatedly. With the help of the Feelings Wheel and some prompting of "What else did you feel?", she was able to identify more specific feelings—anger, shame, and sadness. In addition, it was helpful for the therapist to ask her how her body felt, so that she could identify some of the physical connections to her emotions. For example, her fists were clenched, she was flushed, she had a headache, and she was breathing quickly. After the feelings were labeled, the therapist discussed with her that it is possible to have more than one feeling at a time, and that while this might be confusing occasionally, it is normal.

Example: Petra's Completed Feelings Monitoring Form

Triggering Situation	Feeling	Intensity at Start (0–10)	Duration	Thoughts	Behavior	Intensity Afterward (0–10)	Effective?
Son didn't put his phone away at the table after I asked him to repeatedly.	Anger	10	Several hours	He doesn't respect me, and he thinks he can take advantage of me.	Eating a whole bag of candy	9	No
Same	Shame	10	Same	I'm a bad mother.	Same	10	No
Same	Sadness	7	Same	If he loved me, he would do what I ask, and would not want to upset me.	Same	7	No
Situation	**Feelings**			**Thoughts**	**Behavior**	**Result**	

Identifying Intensity and Duration of Feelings

Together, Petra and her therapist numbered the intensity of each feeling she'd had on a scale of 1–10, where 10 was the most she could ever imagine feeling something (e.g., so angry she could explode, so ashamed she felt like "a total failure," so sad she could not think of anything positive) and 1 was the least. By labeling the intensity, Petra began to develop perspective on the degree of emotions she was experiencing in various situations, rather than having all of her feelings blend into one big, unmanageable, and scary knot. She initially was not sure how long the feelings had lasted, but then remembered that she did not feel any better until she woke up the next morning, so her feelings lasted for several hours (from after dinner until she went to bed).

Identifying Thoughts

The next step, and one of the hardest, was for Petra and her therapist to figure out the thoughts that went along with her emotions. Since Petra had never tried to link her thoughts to her feelings before, the therapist had to help her out with suggestions of things she might have been thinking. In discussing the situation at home, they noticed that Petra felt responsible for her son's behavior, and that when he failed to do something, she felt like a failure too. So, her shame and sadness were coming from thoughts like "I'm a bad mother," and "If he really loved me, he would do what I ask, and would not want to upset me." She was also thinking, "He doesn't respect me . . . ," which led to frustration with her son and with herself. Her anger was connected to thoughts such as ". . . he thinks he can take advantage of me."

Identifying Responses and Coping Strategies

Eventually, Petra and the therapist would work on replacing this kind of thinking with more positive and less self-blaming thoughts, but for now they just tried to identify what she did in response to the feelings. To make herself feel better, Petra ate a whole bag of candy. She had shared earlier in the treatment that she had developed a problem with emotional eating when she was younger, and that she continued to find herself turning to food when she felt particularly distressed. Petra was aware that the comfort and distraction food often provided were temporary. She understood clearly in this example that eating was not an effective coping strategy, and, if anything, it had made her feel worse; this was reflected in her answers when the therapist asked her to rerate the intensity of her feelings after her behavioral response.

Developing Self-Awareness

Once she had learned how to monitor her feelings in session, Petra was able to complete further copies of the Feelings Monitoring Form over the course of the following week. When she came back to session she said to the therapist, "I was going to tell you I'd had a good week, but when I looked back at my forms, I realized I'd felt bad almost every day!" In looking at the forms together, Petra and the therapist not only noticed when and where she was feeling bad, they also noticed that whenever she had strong feelings, she either went on an eating binge, immersed herself in her work, or went to sleep for a long time. Basically, all of her coping responses for strong emotion involved escape tactics. One of the first therapeutic tasks became helping Petra find additional coping responses for managing her feelings.

SUMMARIZE THE GOALS OF THE SESSION

Especially in the first few sessions, it is worthwhile for the therapist to review the key ideas and goals at the end of each session, as many clients will be unfamiliar with these concepts and may be feeling anxious and somewhat distracted. In summary, in this session, the therapist discusses with the client how the client's experience of trauma has impaired their ability to identify and understand their feelings. The client and therapist have worked together to identify the client's emotion regulation difficulties. The three channels of emotion have been introduced: body, thoughts, and behaviors. The therapist and client have practiced using the three channels to help identify how each element is related in a specific emotion (e.g., anger).

To help the client identify their feelings, the therapist has reviewed the rationale for and process of self-monitoring feelings. The therapist and client have filled out Handout 11.3, the Feelings Monitoring Form, together. The therapist has also reviewed two other emotion identification tools with the client: Handout 11.7, the Feelings List, and Handout 11.8, the Feelings Wheel.

PLAN SKILLS PRACTICE

At the end of each session, the therapist presents the rationale for skills practice between sessions. After doing so, the therapist and client collaboratively plan for specific practice related to the session. One primary type of practice after Session 2 is completion of the Feelings Monitoring Form: The client will complete at least one copy of this form per day until the next session. The form will indicate situations the client faced that raised strong feelings, and will also provide data on the client's coping strategies. The therapist and client will benefit from reviewing the completed forms at the beginning of the next session. This way, both can address any practical difficulties or misunderstandings regarding the use of the form, such as what information goes in which column. If necessary, the therapist and client can again complete the Feelings Monitoring Form together (e.g., if the client has not completed the work during the week, or if aspects of the experience are unclear to the client).

Once the client has become more adept at completing these assignments, the therapist can emphasize the utility of this form in providing important data for the therapeutic sessions and allowing the therapist a window into the client's real-world experiences. It is also beneficial for the therapist to stress the importance of recording the details as soon as possible after the moment, perhaps by saying something like this: "Filling this form out soon after the experience or trigger will provide the two of us the most helpful and accurate data." The therapist can mention explicitly that the client can add both positive and negative examples of emotions and outcomes of their feelings. All kinds of emotional experiences can provide information helpful in helping the client meet their therapeutic goals.

In addition, the client is instructed to continue to practice Focused Breathing twice a day. The therapist provides the client with several copies of the Feelings Monitoring Form (Handout 11.3), as well as copies of each of the other handouts from the session (Handouts 11.1, 11.2, and 11.4 through 11.8) for the client's continued review.

The Impact of Childhood Abuse and Neglect on Emotion Regulation

For many people, experiences of abuse and neglect in childhood have a powerful impact on emotional functioning in adulthood. Good parenting provides children with emotion regulation skills, which include the ability to identify feelings, understand their sources, and manage them for optimal functioning. Abuse and neglect elicit a range of powerful and confusing feelings. Often survivors of childhood abuse and neglect have been raised in a family context where caregivers offer poor soothing during times of distress and poor guidance in modulating feelings. Many survivors feel overwhelmed by their emotions, or, in contrast, feel numb and unable to experience many or all emotions.

TYPES OF EMOTION REGULATION DIFFICULTIES

Difficulties in emotion regulation vary by person and sometimes by situation. Some people have trouble labeling and identifying their feelings. They may feel either "bad" or "OK," and have little sense of differences between their emotions (for example, anxiety vs. sadness). Other people lack an understanding of what triggers their feelings. It may seem that their emotions randomly come "out of the blue" and make no sense. Many people can learn to recognize a "triggering situation," but will have more difficulty knowing what to do with the intense feelings that emerge. Such feelings may be experienced as overwhelming or even dangerous, and people often feel ill equipped to handle them.

THE ROLES OF FEELINGS

Learning how to modulate and attend to feelings is a critical skill, because feelings, once managed, serve important roles in effective living. One role of emotions is to serve as guides for action. For example, a feeling of fear can guide you to leave an unsafe situation and take steps to ensure safety. Anxiety can be adaptive, but when chronic and excessive, it floods the ability to differentiate feeling states. It causes people to overreact to situations, or to underreact because they are trying so hard not to overreact.

Feelings also contribute to effectively communicating how you feel and what you need from others. Some people who have experienced trauma are chronically anxious, angry, or sad, or are so numbed that they cannot use this kind of information. By working on attending to your feelings and modulating them, you will be able to make better use of information from your feelings and to express them more effectively.

Lastly, feelings can be used to inform you about your preferences (likes and dislikes) and to help guide you in the selection of valued life goals. Awareness of feelings includes awareness of positive feelings and, in combination with emotion modulation skills, can enhance your experience of life, your creativity, and your appreciation of yourself.

(continued)

FEELINGS MONITORING FORM

One way to begin learning how to identify feeling states and their triggers is to monitor your feelings in different situations. Using the Feelings Monitoring Form, you will practice labeling your feelings and identifying the situations and thoughts that trigger those feelings. With your therapist, you will review your completed copies of this form to increase your skills in identifying feelings and their triggers and to build your awareness of the patterns in your feelings. The completed copies of the form will also serve as important data for developing new coping strategies.

Social Influences on Your Emotional Experiences

What are the messages you have received about emotions throughout your life?

	Growing Up (Examples: your family, teachers, friends)	Current Relationships (Examples: close friends, romantic partner)	Community/Society (Examples: military, culture, religious community)
Which emotions should you feel?			
How should you cope with emotions?			
How should you express your emotions?			

Feelings Monitoring Form

Triggering Situation	Feeling	Intensity at Start (0–10)	Duration	Thoughts	Behavior	Intensity Afterward (0–10)	Effective?
Situation		**Feelings**		**Thoughts**	**Behavior**		**Result**

Examples of Emotion Regulation Coping Skills for the Three Channels of Emotion

THREE CHANNELS OF EMOTION

To help us explore our feelings, we can think of our emotional experiences as expressed through three channels: body, thought, and behavior.

The "body channel" is what we feel physically in our bodies. For example, when we're feeling anxious, we may notice that our breathing quickens, our heart rate increases, and we sweat or shake.

The "thought channel" includes what we say to ourselves, our beliefs, and the attributions we make. For example, when we're feeling anxious, we may think to ourselves, "I'm such a loser," or "I can't trust anyone." These thoughts contribute to and maintain distress.

Finally, the "behavior channel" consists of what we actually do in response to the distress. For example, when we're feeling anxious, we may overeat, get into a fight with someone, or distract ourselves with another activity.

Of course, there are healthier ways to cope and experience emotion in each channel, and that's what this treatment is all about!

EXAMPLES OF COPING SKILLS FOR EACH CHANNEL

Because these channels are interconnected, we can target interventions at any one channel. The bonus effect is that targeting one channel will have an impact on the other channels as well. People differ about which channel feels easiest to tackle first. Not all people feel relief from using each of these coping skills. By trying each one, you'll find which skills work best for you!

In the body channel, Focused Breathing helps to reduce the bodily symptoms of distress. That's why you have learned Focused Breathing first! Other relaxation techniques can also help in this way, so you don't have to stop there.

In the thought channel, Thought Shifting can be effective. Examples of Thought Shifting include cleaning your home, calling a friend, planning a vacation, recalling pleasant past events, watching a funny movie, and counting backward by sevens. Positive Imagery can also intervene in the thought channel. This technique involves calling to mind a situation or setting (real or imagined) in which you feel calm and happy. To get the most benefit from Positive Imagery, you should make the image as clear as possible by imagining how the place looks, smells, feels, and so forth. Another thought channel skill is making Positive Self-Statements. When your thoughts are self-critical, it can be useful to weaken those negative thoughts by formulating positive responses. For example, in response to the thought "I'm a loser," you may tell yourself, "I'm doing my best."

In the behavior channel, Take a Break/Time Out and Replacement Behaviors are helpful. Time Out involves leaving a difficult situation for a period of time to reduce your distress before responding. For example, if you're having a fight with a friend, you can tell your friend that you will finish the discussion in an hour, and then go out for a walk to give yourself time to calm down. Engaging in Replacement Behaviors entails doing pleasurable or neutral activities to distract yourself from distress.

Note that these are all just examples of many options you can select in each of the channels. You and your therapist can select what you think works best for you and what might be appropriate for any given situation.

Three Channels Skills Graphic

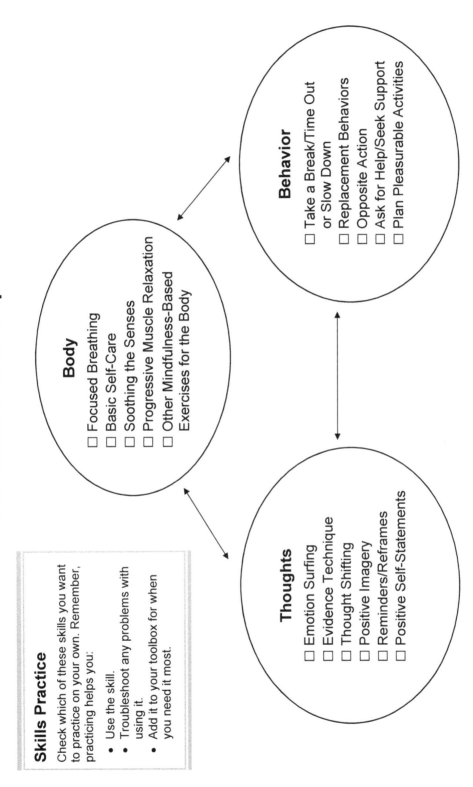

Skills Practice

Check which of these skills you want to practice on your own. Remember, practicing helps you:

- Use the skill.
- Troubleshoot any problems with using it.
- Add it to your toolbox for when you need it most.

Body

☐ Focused Breathing
☐ Basic Self-Care
☐ Soothing the Senses
☐ Progressive Muscle Relaxation
☐ Other Mindfulness-Based Exercises for the Body

Behavior

☐ Take a Break/Time Out or Slow Down
☐ Replacement Behaviors
☐ Opposite Action
☐ Ask for Help/Seek Support
☐ Plan Pleasurable Activities

Thoughts

☐ Emotion Surfing
☐ Evidence Technique
☐ Thought Shifting
☐ Positive Imagery
☐ Reminders/Reframes
☐ Positive Self-Statements

Negative and Positive Emotions as Messengers

Emotion	Purpose
Fear or anxiety	Keeps you safe.
Anger	Provides warning that action may be needed.
Sadness	Provides time to rest and reevaluate.
Guilt	Lets you review what has been done and make amends as appropriate.
Happiness	Reinforces certain actions and relationships; supports engagement in life.
Pride	Indicates a positive action or result; builds self-esteem/sense of worth.
Love	Helps maintain connection with others, even in times of conflict!

Feelings List

Affectionate	Glad	Relaxed
Afraid	Gloomy	Relieved
Amused	Grateful	Resentful
Angry	Great	Resigned
Annoyed	Guilty	Sad
Anxious	Happy	Safe
Apathetic	Hateful	Satisfied
Apprehensive	Helpless	Secure
Ashamed	Hopeless	Sexy
Bitter	Horrified	Shy
Bored	Hostile	Silly
Calm	Impatient	Strong
Capable	Inadequate	Stubborn
Cheerful	Inhibited	Stuck
Comfortable	Irritated	Supportive
Competent	Isolated	Sympathetic
Concerned	Jealous	Tearful
Confident	Joyful	Tender
Confused	Lonely	Terrified
Contemptuous	Loved	Threatened
Controlled	Loving	Thrilled
Curious	Loyal	Touchy
Defeated	Manipulated	Trapped
Dejected	Manipulative	Troubled
Delighted	Melancholy	Unappreciated
Depressed	Miserable	Uncertain
Desirable	Misunderstood	Understood
Despairing	Muddled	Uneasy
Desperate	Needy	Unfulfilled
Determined	Nervous	Unimportant
Devastated	Numb	Unloved
Disappointed	Out of control	Upset
Discouraged	Outraged	Uptight
Disgusted	Overwhelmed	Used
Disillusioned	Panicky	Useless
Distrustful	Passionate	Victimized
Embarrassed	Peaceful	Violated
Enraged	Pessimistic	Vulnerable
Excited	Pleased	Withdrawn
Frantic	Powerful	Wonderful
Frightened	Prejudiced	Worn out
Frustrated	Pressured	Worried
Fulfilled	Proud	Worthwhile
Furious	Provoked	Wronged
Generous	Put down	Yearning

Feelings Wheel

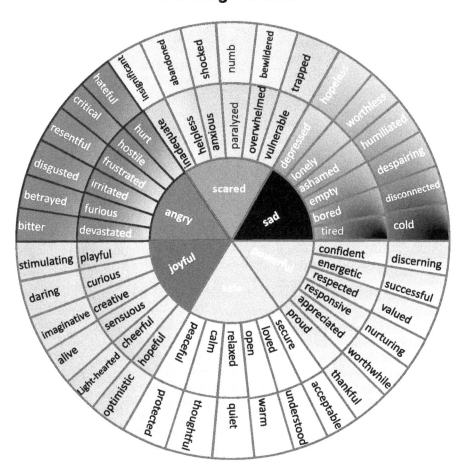

CHAPTER 12

SESSION 3

Emotion Regulation
Focus on the Body

The art of soothing ourselves is a fundamental life skill.
—DANIEL GOLEMAN (1995, p. 57)

Clients who have been traumatized as children appear both to experience more negative feelings and to have more difficulty coping with feelings than those who have not experienced childhood trauma. Often such clients will vacillate between being overwhelmed by distress and feeling nothing or numb. Clients often attempt to cope with overwhelming feelings via strategies that make them feel better in the short run but are ultimately self-destructive. These attempts to cope include using alcohol or other substances and engaging in other self-injurious behaviors (e.g., self-cutting or bingeing and purging). Session 2 has focused on helping clients know what they are experiencing by learning to name and describe their feelings. This exercise allows the clients to begin experiencing greater emotional awareness in daily life. The primary goal of Session 3 is to help clients start the process of developing and strengthening skills that will enable them to regulate feelings without resorting to self-destructive attempts to cope. Developing new, healthy skills will enhance their competence and confidence in the process of exploring emotion-laden experiences, especially for clients who will be going on to the Narrative Therapy module of treatment.

The emotion regulation skills proposed here build on Session 2's organization of emotional responses into three channels or modes of experiencing (body, thought, and behavior). This session focuses on the concept of emotion regulation, with an emphasis on strengthening capacities for self-soothing in the physical ways emotions are felt within the body—what we call the "body channel" of emotion. The exercises presented here aim to strengthen emotion regulation within the body channel as the first target for developing new skills, for several reasons. First, the connection between body and emotions is fundamental from a physiological standpoint. Feeling states often start (if not also end) in the limbic system or the "animal brain." Humans have developed many higher-order ways to interpret and understand feelings, but the foundation often remains in the physical body.

Second, understanding emotions as expressed in the body is key to understanding how early trauma affects the developing person. Children who survive trauma may have their first experiences of their bodies be ones of pain, discomfort, or violation. Connecting with one's body then becomes not only a difficult task, but a trauma trigger. Using one's body to soothe emotions can also be associated with shame. This pattern is especially seen in cases of sexual abuse, where a child's first experiences of their physical body may be tainted by trauma memories. Survivors may implicitly transform the confusion that is often a part of childhood sexual trauma into shame and avoidance of all body sensations, whether these are sexual in nature or not. Even in adult trauma, sometimes neutral or pleasurable sensations in the body can be rewritten as negative ones and thus avoided like any other trauma trigger.

Third, focusing on body channel exercises allows survivors to start with very concrete, simple (if not always easy) skills for healthier coping. Because most Western cultures have undervalued the connection between mind and body, focusing first on this connection as part of healing helps repair broader gaps in popular understanding of feelings. This treatment assumes that body and mind interact with and influence one another as parts of a greater whole. This integrated understanding can shift perspectives of survivors who have neglected one or both sides of their experience of physical and emotional well-being.

CHECK-IN AND REVIEW OF SKILLS PRACTICE

After a brief check-in on the client's current emotional state, the therapist begins reviewing the client's Feelings Monitoring Form entries and inquiring about the client's progress in using Focused Breathing. The client's self-monitoring can provide useful examples of emotion regulation difficulties that the therapist can highlight throughout this and following sessions. If the client did not do either practice, the therapist can take a few moments to review the rationale for between-session work, to problem-solve any practical barriers, and to help the client fill out the form, using at least one example.

IDENTIFY FOCUS OF THE SESSION

This session expands the previous session's introduction to the three channels of emotion and focuses on the body channel. It introduces several body channel skills beyond focused breathing, including basic Self-Care, Soothing the Senses, Progressive Muscle Relaxation, and various forms of mindful awareness. Box 12.1 outlines the contents of this session.

ELABORATE ON CONCEPT OF EMOTION REGULATION

The first step after skills practice review and summarizing the session's focus is for the therapist and client to continue discussing the concept of emotion regulation. Emotion regulation consists of the responses that individuals develop to help them create an emotional

Theme and Curriculum for Session 3
Emotion Regulation: Focus on the Body

Individuals learn emotion regulation early in life in the context of relationships with caregivers. Clients who were traumatized as children often have caregivers who cannot regulate their own feelings. Such caregivers may use alcohol or other substances to make themselves feel better, or may express emotions in frightening ways, such as rage or dissociation. Thus clients may never have learned positive and effective ways to cope with their emotions. Instead, such clients may go to extreme measures to avoid difficult feelings or may adopt ineffective strategies they have observed in their environment (e.g., social withdrawal or substance misuse). Understanding such behaviors as unproductive efforts to cope is a first step in learning new, positive, and more adaptive skills to manage feelings. This session is the first of two sessions that introduce specific, healthy coping skills by the emotion channel each set of skills taps. We start with focusing on how emotions are experienced in the body and how clients can learn to cope by using healthy, body-based skills.

PLANNING AND PREPARATION

Review emotion regulation self-report measures to identify patterns that can guide your work with the client. Bring additional copies of the Feelings Monitoring Form (Handout 11.3) and copies of the Session 3 handouts listed below. Prepare several examples of emotion regulation skills for the body channel of emotion. The work in the session is estimated to take about 60 minutes; a flexible application is assumed (i.e., not every client will need all interventions).

AGENDA

- Check-in and review of skills practice.
- Identify focus of the session.
- Elaborate on concept of emotion regulation.
- Identify and evaluate client's current emotion regulation skills.
- Introduce skills for the body channel of emotions:
  - Basic Self-Care.
  - Soothing the Senses.
  - Progressive Muscle Relaxation.
  - Other mindfulness-based skills for the body channel.
- Review misconceptions about emotion regulation work (as necessary).

(continued)

- Summarize the goals of the session.
- Plan skills practice:
  - Complete Feelings Monitoring Form once a day (note positive and negative emotions). Specify coping skills on the body channel that were used to deal with difficult feelings or situations described in entries.
  - Practice one or more new body channel skills once a day.
  - Practice Focused Breathing twice a day.

SESSION HANDOUTS

Handout 12.1. Healthy and Unhealthy Ways to Cope on the Body Channel

Handout 12.2. Body Channel Coping Skills

Handout 12.3. Basics of Self-Care (A Body Channel Skill)

Handout 12.4. Soothing the Senses (A Body Channel Skill)

Handout 12.5. Progressive Muscle Relaxation (A Body Channel Skill)

Additional copies of Handout 11.3. Feelings Monitoring Form

"comfort zone" that is neither too intensely high nor too low, and that as such allows them to function, to learn, and to stay connected with the environment. A metaphor is often helpful in explaining abstract concepts like the dangers of dampening one's emotions too much. We have found that the easiest one for clients to understand is comparing the mind to a soda bottle and emotions to the soda inside. The therapist can say something like the following:

> "Imagine that your emotions are like the soda inside a soda bottle. Because we're human, our emotions come and go throughout the day. If we try to bottle them up inside and not let them out, though, we might experience a growing pressure. Just like you see in a soda bottle that's been shaken but remains closed. What happens when you finally open that bottle? It explodes and soda gets everywhere. The soda then returns to normal (though perhaps it's a bit flat).
>
> "Now imagine instead that you're able to let out a little pressure at a time. You don't keep the lid on your bottle so tightly, so the pressure doesn't build up as intensely. This approach is what we're talking about when we discuss better ways to manage emotions. Pay attention to them, express them as appropriate, and take care of yourself in the process."

This message is important, as part of learning healthy coping skills is allowing clients to feel, in a manageable way, the emotions they have tried so hard (and often unsuccessfully) to suppress.

A prerequisite to effective emotion regulation is the capacity to be aware of and to monitor one's feelings—skills introduced in Session 2. While the term "emotion regulation" functionally refers to the capacity to manage feelings, it also implies the necessity of a certain degree of emotional awareness. Moreover, emotion regulation is linked to enhanced life engagement, as it directly contributes to improved functioning in interpersonal relationships, parenting activities, and work efforts.

Emotion regulation includes the abilities to self-soothe and to reduce intense emotional states of all kinds, including fear, anger, and sadness. It also includes the ability to raise and sustain feelings that facilitate effective and positive engagement in life. This might include finding humor in a difficult situation, being curious about how things work, yearning to spend time with loved ones, or being satisfied with a job well done. When survivors of interpersonal trauma dampen their feelings, they often dampen all emotions, even positive ones.

The therapist can emphasize that emotion regulation includes both reducing overwhelming or negative emotions and increasing positive and helpful ones. A well-regulated emotional state varies from person to person and from one circumstance to another. The ideally regulated emotional state is one in which a person is "comfortable in their own skin" and effectively and appropriately engages in their environment, with the people in it, and in the tasks being pursued. When positive feelings do come up for some survivors, a reaction of guilt may immediately follow. Helping clients explore positive feelings is just as much a part of recovery as helping them cope with negative feelings.

Review the Development of Emotion Regulation in Childhood

Before proceeding to skills work on emotion regulation, the therapist and client can have a detailed discussion about the ideal course of development of emotion regulation. We have found that understanding how emotion regulation develops helps clients feel less "crazy" and understand why they behave the way they do. In addition, emphasizing that emotion regulation skills are learned behaviors, and not something people are born with, encourages the clients to learn new, more positive, and more effective ways of managing their moods. The developmental perspective also helps clients avoid feeling discouraged by emphasizing that emotion regulation develops over years when children are trying to survive in the environment they have, which for survivors of childhood trauma is far from ideal. Knowing that they learned these behaviors over years also helps clients understand that learning new strategies will also take some time. Understanding that emotions, especially early in life, are often about physical safety can further validate their importance and the need to include physical, body-based strategies in coping with them.

Provide examples of learning to regulate emotions

Throughout development, a child learns emotion regulation strategies in two primary ways: through caregivers' responses to the child's emotions, and through observing caregivers' management of their own moods (modeling). Children who have been abused often have parents with deficits in both areas. Such parents are often unable to respond or ineffective in responding to their children's needs. Sometimes because of their own trauma histories, they are unable to cope with their own emotions in positive and effective ways. It is often helpful to provide clients examples to illustrate how emotion regulation strategies develop in the context of normative child–caregiver relationships. Such examples can easily be linked to the skills clients are learning in the therapy.

The therapist can describe the following (or a similar) scenario. Consider a situation in which a 4-year-old child who is climbing a jungle gym in the playground slips and falls. The child starts crying. Ideally, what does the child's caregiver do? The caregiver runs to the child and helps the child get up. They ask the child, "Did you hurt yourself? Where does it hurt?" and inspects the child for physical injury. Finding no real damage but realizing that the child has a scraped knee and was scared by the fall, the caregiver might say while holding and comforting the child, "I know, I know, it's scary to fall like that. I know your knee hurts. But I'm here; it will be OK." The caregiver might rinse out the scrape with some water. Once the child calms down, the caregiver might ask, "Do you want to climb the jungle gym again?" If the child is hesitant, the caregiver might say, "Do you want me to help you climb?" Then the caregiver might stand behind the child so that the child feels safe while climbing.

This scenario provides an illustration of a caregiver acting as an external regulator of the child's emotional experience. The caregiver's guidance also acts as instruction to the child, who, through this and many similar examples, will learn how to manage their own distress over time. This example includes the prerequisite presence of emotional awareness in the caregiver for the child. The caregiver is aware of the child's feelings/reactions and provides labels for them ("It's scary to fall like that" and "I know your knee hurts"). The caregiver also signals acceptance of the child's expression of these feelings by naming and thus verbally "echoing" them, rather than ignoring or censoring them. The caregiver monitors the child's emotions from the first instant after the fall, as they hold the child (bodily soothing and comforting); evaluates the situation and takes action ("It's not too serious; let's rinse the scrape out"); and finally guides the child back to the situation and monitors any hesitation ("Do you want me to help you climb?"). By encouraging the child to climb on the jungle gym again, the caregiver facilitates reengagement in a pleasurable activity and the resolution of any remaining fear by helping the child confront rather than avoid the source of the misadventure.

A child's capacity for emotion regulation grows out of such experiences. Over time, the child internalizes lessons in managing distress. Children learn various strategies to soothe themselves: body-based strategies to create physiological comfort (e.g., running, jumping, focused breathing, stretching); thought-based strategies (e.g., telling themselves it is going to be all right, planning solutions); and behavior-based strategies (implementing an action plan, confronting rather than avoiding). Finally, the example above illustrates the presence of strong emotional support and attachment, suggesting that requests for help will be met and so encouraging a final behavioral strategy—recruitment of social support when needed. The caregiver is giving the child this message: "If you are upset and need help, someone will listen to you and help you feel better." By asking if the child needs help, the caregiver is also teaching the child, "If you need help, let someone who cares about you know." And, by standing behind the child while they climb, the caregiver is teaching the child recruitment of social support: "You can rely on others to give you help if you ask for it."

Explore the impact of abuse on development of emotion regulation behaviors

How might this example be different for a child whose caregivers are abusive? We can envision a number of scenarios in response to that question. The therapist can provide examples as relevant to the client's own personal experiences in childhood. Often the current patterns of emotion management that the client reports have parallels to those experienced and observed in the client's caregiving environment. If it seems helpful, the therapist can share a couple of common scenarios below.

For example, a child who has been abused is often also neglected. In that case, there may not even be a caregiver around in the playground example. Another possibility is that the child's caregiver, even if present, may respond angrily to the child and say, "Stop being a baby. You're fine. Stop crying." The caregiver is thus neither acknowledging the child's feelings nor helping the child identify these feelings. If the child actually runs to such a caregiver, the caregiver may push the child away. Or the caregiver may dismiss the child because the caregiver is incapacitated by depression or substance use. Yet another maladaptive response by the caregiver may be hitting or punishing the child who is crying in this example. The child then learns that their feelings are not important, and that when feelings are expressed, they will bring negative responses from others. In fact, here a negative emotional state leads directly to another instance of maltreatment. In this way, negative feelings really do become triggers for even deeper trauma reactions.

Because of various experiences like those above, survivors of maltreatment often have not developed the ability to recognize their feelings, or have learned to avoid certain feelings altogether or even to engage in self-destructive behaviors when feelings seem overwhelming or unavoidable. Such clients often do not understand why they behave the way they do and cannot see a connection between their feelings and behaviors. When clients begin to see that many of their behaviors are learned responses from childhood, they begin to feel "sane" and to develop some self-compassion—a theme therapists can preview here before it is explored more fully in the later sessions of STAIR.

Discuss the Impact of Emotion Regulation Problems on Parenting Skills (If Relevant)

Talking about connections between early childhood experiences with caregivers and emotion regulation can be enlightening, if not also very difficult, for survivors of abuse who are now parents themselves. For this reason, another area to explore with clients, if relevant, is their own behavior as caregivers. Clients who have been abused as children are at higher risk of abusing their own children. Although most survivors of abuse do not abuse their children, they often worry about behaving toward their children in ways that their parents behaved toward them. They often struggle with the question of how best to parent their children. They do not want to repeat their own parents' mistakes, but do not know how to behave differently. When their children are distressed and crying, clients may feel overwhelmed and helpless, or may even shut down. When their children are angry, clients may feel vulnerable and victimized. Rather than helping their children learn to regulate their own feelings,

> ### BOX 12.2
> # An Example of How Trauma Can Influence Parenting: Judy
>
> A client named Judy had parents who belittled and made fun of her whenever she cried. Her earliest memory of this experience dated from when she was 5 years old. Judy was an overweight child and would often be teased at school about her weight. One day, walking home from kindergarten, some older boys followed her, teased her for being "fat," and laughed when she tried to run away. She arrived home in tears. Her mother's response was to say angrily, "Look at Judy being such a baby. Boo-hoo-hoo." When Judy cried more, her mother threatened punishment: "If you don't stop crying, I will give you something to cry about." As a result, Judy learned quickly not to cry or to show when she was hurt, afraid, or vulnerable in any way. She learned this lesson so thoroughly that she developed a very "thick skin" and had difficulty recognizing any feelings of vulnerability in herself. She also developed little tolerance for vulnerability in others. She had internalized her mother's punitive coping style and now inflicted it on those around her, including her daughter. When her daughter cried, she found herself getting angry and wanting to yell at her. Knowing that anger was not appropriate, she sometimes shut down and ignored her daughter instead. At other times, she lashed out like her own mother.
>
> When viewed in the context of her developmental history, Judy's response to her daughter was not surprising. Judy was merely repeating what she had learned from her own parents and applying the same rules to her daughter that she applied to herself. By learning in therapy how children develop emotion regulation skills, Judy became able to understand herself and her behavior better. As she learned to recognize her own feelings, she was able to identify how her daughter's behavior triggered her own history. This insight helped foster greater compassion for both herself and her daughter. She was then better equipped to differentiate her daughter's feelings from her own feelings and history. By understanding that emotion regulation skills are something learned, Judy became empowered to respond to her daughter in a way that would teach her emotion regulation skills, rather than feeling victimized and overwhelmed in the face of her daughter's behavior.

clients who were abused as children find themselves reliving their own histories through their role as parents. This pattern may be particularly insidious, because it can trigger not only their own trauma reactions, but also further guilt and/or shame about their role as a parent. To help normalize these challenges, the therapist can provide a case example from our work (or their own) about such a situation. See Box 12.2 for an illustration of this pattern.

IDENTIFY AND EVALUATE CLIENT'S CURRENT EMOTION REGULATION SKILLS

Review Relevant Emotion Regulation Assessment

After reviewing the broader importance of emotion regulation, the next step is to have the client identify their own emotion regulation strategies. Before this session, the therapist will have reviewed the client's results on any measures collected about emotion regulation. Thus the therapist can provide the client with information about their relative strengths and weaknesses in body channel strategies. The therapist and client can use the results on the selected measure(s) as a basis for continuing to build on skills already present and to identify areas of vulnerability.

Review the Feelings Monitoring Form

In addition, the Feelings Monitoring Form (Handout 11.3) informs both the therapist's and the client's understanding of the client's typical emotion management strategies as they relate to the body (e.g., "I pinched myself hard, hoping the pain would distract me from feeling so helpless"). A lot of times clients will not recognize these activities as efforts to regulate emotions, so therapists can highlight this connection. The therapist can talk with the client about each example on the form and help them identify how they respond to each identified feeling. Some clients may have difficulty with this process because their coping strategies are not intentional, but are experienced as automatic and unconscious. In fact, body-based coping strategies are often so ingrained that recognizing and then slowing down the process from trigger to response can be particularly challenging. Gaining insight from the Feelings Monitoring Form often requires gentle guidance from the therapist, alongside reinforcement, to help shape the client's understanding of patterns.

Elicit Examples of Regulation Strategies

If a client has difficulty coming up with examples, it is sometimes helpful to ask, "What do you do to make yourself feel better when you feel bad?" The therapist can then work with the client to make a list of the different things the client does currently to make themselves feel better. These activities are attempts to regulate their feelings. Handout 12.1, Healthy and Unhealthy Ways to Cope on the Body Channel, summarizes common ways these attempts are manifested in survivors of trauma and lists healthy alternatives.

Once the client provides a few examples, the therapist can start from the beginning and help them evaluate the strategies used. This process can be facilitated by asking, "Did doing X make you feel better?" If the client did feel better, the therapist can move on to evaluate the broader consequences of the strategy. How long did the client feel better? Were there any negative consequences to this strategy? Personal short-term and long-term outcomes from the client's life can be used to determine whether this is a useful, effective strategy for regulating emotions.

Identify Timing of Strategies

Identifying and evaluating the client's emotion regulation strategies also involves investigating *when* the client uses the strategies. Timing is especially important, given the automatic nature of body-based efforts to cope. Many clients are very avoidant in directly addressing their emotions. As a result, rather than engaging in conscious emotion regulation strategies when they first start feeling distressed, they suppress their feelings and wait until they are completely overwhelmed and have no choice but to deal with their feelings (often in unhelpful ways at that point). By learning to identify what they are feeling when they start having a feeling, such clients can learn to use coping strategies before becoming overwhelmed. Early identification of emotions often involves mindful awareness of how one's body feels—a signal that can precede more conscious experiencing of feeling. Modern Western society does not frequently emphasize connecting body sensations to emotional states. Thus therapists may need to spend extra time connecting physical experiences (like headaches) to emotional triggers and stress.

For example, a client may be feeling physically exhausted after having a very difficult day at work. If the client recognizes that they are feeling anxious and not just physically tired, they can decide to do something after work that addresses their anxiety and not just their sense of being tired. The client may call a good friend and ask the friend to go for tea or go for a walk in the park. If the client does not recognize the feeling of anxiety, or if they ignore or discount their feelings, they may choose to do something that does not make them feel better (and in fact may make them feel worse). In this example, interpreting their physical tiredness as the core nature of their experience may lead to going to bed early, which may be effective in the short term but may prevent them from consciously addressing their emotional needs when the next day they return to work. Identifying feelings while they are still at relatively low intensities helps the client manage them early and successfully.

INTRODUCE SKILLS FOR THE BODY CHANNEL OF EMOTIONS

Many different skills are effective in targeting the body channel of emotion. These include Focused Breathing (discussed in Session 1), Progressive Muscle Relaxation, Soothing the Senses, and other mindfulness-based techniques. Because each of these skills has been described in detail by other authors, we only briefly summarize their use here, with special emphasis on the interventions we have used most commonly in STAIR.

However, a key aspect of all these regulation strategies is that they must be practiced regularly and in nonstressful circumstances before they can be effectively applied in triggering situations. One of the most common problem clients have in learning body-based regulation exercises is that clients tend to implement them only under stress. This approach is like running a marathon without training with shorter distances first; the result would be likely one of failure instead of empowerment and success. Similarly, with emotion regulation practice in tough situations, clients may be burdened with simultaneously trying to remember how a new skill works while managing their overwhelming feelings. Skills need to be practiced regularly and in relatively relaxed and quiet conditions, so that they become ingrained, relatively automatic behavior patterns that require little effort to initiate under stress. In a triggering situation, a client realistically has only one key task: managing the distress in a healthy way. The skills are intended to be resources clients can immediately recruit and automatically initiate when needed most.

If the therapist has not already done this during the check-in, this session is also a good time to review with the client their practice of Focused Breathing and any difficulties that have come up, since it has been introduced first and is a core example of a body channel coping skill. Handout 12.2, Body Channel Coping Skills, is a graphic that shows additional examples of such skills; therapist and client can check these off for continued practice as they see fit.

Basic Self-Care

Sometimes early trauma disrupts even the most basic skills of daily living. Basic Self-Care includes bathing, eating, sleeping, and exercise, all of which promote both physical and emotional well-being. Barriers to using this basic skill set for people who have experienced trauma may include conscious or unconscious efforts at self-harm (often in response to underlying shame); reduced resources and energy available to be directed toward self-care; and occupation of a "sick role" because of fear of losing out on needed support if the client shows any level of improvement. Modeling for the client the importance of Basic Self-Care as a priority may be particularly important in very severe cases of childhood trauma. It may be necessary to reassure the client that improvement in managing their physical well-being can lead to greater self-confidence and ability to manage their mental state and relationships. Sometimes this change will cause "growing pains" in relationships, but ultimately the results should be stronger, healthier relationships with the self and significant others. Handout 12.3, Basics of Self-Care (A Body Channel Skill), reviews components of self-care that therapists can use with clients to create a simple self-care plan.

Soothing the Senses

Basic human experience often involves various dimensions of sensations in the physical body. Unfortunately, it is easy for clients to get distracted by external and internal stimuli that limit their experience. Survivors of trauma, may routinely ignore or devalue certain senses, because their attention is diverted to avoiding trauma cues or painful emotions or thoughts. Soothing the Senses is a skill that guides clients to attend to each major sensory experience (sight, sound, touch, smell, taste) one at a time, with a special emphasis on pleasurable or relaxing stimuli. Note that for clients with any type of sensory impairment, therapists can collaborate with the clients to make modifications.

Clients ideally will choose at least two senses to focus on. Therapists can give examples of soothing sensations and skills for quickly accessing these sensations in the moment. For example, saving pictures on a smartphone (even as the background or lock screen) may be a quick way to conjure up memories of pleasant sensations, such as warmth (a sunny beach), tactile comfort (a soft blanket), or a preferred taste (a peppermint candy). If possible, actually experiencing the sensations is even better. Clients can bring a small keepsake with them to touch when they want to feel soothed, or bubble gum to chew. Even comfortable, soft clothing can make a big difference during times of distress. Whatever is chosen, it should be specific to the client. See Handout 12.4, Soothing the Senses (A Body Channel Skill), for more guidance and a worksheet that therapists can use with their clients.

Progressive Muscle Relaxation

A staple relaxation skill for decades, Progressive Muscle Relaxation is an excellent tool for learning to attend to the body as a whole and to release tensions that may not enter conscious awareness. The skill involves guiding one's attention slowly and methodically to each major part of the body, usually going from head to toe (or vice versa), while carefully tensing and releasing the relevant muscles. This skill can be practiced anywhere and in many ways. Clients with any chronic pain issues can adjust the exercise to their needs. A client can practice Progressive Muscle Relaxation lying down, sitting, or standing, as long as the person is safe, comfortable, and aware of their surroundings. Handout 12.5, Progressive Muscle Relaxation (A Body Channel Skill), is a written description clients can take home.

Other Mindfulness-Based Skills for the Body Channel

A welcome side effect of practicing body-based skills can be a greater awareness in the moment of sensations both internal and external to the client. Mindfulness has been practiced in some form throughout recorded history, and today it has proven to be a useful skill for gaining insight into the present, fostering a sense of peace and relaxation, and even expanding one's sense of consciousness. Not only is mindfulness a body channel skill itself (it spans all three channels of emotion), but introducing it as such may give clients access to a challenging yet powerful set of practices. For clients who have experience in or enjoy mindfulness, therapists can encourage its use beyond the skills (Focused Breathing, Soothing the Senses, and Progressive Muscle Relaxation) described to this point. Some further examples of mindfulness-based skills include mindful awareness of one's immediate environment (which can be especially grounding during times of internal distress), mindful eating (either a small snack or an entire meal), mindful walking (focusing on the full experience of walking, feeling toes inside shoes as one takes each step), and mindful meditation on a specific object (e.g., watching the flame of a lit candle). Although the practice of mindfulness can be hard, the concept is simple—just being present wherever one is without giving in to distraction from thoughts, memories, and plans. This stance of mind is quite hard for everyone in the modern world, but especially for survivors of trauma, who may have had few experiences of feeling safe and at ease in the present. In fact, for clients who have learned to dissociate to cope with trauma, mindfulness is the exact opposite of their automatic response. As with teaching other new skills, therapists can encourage self-compassion. There is no wrong way to practice mindfulness. Every attempt is a success. Every moment clients realize they are distracted and then choose to bring themselves back to the present moment, they are succeeding in practicing mindfulness.

REVIEW MISCONCEPTIONS ABOUT EMOTION REGULATION WORK (AS NECESSARY)

Some clients resist learning emotion regulation, either as a whole or through specific channels of emotion. This resistance often stems from fears or misconceptions about its nature and consequences. Attempts at healthy emotion regulation do not intend to produce any of the circumstances below. The therapist reviews each point as necessary for each client.

Distress Reduction Requires Rejection or Denial of Feelings

Some clients think that regulating emotions means not having them at all, or not showing them if they have them. The developmental perspective can help clients understand that emotions, both positive and negative, are typical parts of being human. Whether emotions are pleasant or not, we all have them, and that is actually a good thing! What clients are trying to learn, therefore, is not to turn off their emotions, but to learn from them and to cope with them in healthier, more effective ways.

Distress Reduction Trivializes Feelings

Some clients feel as if their pain is so great that using some type of coping skill will merely trivialize it. If so, the therapist can take time to make clear that the aim of distress reduction is to give clients control over their feelings, and some choice in how and when to tolerate distress. We are not suggesting that simply thinking positive thoughts will make everything fine, but it does offer a way out of unproductive ruminating or self-criticism and escalating emotional distress. Once clients can experience emotions at a tolerable level, they can use them to gain insight into their other experiences, their perspectives, and ultimately their personal values.

Distress Reduction Invalidates Trauma

Even if clients come to believe that these skills could make them feel better and improve their lives, they may feel a need to hold onto their suffering as a testament to what was done to them. They may think, "If I feel better, it means that what happened to me was not that bad." The therapist will need to assess this resistance and gently address it, emphasizing that obtaining relief from suffering does not trivialize or invalidate it. In treatment, we commonly use the example of a scraped knee. We ask such clients, "What would you do if you had a scraped knee?" Clients will easily answer that they would clean it, put a bandage on it if necessary, and take an over-the-counter medication for the pain if necessary. We then ask, "What if the reason you had the scraped knee was that someone pushed you? Would you treat your knee any differently? Would you go without relief?" Clients will of course answer that they would not. The therapist can then make the analogy that if a client were pushed and fell and had a scraped knee, putting a bandage on the wound would not take away the right to be angry at the person who pushed them. In fact, later in this treatment, exploring ways to express anger and make sense of such of an event are important areas of focus.

CASE EXAMPLE: MOVING TOWARD HEALTHY EMOTION REGULATION ON THE BODY CHANNEL

Cathy was sexually and physically abused by her mother and stepfather. As an adult, she experienced overwhelming feelings of sadness and anger, often flying into violent rages, which took a toll on her physically as well as on her relationships. She recalled that her mother and other family members regularly invalidated her feelings and denied that the abuse even occurred. On one occasion, Cathy came home crying after being teased at school. Rather than comforting her, Cathy's stepfather slapped her, saying, "No daughter of mine will be a sissy! Next time, you better fight back! Be a grown woman!" Cathy claimed that she never cried in front of anyone in her family again.

THERAPIST: In the last session, we talked about starting to identify your feelings—learning to know what you're feeling when you're feeling it. In this session, we're focusing on emotion regulation—that is, how you cope with your feelings, especially negative or difficult ones. So let's start with a general question: When you feel bad, what do you do to make yourself feel better?

CATHY: I don't know. I feel bad most of the time. Nothing I do really seems to work; that's why I am here. I feel hopeless.

THERAPIST: I can understand why you'd feel that way, given everything you've tried and what you had to go through as a child. Part of what we'll be doing is helping you learn new, more helpful ways of coping with difficult feelings. But before we do that, we need to understand what you do now when you feel bad, whether or not it really helps. Let's start with what you brought up earlier today—the negative evaluation you received at work. On the Feelings Monitoring Form, you said that after you met with your boss, you felt really depressed and hopeless.

CATHY: Yeah, that's how I feel most of the time. But I felt even worse after I got that bad review.

THERAPIST: What was your boss critical about?

CATHY: She said she and other coworkers noticed I had been late for work a lot. She said my work had lots of errors in it, was often overdue, and wasn't the quality they were used to from me.

THERAPIST: Let's start by labeling what you were feeling when your boss said this. Do you remember last week when we talked about the three channels of emotion—body, thought, and behavior? Since we've focused on the body channel first, let's start there. What did you feel in your body while your boss was speaking?

CATHY: I felt anxious as soon as she started, because I knew the review wasn't going to be good. My heart was racing, and I had butterflies in my stomach. It made me sick.

THERAPIST: That sounds really awful to have to feel during a meeting with your boss. What did you end up doing in the meeting?

CATHY: I just sat there and didn't say anything. She even asked if anything was going on with me personally that would explain everything. She actually looked concerned, so I just looked at the floor the whole time so I didn't have to look her in the eyes. I just shook my head no and said, "Everything's fine," and left. I'm afraid now it came across like I didn't care.

THERAPIST: What did you do after you left the meeting?

CATHY: I went back to my office, slammed the door, and punched the wall. It really hurt my hand, and one of my coworkers heard and came by to see what was going on. Then I just told him everything was fine and stormed out. I haven't been to work since then, and that was 2 days ago.

THERAPIST: So it sounds like you were angry, then embarrassed.

CATHY: Yeah, I guess I was.

THERAPIST: And you tried to cope with being upset and express it somehow. You slammed the door, you punched the wall, you stormed out after your coworker checked on you, and you've avoided going to work since.

CATHY: Yeah, it sounds pretty bad when you put it like that.

THERAPIST: I'm just struck with how intense those feelings must have been. I'm sorry you experienced that. Did any of these things you did make you feel better?

CATHY: At the time, I felt so. But maybe I was just overreacting. Now I'm worried that I will get fired because of it. I can't lose this job! And I feel guilty, because I actually like and respect my boss a lot, and she was right about what she said. I haven't been doing my best lately at work

THERAPIST: Well, it's understandable from how you grew up why you responded the way you did. Remember when we talked about the time you were teased at school—the last time you cried in front of your family? What were you told to do?

CATHY: Fight back.

THERAPIST: So, actually, we can be thankful that you had enough self-control not to fight your boss in the meeting. If you had followed your stepfather's example, you would have punched her!

CATHY: I never thought about it that way.

THERAPIST: Right. How about we replay the situation and see if there might be a better way to cope with your feelings? Maybe by using one of the body channel skills we talked about today? Since you started feeling anxious before the meeting, would that have been a time to practice a skill?

CATHY: Yeah, probably because I knew it was only going to get harder.

THERAPIST: I think you're right. What do you think could have helped you calm your body down?

CATHY: I really liked what we were talking about today with Soothing the Senses. I have a keychain from a vacation I took with my wife last year to the beach. I could have brought it out and rubbed it while remembering what it felt like—feeling the waves of the ocean. It makes me feel better now just thinking of it.

THERAPIST: That's a perfect example, and what a great memory to use, too. Maybe if you are able to calm yourself down, using that keychain as a reminder, you can face the stress of going back to work. I'm glad you have that keychain to help in future situations.

SUMMARIZE THE GOALS OF THE SESSION

To segue to the end of the session, briefly remind the client of the overall goals of the session and how the specific skills discussed fit into the bigger framework of STAIR. Not all clients will take to all the coping skills discussed in this chapter, especially given some of the challenges we have mentioned about the body channel of emotions. The therapist can encourage a reluctant client to give things a try, but convey that they can focus on skills they find most helpful first. For the body channel, clients may need extra support in knowing how to feel grounded in their bodies and allowing themselves to experience pleasure and relaxation in physical ways. A therapist may omit certain skills and encourage others, based on their understanding of each client. For example, a very avoidant client may have trouble with Progressive Muscle Relaxation, but can tolerate Soothing the Senses. We have described these healthy skills in the form of handouts for the client, and the therapist can encourage the client to continue reviewing these handouts on their own.

PLAN SKILLS PRACTICE

At the end of the session, the therapist can briefly summarize the body channel skills discussed in the session before talking with the client about ways to practice these new skills before the next session. For skills practice during the week, the therapist requests that the client continue to fill out the Feelings Monitoring Form once a day, and this time include any body channel skills the client may have used to help cope. Outside of these specific situations, the client can choose one or more of the new body channel skills to practice daily. If the client has trouble choosing a skill, the therapist can use their own judgment about which skill may be easiest and/or most effective for the client to practice. Finally, the client also continues to practice Focused Breathing twice a day.

Healthy and Unhealthy Ways to Cope on the Body Channel

Check any of the following if they seem familiar to your own experience. All of them are common among survivors of trauma.

UNHEALTHY EFFORTS TO COPE

☐ Poor sleep habits

☐ Poor diet (examples: fast food only, overeating, undereating)

☐ Use of harmful substances

☐ No or limited exercise

☐ Pushing your body too much or too much exercise

☐ Ignoring your body (examples: not treating illness, not visiting the doctor or dentist, ignoring physical discomfort like being too hot or too cold)

☐ Self-harm to cope with negative feelings or to help with numbness (examples: pinching yourself, cutting, burning, etc.)

☐ Poor hygiene (examples: not showering, not shaving, not combing your hair)

Others?

☐ _____

☐ _____

☐ _____

Check any of the following that you'd like to practice for coping better with your feelings.

HEALTHY EFFORTS TO COPE: BODY CHANNEL SKILLS

☐ Focused Breathing

☐ Basic Self-Care

☐ Soothing the Senses

☐ Progressive Muscle Relaxation

☐ Other mindfulness-based body exercises (sitting meditation, walking meditation, etc.)

Others?

☐ _____

☐ _____

☐ _____

Body Channel Coping Skills

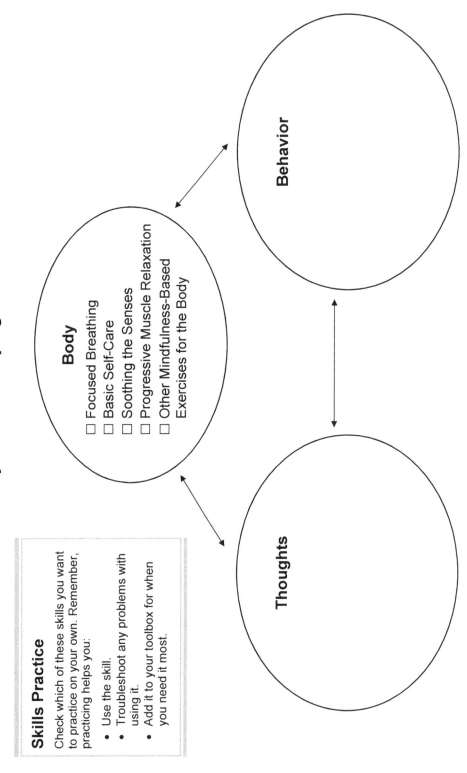

Body

☐ Focused Breathing
☐ Basic Self-Care
☐ Soothing the Senses
☐ Progressive Muscle Relaxation
☐ Other Mindfulness-Based Exercises for the Body

Behavior

Thoughts

Skills Practice

Check which of these skills you want to practice on your own. Remember, practicing helps you:

- Use the skill.
- Troubleshoot any problems with using it.
- Add it to your toolbox for when you need it most.

Basics of Self-Care (A Body Channel Skill)

IMPROVING YOUR EMOTIONAL HEALTH

Your emotional health is like your physical health: It needs nurturing. When it does not get care, you begin to show more strain, and it has an impact on what triggers you, how you respond (thoughts/feelings), and how you behave as a result.

WHAT WOULD IT TAKE TO REFUEL YOUR EMOTIONAL TANK?

- Meet your basic needs.
  - *Stress and lack of attention to your body* (hunger, thirst, rest, illness, discomfort/pain, hygiene, and exercise) can influence your mood.
  - *Routinely refuel your body.* Treat your body well with a good diet, adequate sleep, regular exercise, and other healthy behaviors.
- **Exercise.** Take a walk, run, or stretch.
- **Improve your physical environment to make yourself feel comfortable.** When possible, notice your response to temperature, clothing, colors/textures, sounds/noise, and clutter. Small changes in your surroundings can increase serenity and positive emotions.
- **Create a Basic Self-Care health plan.** Make *one* commitment to do something to improve your physical health, starting today. Schedule and track your activities related to this commitment. You can use the Feelings Monitoring Form to track how specific Basic Self-Care practices you try out affect your mood, thoughts, and behavior.

  ☐ Sleep _____

  ☐ Eating _____

  ☐ Exercise _____

  ☐ Your environment _____

Soothing the Senses (A Body Channel Skill)

In addition to basic refueling and other aspects of self-care, you can learn skills for reducing stress. You have already learned the Focused Breathing exercise, which you should keep on using. The Soothing the Senses skill is about exploring ways that your bodily senses can help calm you. You can pick any or all of the sense experiences below to explore, but pick at least two. For your chosen senses, write down specific soothing examples that come to mind. It helps to choose ones that you can either imagine vividly or actually experience when you want to relax.

GET IN TOUCH WITH THE ENVIRONMENT, USING ALL FIVE SENSES

Sight

- What can you carry with you to **look** at that is soothing? _____

_____

Sound

- What can you **listen** to that is soothing, or which person can you call? _____

_____

Smell

- What can you **smell** that is soothing? _____

_____

Taste

- What can you **taste** that is soothing? _____

_____

Touch

- What can you **touch** that is soothing? _____

_____

Try to target more than one sense at a time, to help you relax more quickly and effectively.

Progressive Muscle Relaxation (A Body Channel Skill)

Brief description: You'll be alternately tensing and relaxing specific groups of muscles. After tension, a muscle will be more relaxed than it was before the tensing. Concentrate on the feel of the muscles—specifically, the contrast between tension and relaxation. In time, you will recognize tension in any specific muscle and will be able to reduce that tension. This exercise may be especially helpful for people with chronic pain and/or dissociation.

How often do you practice it? Do the entire sequence once a day if you can, until you feel you are able to control your muscle tensions.

Before the exercise: Sit in a comfortable chair or lie down on a bed. Get as comfortable as possible—no tight clothes, no shoes. Also, don't cross your legs.

Be careful: If you have problems with pulled muscles, broken bones, or any medical contraindication for physical activities, consult your doctor first. Don't do things that hurt. If you have pain in a specific area, skip that area.

Directions: Take a deep breath; let it out slowly. Again. Don't tense muscles other than the specific group at each step. Don't hold your breath, grit your teeth, or squint! Breathe slowly and evenly and think only about the tension–relaxation contrast.

- Each tensing is for 10 seconds; each relaxing is for 10 or 15 seconds. Count "one-one-thousand, two-one-thousand . . ." until you have a feel for the time span.
- Note that each step is really two steps: one cycle of tension–relaxation for each set of opposing muscles.
    1. Hands.
    2. Biceps and triceps.
    3. Shoulders.
    4. Neck.
    5. Mouth.
    6. Tongue.
    7. Eyes.
    8. Back.
    9. Butt.
    10. Thighs.
    11. Stomach.
    12. Calves and feet.
    13. Toes.

CHAPTER 13

Emotion Regulation
Focus on Thoughts and Behavior

> Human freedom involves our capacity to pause between the stimulus and
> response and, in that pause, to choose the one response toward which we
> wish to throw our weight. The capacity to create ourselves, based upon
> this freedom, is inseparable from consciousness or self-awareness.
> —ROLLO MAY (1975, p. 100)

The focus of this session is expanding on the thought and behavior channels of emotion—first by identifying trauma-driven thoughts and behaviors, and then by exploring alternative ways of coping along these channels. Survivors of trauma often have thought and behavior patterns that are fear-driven and consequently narrow, rigid, and limiting. A primary goal of this session is to help clients learn more flexible ways of thinking. This includes, for example, weighing the evidence for a belief and considering alternatives; learning to approach (vs. automatically avoid) frightening beliefs, as well as to move away from unproductive, ruminative thoughts; and finally learning how to generate and attend to positive thoughts and images. Unlike traditional cognitive restructuring, the work in this early phase of treatment is not primarily about challenging old beliefs and providing alternatives, although indeed some exploration of this type will occur. The focus here, instead, is on helping clients create alternative ways of thinking and experience a sense of agency about what and how they choose to think about things.

In a similar vein, the other primary goal of this session is to introduce flexible behavioral choices in response to emotional triggers. Environments of repeated trauma are typically highly controlling and give individuals very little choice about what happens. For example, a child in an abusive home is told to obey a parent or stop complaining (or even stop feeling sad), "or else." The "or else" punishment can be severe, such as being denied dinner or being shut in a closet, but even the vague threat itself creates an environment of hostility. Threatening environments by definition use fear to shape and direct a person's behaviors and thoughts. In regard to behavior, a person might have found that it was necessary to walk a "straight and narrow" path to survive their environment.

The purpose of this session, thus, is to introduce a client to new ways of thinking and behaving, in order to awaken in them a sense of freedom of choice. The work invites the client to think and do things differently than they might have learned to in their traumatic environment. As a result, they can begin thinking about themselves, others, and the world differently and in ways aligned with their personal values and goals.

CHECK-IN AND REVIEW OF SKILLS PRACTICE

As in previous sessions, the therapist begins with a brief check-in on the client's current emotional state and completion of between-session skills practice. The therapist begins reviewing the client's Feelings Monitoring Form entries, and asks specifically about the client's practice of Focused Breathing and one or more of the body channel skills learned in the previous session. The therapist provides genuine positive feedback for completing skills practice, filling out forms, and sharing any successes the client has had since the last session. The client's self-monitoring may provide useful examples of emotion regulation difficulties that the therapist can highlight throughout this phase of treatment and explore, using different, healthier alternative skills from the previous session and this current one.

If the client did not do one or more agreed-upon practice activities, the therapist reviews the rationale for between-session work and helps the client problem-solve any practical barriers. The therapist broadly reinforces the importance of daily practice of skills by stating, "The more you practice a skill, the better at it you will become." If the client has not completed a Feelings Monitoring Form entry, the therapist can say something like this:

> "Today we will be learning new skills. After we review them, we can take a few minutes to complete a Feelings Monitoring Form entry about a difficult situation and consider ways to apply some of the skills that we are reviewing today. Over time, it'll get easier, almost automatic, to choose skills that will help in a particular situation."

IDENTIFY FOCUS OF THE SESSION

In the previous session, the therapist has introduced the client to various body channel skills, aimed at reducing physical experiences of emotional distress and discomfort. By this session, the client's skills practice has ideally started moving the client away from the often-confining physical experience of intense emotion (e.g., fear or shame) and toward an opening "window of opportunity" where they can deploy resources for engaging in new ways of thinking and behaving. The practical goal of this session is to help the client select, learn, and practice new skills in the thought and behavior channels of emotion that better match their personal and interpersonal aspirations. The therapist and client select tools according to the client's preferences and abilities. Before and throughout the session, the therapist thinks ahead about which tools might resonate most with the client's strengths and therapeutic goals. Box 13.1 outlines the theme and curriculum for Session 4.

Theme and Curriculum for Session 4
Emotion Regulation: Focus on Thoughts and Behaviors

The focus of this session is on introducing and exploring trauma-driven maladaptive thoughts and behaviors, and exploring alternative ways of thinking and behaving. This session completes the introduction and review of the three channels of emotion. The body channel interventions from the previous session ideally help the client move away from a sense of chronic crisis or threat, which in turn opens a window of opportunity for the client to become curious and open about what changes might be of value to them. The goal of the session is to engage and motivate the client to select, test, and practice alternative thoughts and behaviors that match the client's personal and interpersonal aspirations. The tools selected should be based on the client's preferences and strengths. The ultimate goal of the session is to integrate all three channels and demonstrate how they all work together.

PLANNING AND PREPARATION

Bring extra copies of the Feelings Monitoring Form (Handout 11.3) and copies of the Session 4 handouts listed below. Review the skills for the thought and behavior channels, and consider which might be a good match for the client. The work in the session is estimated to take about 60 minutes; a flexible application is assumed (i.e., not every client will need all interventions).

AGENDA

- Check-in and review of skills practice.
- Identify focus of the session.
- Review trauma-related patterns of thinking.
- Review and select thought channel skills.
- Review trauma-related patterns of behaviors.
- Review and select behavior channel skills.
- Explore positive emotions and plan pleasurable activities.
- Complete Summary of Three Channels of Emotion Skills checklist.
- Apply new skills to Feelings Monitoring Form.
- Summarize the goals of the session.

(continued)

- Plan skills practice:
  - Complete Feelings Monitoring Form once a day (note positive and negative emotions). Specify coping skills in any channel that were used to deal with difficult feelings or situations described in entries.
  - Practice at least one skill identified in each of the thought and behavior channels (continue practicing body channel skills as helpful to client).
  - Continue to practice Focused Breathing twice daily
  - Do something pleasurable.

SESSION HANDOUTS

Handout 13.1. Typical Trauma-Related Thought Patterns

Handout 13.2. Thought Channel Skills for Emotion Regulation

Handout 13.3. Emotion Surfing

Handout 13.4. Examples of Positive Self-Statements (Affirmations)

Handout 13.5. Typical Trauma-Related Behaviors

Handout 13.6. Behavior Channel Skills for Emotion Regulation

Handout 13.7. Time Out (A Behavior Channel Skill)

Handout 13.8. Opposite Action (A Behavior Channel Skill)

Handout 13.9. Pleasurable Activities List

Handout 13.10. Summary of Three Channels of Emotion Skills

Additional copies of Handout 11.3. Feelings Monitoring Form

REVIEW TRAUMA-RELATED PATTERNS OF THINKING

The therapist reviews the examples in Handout 13.1, Typical Trauma-Related Thinking Patterns, and uses the client's Feelings Monitoring Form as a way to ground the discussion. This process will facilitate understanding of the client's typical negative thought patterns, such as "black-and-white" thinking or generating "doomsday" scenarios.

REVIEW AND SELECT THOUGHT CHANNEL SKILLS

The client may already have obvious strengths in using the thought channel to regulate their emotions. If so, the therapist notes them and identifies ways in which the client can generalize already existing skills. For example, on the job, a client may recognize how they or others can slip into black-and-white thinking; see that it limits successful communication and problem solving; and then easily shift to an approach that involves evaluating alternatives and asking, "What other way of thinking about this situation might be helpful?" This more flexible approach to problem solving might be harder for the client to apply in more affectively charged situations, such as conflicts at home with loved ones. The therapist makes it clear that the same skills can be applied to different situations and different people, and that practicing across all of these contexts helps build the greatest flexibility in using skills. Later sessions will expand upon this theme of flexibility and context. To aid the discussion in session, the therapist uses Handout 13.2, Thought Channel Tools for Emotion Regulation.

Emotion Surfing

Emotion Surfing is a technique that uses a metaphor of how the experience of an emotion can feel like waves in the ocean. The waves crest, slowly fall, and then may rise again—but by noticing the flow of the experience, the client can realize that no feeling, no matter how distressing and intense, can last forever. Moreover, one wave of emotion may flow into another wave of a different emotion. Clients can visualize riding the waves of their emotions as they "wait for the surge to pass," so to speak. Handout 13.3, Emotion Surfing, provides a step-by-step guide for clients to use after the session.

Evidence Technique

Another skill to explore is the Evidence Technique. The therapist invites the client to consider their belief with an attitude of curiosity and interest (as opposed to one of judgment). The approach to the evidence technique is not confrontational, as it can be in some cognitive-behavioral approaches. The key steps in the process of conducting this inquiry are as follows:

1. Validate initial viewpoint. (Therapist acknowledges that trauma-generated beliefs served a purpose at some point.)
2. Ask, "What other ways of thinking about it are there?" (Therapist invites client to consider alternative beliefs, now that the trauma is over.)
3. Ask, "How strong is the proof for your original viewpoint?", followed by "What about the alternative ways of thinking?" (Therapist listens and balances the original thought with alternatives.)
4. Invite client to consider a more helpful alternative and "try it on for size."
5. Invite client to "let the old belief go" and recognize that it may no longer be helpful.

Material from the client's completed Feelings Monitoring Forms can help highlight areas of negative self-talk that could be countered with more helpful statements. For example, many clients report fearful cognitions about experiencing and expressing feelings. A client may report thoughts such as these:

"If I let myself get angry, I'll lose control and become abusive."
"If I show my true feelings, my partner will think I'm weak and won't love me."
"It doesn't matter what I feel. No one cares."

The therapist can gently ask whether these statements are true and whether there could be alternatives to consider and test in the world. The therapist may need to be very active in proposing alternatives. Here are some examples of alternative statements:

"It's OK to feel angry. It's what I do with my anger that's important."
"I can manage my anger in a positive, effective way."
"Expressing my feelings is courageous."
"By expressing my feelings, I let my partner be more supportive of me."

Therapists can focus on other skills for clients who respond to less elaborate approaches (as compared to the Evidence Technique). Examining evidence can be powerful for clients who are willing to try and open to trying the approach; however, some clients may have either a degree of rigidity that prevents deeply questioning core beliefs, or proclivities to obsessional thinking (which may not respond as readily to the Evidence Technique). In these cases, other skills described below may be more effective.

Thought Shifting

An alternative and complementary thought channel strategy we introduce to clients is Thought (or Attention Shifting). That is, when clients recognize they are having a trauma-related thought or dwelling on a problem, they acknowledge it and then make the decision to shift their attention to something else. Thought Shifting can be particularly valuable as a way to get out of repeating "thought loops" or rumination. These types of thoughts often do not lead to solutions to problems, and may indeed lead to worsening or reinforcing of a negative mood. For many clients, Thought Shifting works best if it involves a change in activity as well. For example, a client has an intrusive thought while in their office writing a report for work. Through therapy, they have learned to acknowledge the thought, but instead of internally arguing with it or diving deep into the thought (and its subsequent chain of related thoughts), they know they have another option. They choose to get up and take a moment to water the nearby office plants. They are not avoiding the thought, because they consciously acknowledge its presence—but they choose to shift attention away from that thought, in a mindful, nonjudgmental way, so that they can act in a more useful way in the moment. Examples of activities that can be used with Thought Shifting include cleaning the house, calling a friend, planning a vacation, recalling pleasant past events, and counting backward from 100 by sevens. Over time and with experimentation, clients will figure out what types of activities or thoughts are most likely to facilitate a helpful shift for them.

Reminders/Reframes

An additional thought channel skill is to counter negative cognitions with predetermined alternatives—Reminders or Reframes—when confronted with a distressing situation that typically provokes an automatic negative thought. Whereas the Evidence Technique can help generate an elaborated, alternative assessment of a distressing situation, this skill is quicker and focuses on the client's reminding themselves of an alternative, positive assessment when confronting a situation similar to one already analyzed. For example, a client who is having a difficult moment and is very self-critical may remind themselves of a counterstatement, such as "I am doing the best I can." In another example, when a client is feeling angry and becomes self-critical, they can remind themselves: "It is OK to feel angry; it is what I do with it that matters."

Positive Self-Statements

For any people who have experienced childhood maltreatment, the maltreatment has included emotional abuse/neglect. This means that a client may never have received acknowledgment of their positive attributes. The presence of positive beliefs about the self is distinct and separate from the resolution of negative beliefs. For example, a client may be able to accept that they have not failed at a particular task, but this acceptance does not automatically fill a void about what is good about them, such as "I am friendly and compassionate toward others." In this exercise, the therapist helps the client identify positive attributes, and in doing so can help shape and reinforce positive perceptions that the client may not be able to see for themselves. The Positive Self-Statements skill provides the client with the experience of positive regard—first from the therapist, and then from the self. The statements that the client can agree with can be committed to memory, as well as written down and posted somewhere the client can easily find them. Obviously, the therapist must help select positive attributes that the client can authentically endorse. Sometimes the client can identify the attributes, and the therapist need only endorse and possibly elaborate on the client's observations. Handout 13.4, Examples of Positive Self-Statements (Affirmations), provides a list the therapist and client can review and add to—either in session or as part of the client's skills practice between sessions.

Positive Imagery

A final important skill along the thought channel is the use of Positive Imagery. Such work has proven useful in effecting positive emotional states. This method requires the evocation of specific memories or images that induce positive (nonhurtful or, preferably, pleasure-producing) thoughts or feelings. These images should be fully elaborated, so that each detail can serve as a retrieval cue, thereby increasing the ease with which clients can recall these images. It is often helpful to cue the client with a question such as "Can you think of a time when you felt content?" or "Picture a situation in which you felt relaxed," and ask the client to try to describe it in as much detail as possible, remembering how it felt as vividly as possible. During times of distress, clients can summon their identified images in order to combat the negative effects of invading thoughts or circumstances, and to induce more positive emotional states.

Using the Feelings Monitoring Form with Thought Channel Skills

All of these techniques can help clients stop negative thoughts from spiraling into fully distressing reminders of their trauma. To prevent this spiraling, clients first must learn to identify the thoughts that accompany their feelings. Doing so involves using the Feelings Monitoring Form. Once clients accomplish this goal, they may then proceed to practice the array of skills described above for addressing these thoughts.

REVIEW TRAUMA-RELATED PATTERNS OF BEHAVIORS

Together, the therapist and client review the examples in Handout 13.5, Typical Trauma-Related Behaviors, and the client adds to the list any behaviors specific to their experience. The goal here is for clients to recognize that survivors of trauma use a range of behaviors as attempts to manage emotions (i.e., efforts at emotion regulation). Some of these behaviors work better than others in the short run, but in the long run all have significant downsides. The therapist can use a recently completed Feelings Monitoring Form or example already discussed by the client to identify which behaviors are most typical of them as emotion regulation strategies. Note that in this treatment, we assume that almost all behaviors have or have had some benefit for emotion regulation (and/or even survival) in the past.

REVIEW AND SELECT BEHAVIOR CHANNEL SKILLS

Behavioral emotion modulation skills are often the easiest for clients to identify, because they include anything people do in everyday life to make themselves feel better. Such strategies may include calling a friend, watching a movie, preparing for a meeting, going for a run, taking a bath, or making a favorite food. To focus the discussion on healthy coping skills, the therapist can use Handout 13.6, Behavior Channel Tools for Emotion Regulation.

Time Out/Take a Break

Time Out/Take a Break means leaving, for a set period of time, the environment that is creating the emotional disturbance. This purposeful break is not to be used as an avoidance strategy, but as a modulation strategy. The distinction lies in the client's intention to return to the setting or goal once their feelings have returned to baseline or have settled to a level that allows them to reengage effectively. In some cases, Time Out lasts for only a few minutes; in other cases, it may last for days or weeks. The therapist reviews the recovery timeline for several emotions and notes how the range in time to recovery depends on the emotion and its context, with the goal of normalizing this variation. High-distress reactions can occur rapidly and unexpectedly. The client's work in emotion awareness can help them identify the type and intensity of feelings, as well as situations, that are likely to lead to a negative interaction or outcome.

The client can combine thought channel and behavior channel tools to prepare particular self-statements, mantras, or behaviors to use on an as-needed basis. Clients may rely on phrases such as "I can't productively continue this conversation right now, but why don't we plan to resume later?" when they feel their distress rising too high. If a reaction is very intense (say, a strong anger reaction), and the words that will spill out will be negative or hurtful, the client can do a short Time Out from the conversation (by counting to 10) or a longer one (by simply keeping quiet and listening). For example, asking for a break to go to the restroom is often an easy, hard-to-argue-with strategy that anyone can use. If a client is beyond words and moving into aggressive action, the client needs to be ready simply to leave the room or location, even without saying a word. The potential embarrassment of such abrupt behavior is far less than that which follows letting loose with a verbal tirade or getting into a fight. Handout 13.7, Time Out (A Behavior Channel Tool), provides an overview to use with clients.

Replacement Behaviors and Opposite Action

Clients often find themselves engaging in old, ingrained emotion modulation strategies automatically and in a fixed, repeated pattern. Such patterns are hard to break, and the drive to move into such an action is nearly unstoppable. These actions include reaching for a drink or a pill, cutting, binge eating, or engaging in impulsive and/or unsafe sex. These strategies are often successful in their initial aim, which is rapid emotional relief. Their often immediate, short-term success greatly reinforces the pattern. Still, a client often pays a high price in the later consequences of such strategies. One method of breaking such a behavioral habit is to replace it with another action pattern that can be speedily introduced and has the same end result (reduced arousal), but does not cause the collateral damage. Rather than engaging in compulsive behaviors, the client can engage in other activities that have their own fixed action patterns. These Replacement Behaviors may include cleaning the house, running a jogging circuit several times, returning items that have been on loan, mowing the lawn, washing the car, jumping rope, taking a bath, or going to the gym.

A variation on Replacement Behaviors is the skill of Opposite Action, in which a person chooses not to give in to an immediate impulse, but instead chooses to do the opposite (if it indeed is a safer, healthier alternative). Examples by type of emotion are provided in Handout 13.8, Opposite Action (A Behavior Channel Tool).

Ask for Help/Seek Support

Social support is a strong predictor of recovery from life's stressors, including traumatic events. In this session, the therapist introduces the importance of reaching out to supportive, caring others when needed. Although access to social support is straightforward for some clients, it can be complicated for others who have years of isolation, experiences of emotional numbness, and/or strong distrust in the motives of others. Still, most people have at least one or two people they can call on during periods of distress. These people can range from mental health professionals to close friends, family members, and romantic partners. In the most extreme situations of distress or lack of access to others, clients should know that crisis hotlines exist for 24/7 support. In noncrisis situations, clients can learn to reach out to others and talk on the phone, go for coffee, or ask to watch a movie. The options for Ask for Help/Seek Support are endless, and the therapist encourages the client to come up with ones that highlight specific people in their lives and that resonate with their interests.

Using the Feelings Monitoring Form with Behavior Channel Skills

All of these skills in the behavior channel aim to intervene directly with observable effects of emotional distress. For this reason, they target a key treatment goal—the improvement of functioning. As with other channels of emotion, the Feelings Monitoring Form can help clarify behavioral patterns and show how they are connected to environmental triggers, physiological experiences, and patterns of thinking. Intervening at the level of behavior is ultimately pragmatic, as long as the client can commit to these fundamental changes. The therapist elaborates on the power of behavioral change in the next part of this session by expanding on the final behavior channel skill—Plan Pleasurable Activities.

EXPLORE POSITIVE EMOTIONS AND PLAN PLEASURABLE ACTIVITIES

Making time for enjoyable activities is an essential part of life and thus an essential behavior channel skill. It is so powerful that we recommend spending extra time with clients reviewing ways to incorporate pleasurable activities as part of their skill practice and treatment plan. This section explores ways to expand upon this topic.

Review Rationale for Experiencing Positive Emotions

As briefly mentioned previously, this session also introduces the goal of experiencing positive emotions through actively seeking out pleasurable activities. Emotional numbing is the flip side of hyperarousal, reflecting the "all-or-nothing" emotional responsivity of some survivors of trauma. Some individuals describe being numb or "emotionally dead" most of the time, with occasional extreme reactions to mild stressors. The final task of this session is to highlight that emotion regulation means not only working toward reducing distress, but increasing opportunities to experience positive emotions. The therapist reviews reasons to engage in pleasurable activities, with the awareness that it may feel uncomfortable or even scary for the client at first.

Positive emotions are rewards for distress reduction efforts

The therapist conveys to the client that emotional numbing may protect them from disabling arousal, but it also decreases or eliminates their opportunities for taking pleasure in ordinary events. People who have experienced chronic trauma often have only a limited capacity to respond to their environment, including the positive aspects of day-to-day life. Increasing skills at distress reduction will make time and energy available to the client to open up and engage in positive events, but this change too will take practice. Practicing skills for feeling positive emotions may provide the client with "rewards" for focusing on more taxing efforts in distress reduction activities.

Positive emotions are a form of distress management

Developing skills in experiencing positive emotions is itself a form of distress reduction. Positive feelings can extinguish, cancel, inhibit, or attenuate negative feelings. Amusement can extinguish anxiety. A joke can soften anger. Feelings of tenderness for someone can modulate disappointment.

Positive emotions direct action

Just as distressing feelings of fear or anxiety do, positive emotions predispose a person to action. Positive feelings also support the development of discipline and perseverance, which are required for the completion of long-term goals. Enthusiasm for a particular goal or accomplishment keeps a person working on a variety of tasks, which may not be of great interest in themselves but are necessary to reach the desired goal.

Positive emotions enhance motivation and a sense of future possibilities

As the preceding point indicates, positive emotions can be motivation enhancers. Indeed, they can ultimately give people the mental and physical energy to tap into their creativity and to begin experiencing the possibility of developing and pursuing long-term life goals. This latter possibility may be overwhelming and intimidating to a person with chronic PTSD who is just trying to get through the day at hand; the therapist considers whether to introduce this idea in a later session once such a client has experienced some initial relief.

Positive emotions produce greater self-awareness and connection to others

Positive emotions inform us about our preferences and give us confidence in our decision making. Feelings of warmth toward certain other people inform us that we might want to spend more time with them. Feelings of enthusiasm for certain activities or places confirm for us what we would like to do or where we would like to go. Positive feelings provide us with a surer sense of who we are and greater certainty about personal decisions. Similarly, access to positive feelings increases our attunement to others' needs and wants, and enhances our capacity to empathize with others more fully. The ability to read others' "social signals" helps us to negotiate the first steps in relationships and to maintain them successfully.

Identify and Plan Pleasurable Activities

A general strategy for modulating mood through enhancing positive emotions is to Plan Pleasurable Activities. The therapist can begin this process by simply asking clients what they enjoy doing or what things they do to make them feel happy. Although many clients can answer this question, doing so may not be as simple as it sounds for other clients. Some individuals may respond, "I don't know," or "I don't really enjoy anything." They may really need to take time in or out of session to reflect more, and can be encouraged to look at this reflection as an experiment. Is there something new they have always wanted to try? If it ends up not being pleasurable, then they can try something else. If such a client cannot imagine enjoying anything, the therapist can ask them if they can think back to a time in their life when they did get pleasure out of activities and start from there. The therapist may provide suggestions or resource guides as a way to get the client thinking about specific activities (see Handout 13.9, Pleasurable Activities List).

Review Misconceptions about Positive Emotions and Pleasurable Activities (as Relevant)

Positive emotions require time and money

In response to being asked to engage in pleasurable activities, some clients respond, "I don't have enough time." For clients who view engaging in pleasurable activities as a luxury, the therapist will need to reframe it as an essential part of recovery from trauma and discuss in more detail how the clients can carve out some time. Other clients may say, "I don't have enough money to do anything nice for myself." For that reason, it is important that at least some of the activities scheduled should not cost money. The therapist works with each client to create a list of at least three pleasurable activities they can incorporate into their life. The client can expand on this list of ideas over the course of treatment and keep it handy. The therapist explains that since the client is doing hard work by facing distressing aspects of their life, they should also take the opportunity to reward themselves by building in positive activities. At first this may feel forced, but if they make the effort in the beginning, it will become easier and more natural. This intervention provides a way for clients to expand their range of feelings, with the idea that by allowing for and tolerating negative feelings, the clients will also become more open to positive feelings that have been cut off as a result of avoidance.

Positive emotions are inconsistent with self-image

It is important to keep in mind that a client may not feel they deserve to enjoy or nurture themselves. If so, the therapist explores this issue with the client and discusses how feeling like a "bad person" or having low self-worth is a common reaction to interpersonal trauma, particularly childhood abuse and/or neglect. Not engaging in pleasurable activities further confirms the client's negative self-image and perpetuates the damaging idea that they are not entitled to positive experiences.

Doing things to create positive emotions feels "fake"

Finally, a client attempting to pursue pleasant activities may report, "It feels fake." If so, the therapist can suggest continuing to do so as an experiment during the treatment. The therapist explains that low self-esteem and poor self-image are common reactions to interpersonal trauma. Some clients find the analogy of friendship helpful. The therapist can ask such a client, "If a friend of yours is going through a hard time, and you want to encourage this friend and make them feel better, what would you do?" The client might answer that they would spend time with the friend doing things they both like to do, maybe buy the friend a small gift, or do something similar. The therapist can suggest that the client think of engaging in pleasurable activities for themselves similarly. The client is learning to encourage and support themselves while they are doing something difficult. Often over time, the client will find that engaging in pleasurable activities begins to feel more natural.

COMPLETE SUMMARY OF THREE CHANNELS OF EMOTION SKILLS

One of the last tasks of the session is to summarize the tools that the client has selected in Handout 13.10, Summary of Three Channels of Emotion Skills, a set of three checklists identifying skills the client can plan on using in the future. While the client is completing this handout, the therapist can highlight several aspects of breaking down problems into the three channels, as well as the benefits of introducing solutions along the three channels.

It is important to make clear to a client that the skills they plan to use are *not* designed to cover over or avoid feelings, but to improve the client's ability to manage emotions in a more positive and effective way. In addition, the therapist can remind the client that they can use different skills in different situations—whichever they think will work. Obviously, most skills will influence more than one channel. Moreover, as one skill is strengthened, others may become easier to develop. Both flexibility and practice in application are key ingredients to improved coping.

The client should be made aware that they can slow down the movement from one mode or channel of experiencing to another, particularly the transition from arousal (body) to action (behavior). This experience is one with which individuals who have had trauma or live in a chronic crisis state tend to be unfamiliar. Lastly, the therapist and client revisit their discussion of positive emotions. For some survivors, strong emotions of any kind can be frightening, even those that are positive. The therapist highlights again (if necessary) the functional value of positive emotion, as well as assurances that emotion regulation skills apply to managing positive as well as negative emotions.

APPLY NEW SKILLS TO FEELINGS MONITORING FORM

The therapist can consolidate the work of the session by using a Feelings Monitoring Form to rework one of the problems already described on a previous copy of this form or reported by the client. This reworking also gives clients who did not complete this form during the week an opportunity to do so. Below is an example of how this might go.

CASE EXAMPLE

Varnella was a survivor of human sex trafficking that occurred when she was between the ages of 15 and 19. She quickly learned to avoid her feelings and numb herself in order to function. In treatment, Varnella was beginning to identify her feelings as well as healthy coping strategies for the first time in her life. She completed several entries on her Feelings Monitoring Form, and together she and the therapist decided to begin with Varnella's difficulties completing an assignment she needed to do for her adult continuing education class.

THERAPIST: I see from your Feelings Monitoring Form that you really struggled to work on the assignment that Professor Brown gave you, and it's due the end of this week.

VARNELLA: Yes, I just felt completely terrified and frozen. Maybe I should just drop this class. I don't really have anything valuable to contribute anyway.

THERAPIST: Well, earlier today we were talking about how when you feel distressed, you often have negative thoughts about yourself. Let's spend some time working through this together, and see if we can call upon skills from all of the three channels to help reduce the intensity of your distress. Then we can see what might be feasible as well as consistent with your goals. You've told me before that obtaining your associate's degree is very important to you. But on the Feelings Monitoring Form for this week, you wrote that your thoughts were "I'm never going to be able to do this. No one will want to read what I write anyway. I am too dumb to do this."

VARNELLA: When I see it all written out like that, I realize I really do have a lot of negative thoughts. It's kind of hard seeing how mean I can be to myself.

THERAPIST: Yes, it can be very difficult to realize that, but one of the important purposes of the Feelings Monitoring Form is that it helps make you aware of negative thinking styles that might be impacting your emotions. So let's start with the thought channel. What are some coping skills from the thought channel that might be helpful here?

VARNELLA: I really liked the Positive Self-Statements. I could say to myself, "I have been through hard things before and I can do this."

THERAPIST: Yes, that sounds great! Encouraging statements like that can really help. Also, I wonder if we might use the Evidence Technique here to examine the thought "I am too dumb to do this."

VARNELLA: It's hard for me to believe it, but I do have some evidence that I can do things. I passed the qualifying exam, and my grades have been pretty good so far this semester.

THERAPIST: Nice! So you're able to acknowledge some compelling evidence to counter the belief that you're not smart enough to do your assignment. That is really excellent! . . . Let's bring in skills from the other channels now. I see that on your Feelings Monitoring Form you listed crying and going to sleep as efforts to cope.

VARNELLA: Yeah, that tends to be what I do—just give up and shut down.

THERAPIST: So let's move over to the behavior channel. What are some tools we discussed today that you could see yourself trying?

VARNELLA: I could try putting on music. I always forget how helpful that is for me. Sometimes I even find myself singing along, and I feel inspired to do things. I can also go for a walk. I guess that's kind of Opposite Action to my urge to go to sleep and just shut down. That might even help me come up with more ideas of what to write about for my assignment. I don't need to give up; other ideas might come to me if I get moving. Wow, sometimes I can really be my own worst enemy!

THERAPIST: You identified some great options from the behavior channel. And remember to give yourself a bit of time to learn these new ways of coping. It can be really empowering to see how healthy coping skills can reduce the intensity of feelings, or even change the feeling entirely. But it takes time and practice. Let's finish with the body channel that we discussed last week. What are some skills from that channel that might be helpful?

VARNELLA: I have been practicing the Focused Breathing. It really helps. If I had just remembered to breathe, maybe I wouldn't have been so frozen and terrified.

THERAPIST: Yes, Focused Breathing can really work nicely with skills from the other channels. It can help your body and mind slow down a bit so that you have space to incorporate other approaches. Anything else from the body channel?

VARNELLA: Lavender. I love to smell it. I have some lavender incense, and I'll keep it on my desk to remind me to use it when I'm doing schoolwork. I think that will really help me to relax and focus.

THERAPIST: This is a terrific example of Soothing the Senses! We've discussed skills from each of the three channels that you can use together to help you manage your feelings. These will enable you to do this class assignment, which I know is very important to you.

VARNELLA: Yes, it's very important. I really want my degree, and, truthfully, I don't want to give up. I just felt desperate. But now I'm actually sort of eager to try putting all these skills together.

SUMMARIZE GOALS OF THE SESSION

As part of the final moments of the session, the therapist briefly reminds the client of the session's overall goal and notes how the specific skills discussed fit into the larger treatment approach. The ultimate goal of this session has been to put all three channels of emotion together and demonstrate how each can support the others in a multidirectional fashion. The therapist can note that some of the tools the client has learned today may help them with the previous session's body channel skills, as all three channels interact and support each other. Also, the therapist may predict that new skills from the past two sessions can further help with approaching challenges. Not all clients will take to all coping strategies, but now that a large array of options are available, the therapist encourages the client to choose what skills they want to practice the most. The therapist encourages a reluctant client to give new skills a try, but convey that they can focus on ones they find easiest first. For example, although a very intellectually driven client may prefer thought channel skills, the therapist may want to suggest behavior channel skills to balance out the client's internally oriented tendencies. In other cases, a therapist and client may choose to ease the path toward mastery by narrowing the focus to the client's innate strengths in one or more channels. Because we have described several healthy skills in each channel of emotion in handouts for the client, the therapist empowers the client to choose for themselves which handouts to review in more detail, alongside their actual practicing of the skills on their own. In most cases, though, the therapist gives the client copies of all handouts so they can review them as needed.

PLAN SKILLS PRACTICE

The therapist and client should decide collaboratively what new skills the client will practice before the next session. The therapist should ask the client to continue to complete the Feelings Monitoring Form once a day, but now include any thought or behavior channel skills they use to help them cope, in addition to any of the body channel skills they choose to continue using. As part of their routine, planned skills practice, the client can choose to practice daily at least one thought channel skill and at least one behavior channel skill. If the client has expressed interest and benefit, then they certainly should be encouraged to continue doing any body channel skills they have found helpful (in addition to the twice-daily Focused Breathing, which should be maintained). If the client has trouble choosing a skill from the thought and/or behavior channels, the therapist can use their own judgment about which skill may be easiest and/or most effective for the client to practice. In addition to this practice of new and previously learned skills, the therapist should remind the client to engage in at least one of the enjoyable activities from the Pleasurable Activities List that they chose earlier in the session.

Typical Trauma-Related Thinking Patterns

☐ Assuming that you are not safe

☐ Assuming that no one is there for you or won't help you

☐ Avoiding thinking about your own negative emotions

☐ Refusing to trust others and/or yourself

☐ Tuning in the negative and tuning out the positive

☐ "Black-and-white" thinking (everything is either one way or the other; there are no in-betweens)

☐ "Doomsday" thinking ("What's the use?")

☐ Being tyrannized by the "shoulds" ("shoulda, woulda, coulda . . .")

☐ Avoiding thoughts and memories

☐ Thinking nonstop about problems; trying to prolong negative feelings

☐ "Blanking out" or dissociating

Thought Channel Skills for Emotion Regulation

- **Emotion Surfing**
  - Imagine your emotions are waves in the ocean, rising and falling; notice how they change naturally over time.
  - Be aware of your feelings, but just "ride on top" of them.

- **Evidence Technique**
  - *What's the proof?* List the evidence for and against the accuracy of a negative thought.
  - *How strong is the proof?* Compare the evidence for and against the accuracy of the thought, to determine how realistic or valid it is.
  - *What else could it be?* Consider alternatives; ask friends or people you trust for ideas.
  - *Try it on for size.* Live with each alternative for a while, and consider the benefits.
  - *Let go.* Be willing to let go of inaccurate or unhelpful automatic thoughts.

- **Thought Shifting**
  - *Temporarily shift your attention,* rather than focusing on your worries, until your distress is down to a level where you can think clearly and act appropriately.
  - *Shift to another thought:* Focus on something else in the room (e.g., colors, lights, smells), or replace your thought with another thought—a positive thought/statement, memory, or image.
  - *Shift to a healthy activity:* To help change your focus, go for a walk, listen to music, watch a video, clean/organize, call a friend, or complete some easy tasks that remain unfinished.

- **Reminders/Reframes**
  - These are predetermined positive interpretations. Especially good are ones about accepting your feelings, such as these:
    "Feelings are just feelings, and thoughts are just thoughts; they are not facts, and they don't have to control my behavior."
    "Feelings are short-term and will not be there forever."
    "Stuffing feelings inside only makes it harder."

- **Positive Self-Statements**
  - These are positive thoughts, mantras, or goals to repeat regularly and commit to practicing.

- **Positive Imagery**
  - *Imagine/visualize a situation or setting* (real or imagined) where you feel calm and good.
  - *Make that image as clear and vivid as possible* by imagining how the place looks, smells, sounds, etc.
  - *Keep it handy.* Keep pictures or symbols to remind you of the image/memory (in your phone or wallet, or on a keychain) to help remind you of the positive setting when you're distressed.

Emotion Surfing

1. Notice your emotion.

2. Notice how it feels in your body.

3. Notice your thoughts.

4. Notice your behavior.

5. Notice the intensity of the emotion.

6. Notice how the emotion crests, like a wave.

7. Notice how the emotion (body, thoughts, behavior) slowly changes and diminishes over time.

Examples of Positive Self-Statements (Affirmations)

- "I choose to LIVE!"

- "Excellence does not require perfection."

- "I am letting my feelings drive my actions and beliefs. I don't have to."

- "If I try, I can succeed."

- "I can ask for help."

- "I am willing to forgive."

- "I don't have to act on this feeling. I can make choices about how I behave."

- "The most common way people give up their power is thinking they don't have any."

- "This too shall pass."

- "One day at a time."

- "I write my own story."

Your own personal mantra:

Typical Trauma-Related Behaviors

Check which of these behaviors are true for you:

☐ Avoiding necessary daily activities to avoid anxiety (example: not opening mail or paying bills because doing so feels like "too much")

☐ Getting stuck in addictive behaviors: alcohol, drugs, food, gambling, pornography, shopping, video games

☐ Purposefully avoiding taking care of yourself: restricting food intake, stopping self-care

☐ Acting aggressively to distance others

☐ Avoiding family and friends

☐ Taking care of other people to avoid your own problems

☐ Avoiding having experiences that are positive or pleasurable

☐ Using controlling behavior to avoid feeling unsafe in situations and in relationships

☐ Treating people badly when you are struggling with negative feelings

☐ Other: _____

Behavior Channel Skills for Emotion Regulation

- **Take a Break/Time Out**
  - Take a Break/Time Out:
    - Remove yourself from the situation.
    - Identify and communicate (if possible) a time you will return.

- **Replacement Behaviors and Opposite Actions**
  - Replacement Behaviors:
    - Plan to do something as a replacement for a less helpful habit or addictive behavior.
    - Choose (ahead of time) options that are enjoyable.
  - Opposite Actions:
    - Don't give in automatically to your initial impulse when under stress.
    - Choose a healthy action to counter your emotional urge.

- **Ask for Help/Seek Support**
  - Call or text a friend/family member/sponsor/provider, and share your frustrations or ask for help.
  - Attend a meeting or group.
  - If in crisis, call a 24/7 hotline (identify your local number).

- **Plan Pleasurable Activities (see Handout 13.9, Pleasurable Activities List)**
  - Routinely engage in meaningful and pleasant activities to increase your enjoyment.
    - When distressed, use pleasant activities to improve your mood.

Time Out (A Behavior Channel Skill)

- **Goal:** Allowing yourself to take a break from a stressful situation until your emotional level has decreased and you are less upset. This is deliberately choosing to take a break, not avoidance that is automatic and unhelpful.

- **When to use it**
  - You are struggling with an automatic response that feels overwhelming.
  - You think you may make the situation worse.
  - You are so worked up that you cannot think clearly enough to be effective in the situation.
  - Example: You become very angry while arguing with a family member and think you may say hurtful things or become violent.

- **How to use it effectively**
  - **Simply stop** the discussion that is provoking your increased distress, and/or leave the situation that is causing your escalation.
  - **Communicate** to others what you are doing, why, and when you will be back.
  - **Example:** "I am feeling really angry, and I need a Time Out before I say or do something I will regret. I'm going to take the day to cool down. When I come back and you are willing, I would like to continue this conversation."
  - **During Time Out:**
    - Do not try to purposefully hold on to the negative emotion, increase the emotion, or try to suppress/avoid it.
    - Notice the emotion and watch it slowly ebb away.
    - Engage in an activity (like a walk) or other coping strategies that will help you deescalate your distress. Time Out can also be used with other strategies, and you may want to think about activities that would best suit you and your needs.

Opposite Action (A Behavior Channel Skill)

Your Emotion	Your Urge	Opposite Action
Anxiety	Avoid	☐ Approach. ☐ Do it anyway (repeatedly). ☐ Start small.
Anger	Attack/punish	☐ Practice empathy and sympathy. ☐ Do something nice. ☐ Disengage from conflict or stressor.
Sadness	Isolate/withdraw	☐ Be active. ☐ Do things that make you feel competent. ☐ Do things that you enjoy.
Guilt	Hide/punish self or others	☐ Understand whether this feeling is justified or not. ☐ Identify and repair wrong as needed. ☐ Commit to doing things differently in future, accept consequences, and let go.
Shame	Hide	☐ Understand whether this feeling is justified or not. ☐ Accept and have compassion for self. ☐ Commit to doing things differently in the future, accept consequences, and let go.
Feeling overwhelmed	Shut down/avoid	☐ Slow things down. ☐ Be present in the current moment. ☐ Make a list. ☐ Start with small steps. ☐ Do it anyway (repeatedly).
Hopelessness	Give up	☐ Do it anyway (repeatedly). ☐ Start small.

Pleasurable Activities List

Arts and crafts	Listening to music
Bike riding	Meditating
Browsing in a bookstore	Painting
Camping	Pampering yourself (haircut, shave, manicure/pedicure, facial, etc.)
Cooking	
Dancing	People watching
Drawing	Photography
Exercising	Playing music
Fishing	Playing board games/cards with friends or family
Gardening	Playing with pets or kids
Getting a massage	Reading a book
Going for a drive	Relaxing in the park
Going hiking	Sitting in a coffee shop
Going on a picnic	Supporting a cause
Going to church	Swimming
Going to a library	Taking a long hot bath
Going to a play or concert	Taking an interesting class
Going to a museum	Taking a walk
Having lunch/dinner with a friend	Talking on the phone with a friend
Hanging out with a good friend	Visiting friends
Helping a friend	Viewing beautiful scenery
Jogging	Volunteering
Journal writing	Watching a game on TV
Lifting weights	Watching a favorite movie

Others:

Summary of Three Channels of Emotion Skills

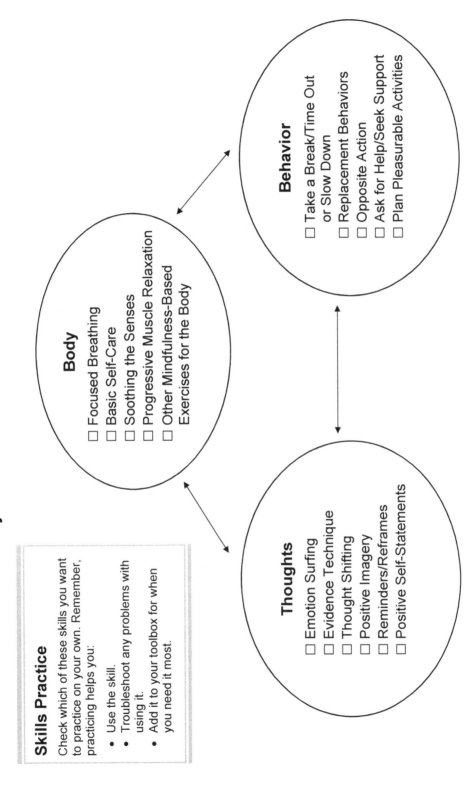

Skills Practice

Check which of these skills you want to practice on your own. Remember, practicing helps you:

- Use the skill.
- Troubleshoot any problems with using it.
- Add it to your toolbox for when you need it most.

Body

- ☐ Focused Breathing
- ☐ Basic Self-Care
- ☐ Soothing the Senses
- ☐ Progressive Muscle Relaxation
- ☐ Other Mindfulness-Based Exercises for the Body

Behavior

- ☐ Take a Break/Time Out or Slow Down
- ☐ Replacement Behaviors
- ☐ Opposite Action
- ☐ Ask for Help/Seek Support
- ☐ Plan Pleasurable Activities

Thoughts

- ☐ Emotion Surfing
- ☐ Evidence Technique
- ☐ Thought Shifting
- ☐ Positive Imagery
- ☐ Reminders/Reframes
- ☐ Positive Self-Statements

CHAPTER 14

Emotionally Engaged Living

Distress Tolerance

> To the degree that our emotions get in the way of or enhance
> our ability to think and plan, to pursue . . . a distant goal,
> to solve problems and the like, they define the limits of our
> capacity . . . and so determine how we do in life.
> —DANIEL GOLEMAN (1995, p. 80)

For many survivors of abuse, the only alternatives to living painful and out-of-control lives are emotional avoidance, social withdrawal, and limited pleasure in daily activities, all of which severely limit actualization of their potential. In this session, therapists encourage clients to identify positive goals for themselves, to articulate their desires and wishes, and to consider ways in which they may realize them. Starting to break away from the familiarity of an avoidant lifestyle will raise anxiety and distress in the short term. Clients will need support from their therapists as they develop skills centered around choosing which goals to attempt, pacing the pursuit of goals, weighing the costs and benefits of any new experiencea, and planning for managing any expected distress that may emerge. This concept of "distress tolerance" and the skills associated with it are key interventions in this effort.

The concept of distress tolerance may seem counterintuitive to both therapists and clients. As one client said, "I have spent my whole life being distressed. I don't want to tolerate it any more. I want to learn to stop it!" What we have found, however, is that clients are often not tolerating distress when doing so would actually be most helpful to them. Rather, they have developed ways of avoiding distress that feels overwhelming and out of control. The primary goal of Sessions 3 and 4 has been to help clients feel empowered by developing coping strategies for emotion regulation. Now that clients are learning to manage their emotions, this session focuses on enabling clients to accept their feelings and tolerate distress for an important purpose: *the pursuit of valued goals.*

Clients will often balk at this idea, for the reasons mentioned above. It is therefore very important to link the introduction of distress tolerance to the pursuit of valued goals. Clients have often lived with distress that had no discernible purpose or personal value, but was simply the result of having the impulses and the will of others imposed upon them. Now clients learn that tolerating distress does not have to be revictimizing, but that it can, at times, be adaptive and can even help them reach *goals they have set* (instead of goals others have set for them). Rather than being victims of their distress, clients can choose distress tolerance with a purpose and as a form of empowerment. In addition, and as an extension of the previous sessions' introduction to positive emotions, this session encourages clients to value positive feelings as a guide to goal identification, and to engage in "approach behaviors" toward positive life experiences.

CHECK-IN AND REVIEW OF SKILLS PRACTICE

As in other sessions, the therapist begins with a brief check-in on the client's current emotional state, followed by a review of the client's between-session skills practice. The Feelings Monitoring Form entries provide the best overview of the client's use of applied skills. The therapist also asks about the client's progress in practicing any specific skills in the three channels of emotion agreed upon in the last session, as well as their continued use of Focused Breathing. The client's report may prove useful in this session when considering the match between goals and skills to tolerate distress. If the client is having difficulty, the therapist can say that today they will talk about how to match skills to efforts at reaching a particular goal the client wants to reach. If the client did not complete any part of the practice, the therapist helps problem-solve any practical barriers and reviews the rationale for between-session skills practice (as needed). If the client has not completed an entry in the Feelings Monitoring Form, the therapist can say something like: "Today we'll be identifying a goal that's important to you right now. Doing this might help you use the form to keep track of how working toward that goal is going."

IDENTIFY FOCUS OF THE SESSION

This session integrates the previous four sessions by introducing the concept of distress tolerance and the importance of making conscious choices about when to use newly acquired skills to help reach valued goals. A key element of the session is thus the consolidation of skills learned thus far in STAIR. Box 14.1 outlines the session's overall content, major tasks and topic areas.

PRESENT CONCEPT OF DISTRESS TOLERANCE

The therapist can introduce the idea of distress tolerance as follows:

"Distress tolerance is the ability to endure pain or hardship without resorting to actions or behaviors that are damaging to yourself or others. Distress tolerance is a necessary

BOX 14.1

Theme and Curriculum for Session 5
Emotionally Engaged Living: Distress Tolerance

This session introduces the counterintuitive idea that tolerating and even accepting some emotional distress can be healthy and can advance the client toward improved life functioning. A clear distinction is made between distress that results from trauma, and necessary distress that emerges as part of reaching one's chosen goals. This session provides clients with practice in identifying goals, determining the value of each goal in relation to unavoidable distress, and deciding to reject or accept the goal and attendant distress. A key task in this session is to identify and consolidate skills from each of the three channels that are working well for the client, and to highlight ways the skills can be integrated to help manage a single situation. The selection of valued goals provides an opportunity for the client and therapist to consolidate the client's mastery of skills and integrate their use into daily life. Each of the previous sessions has introduced new skills. This session provides an opportunity to take a "step back" and review which skills have been working well for the client, and consciously and purposefully to review their potential value in reaching a valued goal. Lastly, the therapist encourages the client to value positive feelings as a guide to goal identification, and to engage in "approach behaviors" toward positive life experiences.

PLANNING AND PREPARATION

Review concept of distress tolerance. Bring extra copies of the Feelings Monitoring Form (Handout 11.3) and a copy of each of the two handouts for this session. Prepare several examples of tolerating distress in pursuit of valued goals that may be relevant to your client in the treatment. The work in the session is estimated to take about 60 minutes; a flexible application is assumed (i.e., not every client will need all interventions).

AGENDA

- Check-in and review of skills practice.
- Identify focus of the session.
- Present concept of distress tolerance.
- Assess the client's distress tolerance skills.
- Connect distress tolerance to client's goals.
- Present and practice skill of assessing Pros and Cons.
- Match distress reduction strategies to goals.

(continued)

- Introduce practice of distress tolerance during life's "random moments."
- Discuss role of positive feelings in pursuing goals.
- Prepare client for work on interpersonal problems.
- Summarize the goals of the session.
- Plan skills practice:
  - Complete Feelings Monitoring Form once a day (note positive and negative emotions). Specify coping skills in any channel that were used to deal with difficult feelings or situations described in entries.
  - Identify three emotion regulation skills relevant to client's needs and practice one each day, especially in situations where tolerating distress is helpful.
  - Continue to practice Focused Breathing twice daily.
  - Schedule at least one pleasurable activity per week.

SESSION HANDOUTS

Handout 14.1. What Is Distress Tolerance and Why Should I Do It?

Handout 14.2. Using Three Channels of Emotion Skills to Reach Goals

Additional copies of Handout 11.3. Feelings Monitoring Form

skill that most of us practice on a daily basis. For example, you practice distress tolerance when you effectively control your anger in confronting a friend who you feel has wronged you. In your work life, successful distress tolerance may involve managing your anxiety when you are receiving a performance review from your supervisor. By managing your anxiety, you can be open to what your supervisor says and can calmly assert yourself when you feel they're mistaken. Skillful distress tolerance is particularly important during periods when we want to make changes in our lives. Change, by its nature, often creates some level of anxiety, fear, or other strong feelings in ourselves and in those around us. That's normal. Managing these feelings so that we can make the changes most important to us requires distress tolerance."

Once the therapist has explained what distress tolerance is, the next step is to work with the client to help them understand why it is beneficial to learn to recognize and tolerate distress. Below, we have outlined some of the reasons we talk about distress tolerance with clients. The therapist can also use Handout 14.1, What Is Distress Tolerance and Why Should I Do It?, to help guide the discussion with the client.

1. *Distress is a catalyst.* Distress is a catalyst for change in recovering from childhood trauma. For example, it is often distress that prompts clients to come for treatment. These feelings of distress are signals that something is wrong; they indicate areas of the clients' lives that they need to attend to or change. It is important to help clients understand that

preparing to make significant changes in life is very likely to involve some anticipatory anxiety and discomfort. If clients do not allow themselves to be in touch with this distress, there will be no motivation to make important changes.

2. *Avoiding distress saps energy.* Clients who were abused as young children have often developed fairly elaborate ways of avoiding distress that require a great deal of energy to maintain. For example, one client who became very distressed when alone at night always worked the night shift. Not only was this strategy draining to her physically; it forced her into a schedule that impeded her from developing relationships. She spent her energy organizing her life around avoiding uncomfortable feelings, rather than spending it pursuing things that were important to her.

3. *Avoiding distress restricts positive feelings.* Learning to tolerate more negative, difficult feelings has the benefit of allowing a person to be more open to experiencing positive feelings as well. It is impossible to avoid only negative feelings, so when clients try to do so, they also end up restricting positive ones as well. As a result, many survivors of trauma have a very restricted range of emotions; they often report feeling "numb" and unable to enjoy things in their lives even when they consciously want to do so. This pattern, unfortunately, also disrupts their ability to connect with loved ones.

4. *Avoiding distress interferes with achieving desired goals.* Enduring some degree of distress is necessary if people want to accomplish goals that are important to them. Clients coming to treatment will often have limited their lives and experiences in many ways, in order to avoid distress—and, in the backs of their minds, to reduce their chances of being hurt again as they were hurt as children. This pattern is often most apparent in their interpersonal relationships, particularly their romantic relationships. Survivors of childhood maltreatment were often hurt by caregivers on whom they most depended and with whom they were most vulnerable. Being in an intimate relationship raises these feelings of vulnerability and fears that if they let themselves trust someone, they will be hurt again. In fact, this transferring of early experiences with caregivers to later close relationships is the primary impact of attachment across the lifespan.

5. *Avoiding distress contributes to PTSD symptoms.* Many clients have come to treatment with a primary goal of decreasing or getting rid of their PTSD symptoms. Given that many therapists and clients will follow the STAIR module with the Narrative Therapy module, which involves discussion and analyses of traumatic experiences, therapists can remind these clients of the value of distress tolerance in reaching this goal. Avoiding trauma memories contributes to the continued presence of PTSD symptoms. Distress about childhood trauma is inevitable, but ignoring or denying this distress or the trauma fails to make the distress go away. Although attempts to avoid or escape the distress are understandable, they unfortunately typically result in prolonging and exacerbating pain and suffering. Not having early opportunities to develop healthy coping skills certainly fosters both more severe and chronic distress. Learning distress tolerance strategies while confronting the emotional

pain of the trauma will lead to an alleviation of this suffering. Indeed, this healthy tolerating and confronting of trauma is what makes the Narrative Therapy component of this treatment program so powerful in resolving PTSD symptoms.

ASSESS CLIENT'S DISTRESS TOLERANCE SKILLS

Identify Successes

The therapist works with the client to identify specific situations in their life where they chose to tolerate distress and where doing so produced a positive outcome. All clients have tolerated distress successfully in some aspects of their lives at some time. Often clients can easily identify the areas of their lives where they need work, but have little awareness of areas where they are successful. For example, a client who has managed to complete education or training in a demanding area has had to tolerate and manage their anxiety related to performing well on exams. Or a client who has carried a child *in utero* has had to tolerate the distress of pregnancy and childbirth. In coming to therapy, clients have tolerated the distress of sharing their trauma history and some of their most intimate feelings with a stranger, in the hopes of feeling better and improving their lives. Linking the concept of distress tolerance to clients' past successes will make the concept seem less frightening.

Identify Maladaptive Strategies

Once the therapist and client have identified how the client has successfully tolerated distress in the past, they can work together to identify ways in which the client has experienced problems resulting from avoiding distress unsuccessfully. Examples can be drawn from Sessions 3 and 4, in which the therapist and client have reviewed ineffective or harmful coping strategies for negative mood regulation. In our experience, clients tend to move among several unhelpful approaches: externalization, internalization, and avoidance.

Externalization

Common externalizing behaviors include using alcohol or other substances; yelling and screaming at others; and behaving in unsafe, violent, or aggressive ways. Clients whose externalizing behaviors are extreme enough that they put their safety or that of others at risk—such as current alcohol misuse, physical violence, or serious risk taking—will need to have those issues addressed first. However, even clients who exhibit some of these behaviors can benefit from this treatment as a means by which to resolve these problems. As an example, one client came to treatment with a history of getting into "screaming matches" with his husband, often triggered by his implicit feelings of not feeling valued or prioritized in their relationship. Over time, he was able to diffuse his explosive reactions and redirect the energy into communicating his more vulnerable feelings in a calm, collaborative way. This example also previews the role of communication skills, which are the focus of STAIR Sessions 6–9.

Internalization

A natural alternative to externalization is, of course, internalization. Often considered a redirection of anger and fear inward, examples of internalizing behaviors include self-injury (e.g., cutting, burning, or hitting oneself) and eating disturbances (binge eating, purging, or self-starvation). For example, a client in one of our studies had the tendency to binge-eat when she became very anxious, including in anticipation of or following a date. Because her binge eating was clearly a reaction to a specific trigger and was not frequent enough to pose a risk to her health, this treatment was appropriate for her. Work on emotion regulation helped her replace binge eating with healthy behaviors, including exercising moderately and calling supportive friends. In addition, she accepted that the distress she experienced, if managed in a healthy way, was worth the opportunity to have a social life.

Avoidance

Clients who have experienced trauma, especially in childhood, often try to protect themselves by arranging their lives to avoid reminders (e.g., particular thoughts, feelings, or places) of what happened. Avoidance of these generalized triggers also enables them to avoid confronting distressing feelings associated with the trauma memories themselves. For example, clients may report prematurely breaking off relationships when conflict arises, because it makes them so distressed. Clients may also have limited their professional lives by not taking advantage of opportunities or by not advocating for themselves, because of the fear that if they assert themselves, they will be harmed. In many cases, avoidance has become so integral to these clients' lives that they do not recognize it or see it as effortful any more. Clients must recognize how they are relying on avoidance, learn to tolerate distress, and take appropriate emotional risks in order to make important changes and reach their goals.

CONNECT DISTRESS TOLERANCE TO CLIENT'S GOALS

As already mentioned, one of the main aims of this treatment is to teach skills for distress tolerance in relationship to identified goals, instead of having clients learn to tolerate distress for its own sake. The emphasis is on determining whether a client's goals are important or beneficial enough that tolerating some discomfort and distress in the process of attaining them is manageable and worthwhile.

Identify Specific Goals

At this point, the therapist will have a good idea of what brought the client to treatment and what their long- and short-term goals might be. In this session, it is important to identify a couple of goals the client can accomplish or begin to address substantially in the time frame of treatment.

Some clients may have difficulty identifying specific goals. For example, it is not uncommon for a client to say, "I just want to feel better." Although the client will likely feel better by the end of the treatment, it is important to identify specific goals, so that both the

BOX 14.2

Examples of Specific Personal Goals

Completing therapy

Asking for a raise

Performing music in front of an audience

Beginning to date or entering a romantic relationship

Searching for a new job

Creating better boundaries with a parent

Improving parenting skills

Reaching or maintaining a healthy weight range

Discussing with a partner their poor spending habits

Establishing a regular sleep schedule

Sharing history of trauma with a close friend

Reading personal poetry in public

Going back to school

Starting an exercise program

Asking someone out for coffee

Recontacting an estranged child

Reestablishing an old friendship

Attending a high school reunion

Helping other survivors of trauma

Meeting with a lawyer about custody issues

---

therapist and the client can evaluate whether the treatment is succeeding. If the client is being vague, the therapist might ask, "Why do you want to feel better?", "What would be different in your life if you felt better?", or "Describe what you would be doing [or who you would be] if you felt better." Most clients will have unspoken ideas about specific ways in which their lives would be different if they "felt better." By verbalizing what they hope for, a client can begin to brainstorm goals. The client's goals can be of any type in any area of life. Box 14.2 contains some examples of specific goals our clients have worked on during and after treatment.

Clients often have many things they would like to change about themselves and their lives. It is one of the reasons they are in therapy. The greater difficulty will be choosing which goals they want to prioritize. The first priorities in choosing a goal are (1) its importance to a client, and (2) the positive consequences of pursuing the goal. To identify which goal is most important, the therapist can have the client identify what they would change first, which goal is most immediate, or which goal would have the greatest impact on other areas of their life.

PRESENT AND PRACTICE SKILL OF ASSESSING PROS AND CONS

Introduce Skill and Its Purpose

The skill of Assessing Pros and Cons is a strategy that can aid in determining whether reaching a specific goal is worth tolerating distress. This skill involves (1) selecting a situation related to reaching an important goal, (2) evaluating the necessity of distress tolerance in pursuing this goal, and (3) identifying a comprehensive list of the advantages and disadvantages of tolerating the situation and its associated feelings. The point of this exercise is for the client to recognize that they do not have to tolerate distress if it does not serve a purpose. Rather, the client is learning to tolerate distress because it is inevitable and worth the effort in the context of working toward a life goal. The concept of linking the presence of distress with identified goals is particularly important when goals require long-term work and when working toward them does not offer an immediate benefit or sense of relief.

Identify the Goal

Sometimes a goal a client proposes will need to be reworked or broken down into more focused goals for which the therapist and client can identify specific implementation strategies. For example, a client named Alice reported, "I become very scared when I am asked to show my artwork. When I get scared, I stop working, start avoiding appointments, act irresponsibly, become depressed, and ruin the show." Her goal: "I want to be a famous artist." Alice's desire to be a famous artist was problematic for the treatment, because it was not within her direct control and was dependent on too many outside forces, including luck. Through discussion with her therapist, Alice was able to restate the goal more concretely: "I want to show my artwork publicly, and ultimately be able to support myself financially as a full-time artist." This goal could then be broken down into smaller steps that the client and therapist could address in the treatment, including finding a studio space, joining a support group for local artists, contacting gallery owners who had shown interest in her work, and working regularly to prepare for a show.

Evaluate the Necessity for Distress Tolerance

Before working through specific Pros and Cons to evaluate a goal, the client may first consider whether there is indeed any distress tolerance necessarily involved in reaching the goal. The concept of "necessary suffering" can help clients evaluate whether they are tolerating distress that is required to reach a goal, or whether they are tolerating unwarranted distress. Clients can ask themselves, "Is it really necessary to tolerate distress to reach this goal?"

Clients who are unclear about the answer to this question might ask a friend for their thoughts on the situation. An alternative strategy is to use displacement. A client can imagine that someone they care about is tolerating a distressing situation to reach a valued goal. Do they see an alternative way for their friend to reach the goal? Do they think their friend has to stay in the situation to reach the goal?

For example, one client wanted to become an architect. Part of the training involved an extensive apprenticeship with someone in the field. This particular client was elated when she got a placement with a very prominent architect. Quickly after starting the work, however, it became apparent that the architect was very abusive. The situation only became worse over time. Initially, the client thought she had to tolerate the distressing situation to reach her goal of becoming an architect. After discussing her situation in therapy, though, the client realized that she might be tolerating unnecessary suffering. She decided to explore getting another placement with someone who was known to be a good mentor.

Identify Advantages and Disadvantages

The therapist can write out the identified goal at the top of a clean sheet of paper and divide the sheet into two columns, headed "Pros" and "Cons." In reviewing the Pros and Cons, the client determines first the level of distress they expect to experience, and then the strategies they have for managing or reducing the distress. Afterward, the client determines whether the remaining distress is worthwhile. In addition to providing a specific example of how to use skills, this exercise is a productive way to prepare and enlist the client in facing challenges inherent in the treatment.

If the client has difficulty with generating Pros and Cons for an identified goal, the therapist can review a specific goal of the treatment—for example, reducing PTSD symptoms. Therapists can prompt clients to ask themselves questions such as: "Why am I putting myself through this?", "What is my ultimate goal here?", and "Will I get enough positive results out of this situation that tolerating these distressing feelings will be worth it?" The associated Pros might be better daily functioning, improvement in relationships, and better sleep, while the Cons might be reliving painful memories.

CASE EXAMPLE: IDENTIFYING GOALS AND GENERATING PROS AND CONS

Beth was a 40-year-old woman with a history of sexual abuse and violations in the context of intimate relationships. In childhood, her uncle, a central caregiver, had repeatedly molested her. She described a "special" relationship with him and noted that prior to the abuse, she had trusted and loved him very much. In college, she was raped by a boyfriend—again, a person with whom she had previously felt closeness and trust. Beth felt that these experiences influenced her choice at age 26 to marry a man whom she did not find sexually attractive and who did not express much interest or initiative in a sexual relationship with her. She divorced him several years later, and since that time had not been involved in any romantic relationships. Although she had felt unfulfilled in many ways over the past 10 years, she also described feeling safe and well protected by the "wall" that she had built to keep others (regardless of gender) from getting too close.

At the beginning of treatment, Beth shared that Doug, a friend she had known for a few years, had recently told her he was romantically interested in her. She expressed tremendous ambivalence and anxiety about this situation. Beth was aware that getting closer to Doug would create anxiety and upheaval in her life. She also stated that she liked and felt comfortable with Doug and feared that if she didn't try to get closer to him, she would regret it and might not get another chance. As part of treatment, her therapist suggested that Beth assess the Pros and Cons to help her decide whether it would be worthwhile and manageable for her to tolerate the distress and anxiety that would arise if she accepted his request for a date.

Beth initially identified that her most ambitious goal would be to develop a wonderful relationship with Doug and maybe get married. The therapist suggested that they shift the

---

BOX 14.3
Beth's Pros and Cons List

Goals: *Developing a more intimate relationship with Doug, learning to open up, becoming close to someone in a healthy way*

Pros	**Cons**
Having companionship	*Making myself vulnerable*
Developing an important connection	*Risking getting hurt*
Having somebody to depend on	*Feeling foolish and anxious*
Learning to enjoy sex	*Having to deal with sexual problems*
Being with someone who is supportive	*Having to confront the abuse*
Developing a deeper relationship	*Risking a good friendship*

---

focus away from this overwhelming, uncontrollable, and distant goal to a more realistic and manageable set of smaller subgoals. These subgoals included going on a first date, developing more intimacy with Doug, learning to be more open, and becoming close to another person in a healthy way. Breaking down the larger goal into more realistic, immediate subgoals was an intervention in itself, as it helped reduce Beth's anxiety. She was then able to generate a useful list of Pros and Cons about committing herself to these smaller goals (presented in Box 14.3).

Beth's Pros and Cons list helped her to identify how her history of abuse was getting in the way of potentially having a rewarding relationship with Doug. She decided it was worth tolerating some distress for the possibility of developing a closer relationship with him. For the next week, she chose the first step as asking him to go see a movie he had mentioned wanting to see together.

MATCH DISTRESS REDUCTION STRATEGIES TO GOALS

A key task in this session is to identify and consolidate skills from each of the three channels of emotion that are working well for the client, and to highlight ways in which these skills can be integrated to help manage a single situation. The selection of a valued goal provides an opportunity for the client and therapist to consolidate skills strength and integrate their use. Each of the previous sessions has introduced new skills. This session provides an opportunity to take a "step back" and review what skills have been working well for the client, and then consciously and purpose review their potential value in reaching a valued goal. Handout 14.2, Using the Three Channels of Emotion Skills to Reach Goals, provides a checklist of skills for the therapist and client to use together to tailor strategies to the client's needs and goals.

The case below describes a way in which a client and therapist organized skills to meet a valued goal. In addition, David's case demonstrates a situation where the client was not clear about what his goals could or should be. In such a circumstance, a default goal can always be completing the therapy. This goal is inherently worthwhile and concrete, and identifying skills in the three channels to support this goal can reinforce the client's sense of mastery, focus, and commitment.

CASE EXAMPLE: CONSOLIDATING SKILLS TO SUPPORT THE GOAL OF COMPLETING THERAPY

David was a young U.S. Army veteran who had served in Iraq. One of his close friends who served with him in combat was killed in an explosion, and David witnessed his death. David had also experienced childhood physical abuse at the hands of his father, who would punish him for any displays of vulnerability. As a child, he quickly learned to put on a brave face no matter what he was feeling inside. Adopting such a brave face was exactly what he did when he lost one of his best friends and had to continue performing in the line of duty despite his grief.

David had a previous history of dropping out of psychotherapy, and he had been ambivalent so far in this treatment as well, sometimes canceling sessions and rarely doing the between-session skills practice. As he and the therapist began to work through the topic of distress tolerance, David was able to articulate some of his concerns about completing STAIR Narrative Therapy, and he agreed to analyze the Pros and Cons of staying in treatment and completing the program.

THERAPIST: I'm really glad we're talking about this. It is absolutely true that engaging in therapy can be extremely challenging, and it is important that we acknowledge those challenges as well as the potential benefits, so that you can feel empowered about continuing in therapy or not. Let's begin by writing down the Pros and Cons of completing STAIR Narrative Therapy.

DAVID: Well, my wife is the one who pushed me to come here, so one Pro is that she will be happy.

THERAPIST: That's good, but what impact would that have on you?

DAVID: Well, she is always telling me that I keep everything inside and it drives her crazy. I really do care about her, and I would like to be able to share things with her.

THERAPIST: Great. Let's put that down as a Pro. What other Pros and Cons come to mind?

DAVID: Honestly, a Con is that I feel nervous about completing the practice outside of our sessions. When I stare at the blank sheet of paper, I feel overwhelmed. It is really scary to share my feelings, even on a piece of paper. In my life, expressing my feelings hasn't been such a good thing to do.

THERAPIST: Yes, that has been your experience at times in the past, so it makes sense that you would feel that way now. I think you have actually named two cons—feeling overwhelmed about doing the skills practice of completing the Feelings Monitoring Form, and fear related to identifying feelings.

DAVID: It has been very weird to talk so much about feelings. But I've already learned that a lot of times when I'm feeling angry, it's really something else underneath, like sadness or fear, or especially guilt.

THERAPIST: Excellent. So this is another Pro—increasing your emotional awareness. And why might increasing your emotional awareness be a good thing?

DAVID: Because anger just covers everything up. I wish there was an easier way, but I know the first step to healing is allowing myself to feel sadness and other emotions that are so hard to feel. And I know you said emotions are messengers, so I guess I'm missing out on some things that might be important for me to know.

THERAPIST: Very good point, David. What other Pros and Cons come to mind?

DAVID: I need to get my PTSD under control. I've just been spinning my wheels since I got back from Iraq. I want to be a good husband. I want to get a job I like. I used to enjoy doing fun things, and I would love to get back to that.

THERAPIST: These are all terrific Pros. Now that you have a complete list, take a look. Compare the Pros and Cons. Based upon what you have outlined, is the goal of completing this treatment worth pursuing?

DAVID: Absolutely, when I look at it this way! I have to say I've never really acknowledged all the challenges of addressing my PTSD. It's just something I know I'm supposed to do. But being very open with the Cons of doing it, and knowing that I have some tools to manage those Cons and the distress that comes with them—this all makes me feel more confident.

THERAPIST: Terrific, David. Now let's talk about some of the coping skills from each of the three channels you can use to tolerate the distress that might come up.

DAVID: I really like the Focused Breathing. Even though I haven't been practicing it as much as I should, it's already helping.

THERAPIST: Very good. What other body-based skills could you use?

DAVID: I really love petting my dog. In fact, I'm thinking about getting her certified as a service animal.

THERAPIST: Sounds like petting your dog is a good example of Soothing the Senses. Let's move on to thought channel coping skills.

DAVID: When I get overwhelmed with the feelings monitoring, I can use a positive self-statement and encourage myself to keep going. I can also list all the reasons that doing the worksheets and coming to appointments too are so important. This includes a better relationship with my wife, feeling better about myself, and so on. I can also look at the evidence and see that I've been through much, much harder and worse things, and I survived after all of that.

THERAPIST: Excellent ideas, David. And let's add "feeling better about myself" as a Pro for completing the treatment. Let's finish up with behavior channel tools.

DAVID: The first one that comes to mind is that I can take a Time Out if I am doing a Feelings Monitoring Form and get overwhelmed. Probably the hardest one is that I can try to reach out for help or support. I know that I can reach out to you, and I know I can get help from my wife, too.

David and his therapist went on to generate strategies that he could employ to help him complete his between-session assignments, as well as ways the therapist can help him accomplish that. The Pros and Cons for completing STAIR Narrative Therapy that David and his therapist identified are listed in Box 14.4. The therapist helped clarify that the Cons David identified in regard to completing treatment had mostly to do with fearing being overwhelmed by the feelings that came up, particularly during skills practice. David was able to identify several skills he could use to manage his fear of being overwhelmed by his feelings (see Box 14.5).

Flexible Application of Skills

Clients can also become aware that they prefer certain emotion regulation strategies for specific situations and may not choose these skills in others. For example, if a client is anxious before a meeting with their boss, they might use Focused Breathing several times during the preceding days to reach and maintain a calmer state. They might also keep their anxiety in check by engaging in anxiety-reducing activities consistent with their goals, such as taking a relaxing bath, preparing/writing out what they plan to say, and doing laundry or otherwise making sure they have clean and appropriate clothes for the meeting. Talking late

---

BOX 14.4

David's Pros and Cons List

Goal: *Completing STAIR Narrative Therapy*

Pros	Cons
Make my wife happy	Feel overwhelmed by doing feelings monitoring
Share things with my wife	
Increase emotional awareness	Fear of identifying feelings (and what I will find)
Get my PTSD under control so that I can:	
Be a good husband	
Get a job I like	
Enjoy doing fun things again	
Feel better about myself	

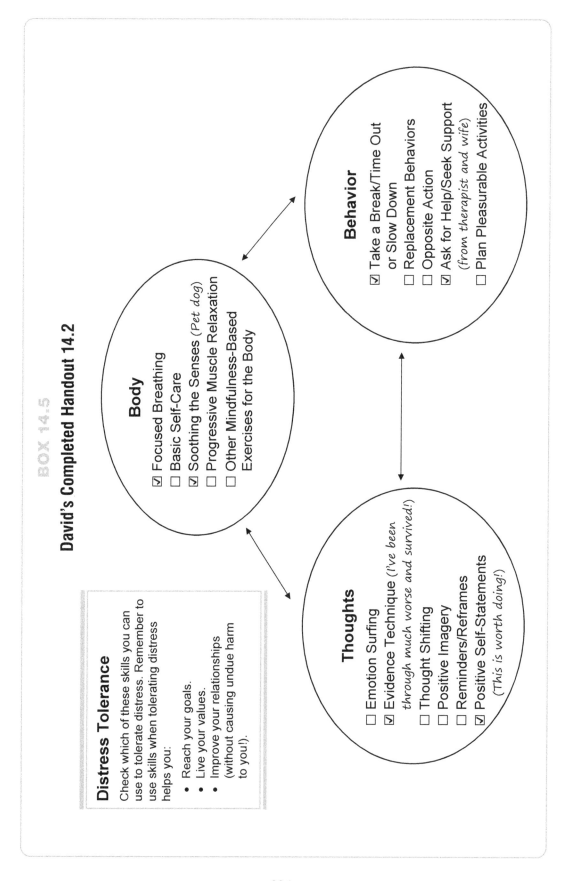

BOX 14.5

David's Completed Handout 14.2

Distress Tolerance

Check which of these skills you can use to tolerate distress. Remember to use skills when tolerating distress helps you:

- Reach your goals.
- Live your values.
- Improve your relationships (without causing undue harm to you!).

Body

☑ Focused Breathing
☐ Basic Self-Care
☑ Soothing the Senses (*Pet dog*)
☐ Progressive Muscle Relaxation
☐ Other Mindfulness-Based Exercises for the Body

Behavior

☑ Take a Break/Time Out or Slow Down
☐ Replacement Behaviors
☐ Opposite Action
☑ Ask for Help/Seek Support (*from therapist and wife*)
☐ Plan Pleasurable Activities

Thoughts

☐ Emotion Surfing
☑ Evidence Technique (*I've been through much worse and survived!*)
☐ Thought Shifting
☐ Positive Imagery
☐ Reminders/Reframes
☑ Positive Self-Statements (*This is worth doing!*)

into the night on the phone with friends might reduce the client's distress but might not be consistent with their goal, which includes being alert and attentive at the meeting. Handout 14.2 provides a checklist of skills for a therapist and client to use together to tailor strategies to the client's needs and goals.

INTRODUCE PRACTICE OF DISTRESS TOLERANCE DURING LIFE'S "RANDOM MOMENTS"

Describe Rationale for Acceptance of Negative Feelings

Up to this point, the emphasis of this session has been on tolerating distress associated with the client's active pursuit of specific, identifiable goals. However, the therapist can note that feelings of distress also frequently emerge during more or less "random moments" in people's lives. They may experience episodic anxiety, sadness, and frustration during everyday unexpected hassles, during difficult interactions with others, or simply as a result of dysregulated biological rhythms (e.g., disrupted sleep–wake cycles). Also, despite efforts at proactive management of symptoms, there will be inevitable occasions where symptoms occur unexpectedly and are not controllable. For example, a client's reliving and hyperarousal symptoms may be triggered automatically by environmental stimuli that unconsciously remind them of their traumatic experiences.

In these and other similar circumstances, the therapist can note that it is not always possible to change or decrease negative emotions. Indeed, there are occasions where it may be preferable *not* to work toward changing the negative feelings. Rather, some negative emotional states can be accepted as common, typical, and necessary parts of human life. Indeed, exercising acceptance of negative emotions during difficult events often paradoxically culminates in clients' feeling less distress. If it seems helpful in this session, the therapist can refer back to previous work on acknowledging the important messages that each emotion can tell us about our experience.

Provide Examples of Accepting Negative Feelings in Everyday Life

The therapist can identify situations where acceptance may work well for the client. For example, it is easy to feel anger or anxiety while having to wait in a long line of customers at a grocery store or bank. In this situation, through simply being mindful of feelings of anger and anxiety, the client can learn to tolerate increasing levels of this type of everyday life distress. The therapist can suggest that the client explore this option of practicing mindfulness. The client can perceive or simply be aware that "this experience is what anger (or anxiety) feels like," but can do so without directly responding to, acting on, or overidentifying with the feeling state. Acceptance is an experience of being aware of feelings without trying to change, reject, or suppress them. It may also be important to note that acceptance does not mean having to welcome the feelings or trying not to be bothered by them. In fact, sometimes stating to themselves matter-of-factly, "I don't like it when I feel this way," or "It's hard to feel this way," can be helpful as well. When the client is not putting energy into pushing away feelings, it will be easier for them to work on trying to be kinder and less self-critical to themselves while dealing with unavoidable, difficult feelings.

Clients may find that if they simply observe their emotional symptoms with a sense of nonjudgmental awareness, their symptoms will often be more short-lived than if they try to avoid their feelings altogether or engage in self-destructive behaviors in an attempt to make their feelings go away. In fact, by observing and accepting a certain degree of negative affect, clients will typically find that negative emotions will abate on their own.

Provide Examples of Accepting Intense Feelings and Moods

The therapist can also note that survivors of trauma often experience intense feelings and then engage in behaviors to minimize or rid themselves of such feelings—behaviors that result in perpetuating the negative feelings or putting them into worse circumstances. For example, a client may wake up in an intensely sad state, and in response to it may stay in bed all day, missing work and other responsibilities. This client may then feel guilty and berate themselves for missing work. They may also be in trouble with their boss. As a result, they may start feeling depressed. The client's response to their initial feelings may thus make them feel worse instead of better.

An alternative approach is for the client to accept their feeling state. If the client can tolerate their sadness and go to work, they will not experience the cascade of guilt and depression that may follow the decision to stay in bed. The therapist can remind the client that intense feelings are often temporary; no matter what mood they experience at any given time, their mood will eventually change. As explored in the Emotion Surfing skill, primary, basic emotions are sometimes akin to waves that crest and then eventually fall. This image may be helpful to the client, because what they are feeling at any one moment may seem unbearable—but the feeling will not last forever.

Identify Long-Term Benefits of Healthy Distress Tolerance: Increased Well-Being

Lastly, the therapist can note that the more clients feels able to tolerate negative emotions during random moments of their everyday lives, the more confident they are likely to be in their ability to tolerate distress while actively pursuing their newly set positive goals. In keeping with this session's theme of working toward goals, exercising distress tolerance during random moments is itself consistent with a major therapeutic goal: that of increasing overall psychological health and well-being.

DISCUSS ROLE OF POSITIVE FEELINGS IN PURSUING GOALS

Although negative emotions can sometimes disrupt the pursuit of important goals, positive emotions can *enhance* motivation in moving toward goals. Therapists can discuss this point as an extension of the work from previous sessions, in which they have invited clients to engage in pleasurable activities and to explore, accept, and modulate (as necessary) positive feelings. Increasing exposure to novel and positive experiences can improve functioning, akin to more general behavioral activation strategies. This viewpoint may be somewhat foreign to survivors of interpersonal trauma, especially childhood abuse. The tendency to engage in "approach behaviors"—even toward things, situations, or people that appear interesting, elicit curiosity, or generate warmth—may have been undermined by repeated negative/hostile feedback in the past and by an inadequate attachment system that discouraged healthy exploration of the world. However, positive feelings can guide a person toward discovering more of their interests, likes, and sometimes even hidden talents. By recognizing and following feelings of pleasure and excitement, clients can discover activities they truly enjoy and even previously dormant talents and abilities. In addition, acknowledging the satisfaction that results from making steps toward a goal can reinforce and sustain a person's commitment and discipline during more difficult times.

The therapist can ask the client what skills or activities attract them or spontaneously engage them. If they do not know, the therapist can encourage continued exploration and reassure the client that some initial confusion is understandable, given that they are thinking in a new way and have less experience in paying attention to their own preferences. The goal is for them to try things out and practice paying attention to their reactions, whatever they are; their responses can then inform what they might want to try next. Eliciting excitement and interest about an idea, problem, activity, or circumstance can help confirm a goal as important and motivate the client to persist in the face of setbacks. Positive emotions have another function as well: They provide the client with feedback about what they like or value about themselves. This growing insight supports the client's movement toward becoming a more integrated, substantial, and specific person in their own eyes—even one who deserves to love and be loved. Selecting a goal in which the client has a positive interest is also likely to lead to greater skills practice and mastery. Such goals can be any number of things: learning to dance, fix a bike, play music, or write poetry. Moreover, if the client experiences some success, a more profound benefit emerges—the experience of feeling engaged in living.

PREPARE CLIENT FOR WORK ON INTERPERSONAL PROBLEMS

The next several sessions will focus on the client's interpersonal relationships. At first glance, it may seem challenging to help the client develop their emotion regulation and distress tolerance skills while at the same time helping them work on their relationships. However, as becomes obvious from examining Box 14.2, almost all clients' goals involve some interpersonal aspects, even if their goals are not specifically focused on a relationship. For example, a client's goal of receiving a raise does not seem on the surface to be an interpersonal goal. However, actually talking to their boss about a raise requires that the client manage their feelings toward their boss, tolerate their anxiety about asking for the raise, and practice their communication skills so that they can ask their boss for a raise in an appropriate and effective way.

SUMMARIZE THE GOALS OF THE SESSION

The therapist can help consolidate the information shared in this session by briefly reviewing the overall theme of using distress tolerance to meet personal goals and determining how it fits within the larger treatment framework. Does the idea make sense? Does it sound doable? Is the Pros and Cons skill useful? The therapist can determine whether any concepts or examples need clarification, and ask the client if they think they will be able to assess the Pros and Cons of tolerating distress, as relevant, in their daily lives. If the client seems hesitant, the therapist can help them come up with examples of possible situations to use. Some of the situations can be relatively mundane (e.g., asking a friend for a ride to the airport) or simple (e.g., waiting in line for ordering lunch), as the important thing is to practice the skill.

The therapist can review which skills seem to be a good match to the client's abilities, valued goals, and day-to-day needs. With continued practice, the client can learn that they have a choice when it comes to feeling distress, and that they can manage distress when they deem it necessary and worthwhile to meet their personal goals and live their values.

PLAN SKILLS PRACTICE

The client will continue to use the Feelings Monitoring Form to chart progress on the goal they have selected in this session, as well as any other activities that occur during the week (either positive or negative). For each entry, they will also examine which coping skills they used and how effective the skills were in helping them reach their goal. The therapist can remind the client to pay attention to using skills from all three emotion channels and seeing how well they work together. The client may select at least three skills to practice daily, especially in relation to distress tolerance. The client can continue practicing Focused Breathing twice daily and can schedule at least one pleasurable activity during the week.

The therapist may spend some time planning how the client might practice using Pros and Cons, encouraging them to be specific about when they will do the designated "steps" to reaching a goal, and helping them decide which coping strategies they will practice. In addition, therapists can suggest that clients allow themselves to be simply aware and accepting of feelings as they plan their goals. To the extent that a client experiences anxiety at "random moments" or in situations they have no power to change right now, they can simply be interested in the feeling and note when it happens and why.

What Is Distress Tolerance and Why Should I Do It?

Distress tolerance is . . .

- The ability to endure pain or hardship without resorting to unhelpful actions that are damaging to yourself or others.

- Distress tolerance is a necessary life skill that most of us practice daily.

- It requires us to weigh the **Pros and Cons** of tolerating stress when it's necessary to reach our goals.

- Examples:
  - Effectively controlling your anger when you feel a friend or family member has wronged you.
  - Managing anxiety when you are receiving a performance review from your work supervisor.
  - What are other examples?

Why tolerate unpleasant emotions? Because doing so . . .

- **Allows us to act in a crisis,** instead of giving up or freezing.

- **Frees up energy we use for avoidance.** Avoiding stress saps energy.

- **Enables us to make positive changes.** If you don't allow yourself to be in touch with distress, there'll be no motivation to make important changes. Distress can tell you that something is wrong, as well as which areas in your life you need to pay attention to and change.

- **Allows us to experience positive emotions.** Avoiding feelings means that most or many feelings are cut off, not just negative ones. Tolerating more difficult feelings has an important benefit: It allows us to be more open to having positive feelings as well.

- **Allows us to achieve goals.** It allows us to do difficult but worthwhile things (such as interviewing for a job). Preparing to make any major life change involves some anxiety and discomfort. By tolerating distress, we allow ourselves to achieve goals important to us.

Use your new skills to tolerate what you need to and live the life you want to live!

Using Three Channels of Emotion Skills to Reach Goals

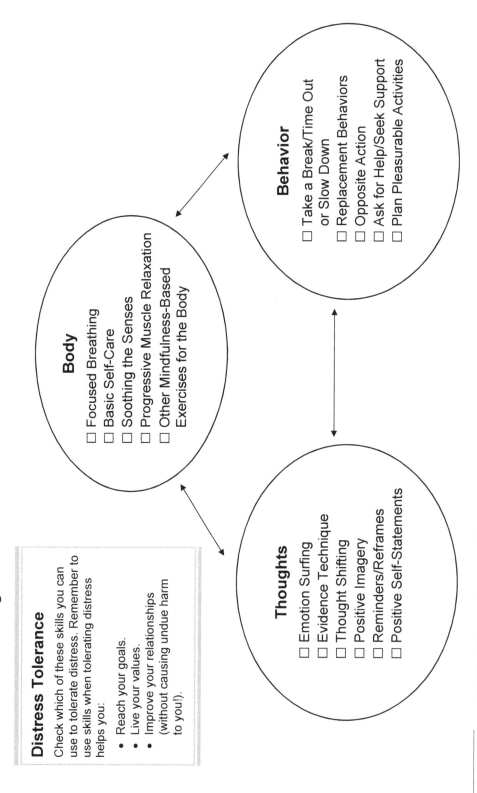

Distress Tolerance

Check which of these skills you can use to tolerate distress. Remember to use skills when tolerating distress helps you:

- Reach your goals.
- Live your values.
- Improve your relationships (without causing undue harm to you!).

Body

☐ Focused Breathing
☐ Basic Self-Care
☐ Soothing the Senses
☐ Progressive Muscle Relaxation
☐ Other Mindfulness-Based Exercises for the Body

Behavior

☐ Take a Break/Time Out or Slow Down
☐ Replacement Behaviors
☐ Opposite Action
☐ Ask for Help/Seek Support
☐ Plan Pleasurable Activities

Thoughts

☐ Emotion Surfing
☐ Evidence Technique
☐ Thought Shifting
☐ Positive Imagery
☐ Reminders/Reframes
☐ Positive Self-Statements

CHAPTER 15

The Resource of Connection
Understanding Relationship Patterns

> Through our relationship with the [caregiving person] . . . , we develop
> a working model of ourselves and our parents . . . that gives a model
> for how we treat each other and ourselves. This model determines
> what information is attended to, which memories are evoked, what
> behaviors are employable. It is the basis for our sense of self and other.
> —SANDRA L. BLOOM AND MICHAEL REICHERT (1998, p. 135)

Interactions with other people shape how we see ourselves in the world and what we come to expect from our environments. From infancy through adulthood, our relationships and our beliefs about these relationships are constantly influencing our thoughts, feelings, and behaviors, even when we are not aware of their impact. Based on our early experiences, we develop models of relationships and test these over time, continually elaborating and adapting them to fit our current realities. Among survivors of trauma, the process of using past experience to guide current expectations can often lead to negative outcomes. The primary focus of Session 6 is on helping a client understand how models of relationships developed in their early life, continue to influence their feelings and interactions with others as an adult.

The first component of this session involves introducing the idea of relationship models and describing how they become relationship patterns over time, in ways that are understandable and relevant to the client. The second component of this session entails introducing and working with a specific tool (Handout 15.3, Relationship Patterns Worksheet–1) to help the client draw out from their life experiences the core relationship models that effectively describe their beliefs in interpersonal situations. Given that many survivors of trauma have difficulty remembering or keeping hold of insights from one week to the next, this tool creates a record of distilled insights that can be referred to in later sessions. Box 15.1 outlines the theme and curriculum for Session 6 of treatment.

The therapist will want to be familiar with the basic principles of attachment theory, which are elucidated in Chapter 2. It may be useful to review this chapter before this session.

Theme and Curriculum for Session 6
The Resource of Connection: Understanding Relationship Patterns

Relationship models are templates for how we expect relationships to work. Originally described by John Bowlby, the father of attachment theory, relationship models arise from actual experiences with caregivers and other important persons in our lives. They represent ideas about who we are, what we expect of others, how relationships work, and what outcomes we expect. Relationship models that arise in the context of childhood interpersonal trauma are typically adaptive in the traumatic context, but once the trauma is over or life conditions have changed, they may no longer be effective for happy and healthy living. The goal of this session is to help clients identify trauma-generated relationship models by reviewing current relationship problems and having the client consider whether they may have "outgrown" their old models. The next session will invite the client to consider developing and testing new relationship models.

PLANNING AND PREPARATION

Review interpersonal situations described in past Feelings Monitoring Forms as a guide to formulating potential relationship models that can be shared and discussed with the client. Bring several copies of Handout 15.3, and a copy of each of the other handouts listed below. The work in the session is estimated to take about 60 minutes; a flexible application is assumed (i.e., not every client will need all interventions).

AGENDA

- Check-in and review of skills practice.
- Identify focus of the session.
- Introduce concept of relationship models and patterns.
- Explore and identify client's relationship patterns.
- Review common relationship beliefs among survivors of trauma.
- Introduce Relationship Patterns Worksheet–1.
- Practice using Relationship Patterns Worksheet–1.
- Summarize the goals of the session.

(continued)

- Plan skills practice:
  - Complete a copy of Relationship Patterns Worksheet–1 once daily.
  - Include emotion regulation skills as relevant to the situation, and keep practicing Focused Breathing.
  - Engage in one pleasurable activity.

SESSION HANDOUTS

Handout 15.1. Relationship Models: Instruction Manuals for Relationships

Handout 15.2. Common Relationship Beliefs among Survivors of Trauma

Handout 15.3. Relationship Patterns Worksheet–1 (several copies)

Handout 15.4. How to Complete Relationship Patterns Worksheet–1

Repetition of Relationship Patterns

Clients will often present for treatment with tremendous distress and confusion about repeated negative relationship patterns with friends, coworkers, and partners. Though they may be well aware of the cyclical nature of their relationships, they often describe being bewildered about why similar situations recur with different people and feeling helpless about how they can break this cycle, which has come to feel inevitable.

People's expectations about relationships, and about the responses they are likely to receive from others, lead them to behave in ways to prepare for the imagined outcomes. Consequently, relationship models are often self-fulfilling, even when the relationship result is one that a person does not want. For example, a young woman from an abusive family who has developed the understanding that interpersonal relatedness is contingent on sexual behavior may be likely to engage in or initiate sexual activity as a way of emotionally connecting to others, whether she is interested in sex or not and whether or not her partner is actually expecting sex.

Individuals often erroneously use relationship outcomes as confirmatory evidence that their original expectations were well founded and accurate. In this way, they form and perpetuate relationship models and patterns with little awareness of how the expectations themselves, which may or may not be based in current reality, are influencing interpersonal sequences. One useful and common example a therapist can share to illustrate this point with a client involves expectations of rejection, which often lead to perceived and even actual rejection. If a client typically expects to be rejected in relationships, they are less willing to engage with others and generally behave in a self-protective manner by maintaining distance and avoiding intimacy. Others interacting with them will be unaware of this basic assumption and are likely to interpret their behavior as lack of interest or of openness to interpersonal contact. As a result, most people will not initiate or pursue involvement with them. They in turn will see this as confirming evidence of rejection in relationships, and will remain unaware of their own role in perpetuating this negative cycle.

Limited and Rigid Interpersonal Repertoires

Not only do individuals with histories of interpersonal trauma, especially childhood abuse and neglect, tend to have negative expectations in relationships; they also often have a limited and rigid repertoire of relationship models from which to select. They may say something like this: "I can't move out of this pattern, because I don't know where to go next." When individuals are not exposed to varying interactions, there is a higher degree of redundancy in their interpersonal relationships, and maladaptive relationship models are especially difficult to disconfirm (Carson, 1969). Thus having a constricted range of models, and engaging in these regardless of the actual situation, further perpetuate the self-confirming cycle and limit possible responses from others.

One common maladaptive model is the victim–perpetrator relationship, which can be reflected in domestic violence situations and even in the therapy relationship. Sometimes the client takes on the victim role, experiencing mistreatment at the hands of a partner, boss, friend, or therapist. At other times, the client can take on the role of the aggressor with significant others. Many clients fear falling into the trap of taking on either role, but the problem is that they have very few alternative ways of thinking about themselves and others.

In sum, attachment theory and research indicate that the tendency to generalize the application of predominant relationship models to new experiences should be viewed as a general principle of interpersonal functioning, rather than as a pathological process associated with survivors of trauma.

CHECK-IN AND REVIEW OF SKILLS PRACTICE

The therapist will review the Feelings Monitoring Form and any patterns or notable situations that came up over the past week with the client. The therapist will also follow up on whether the client completed the practice exercises. Did they use any of the distress tolerance skills that were discussed during the previous session? Did they try to increase positive emotional experiences over the past week? If they did experiment with some of the emotion channel skills, what did they notice, what worked, and what did not work? If they did not experiment with any skills, what obstacles did they encounter?

IDENTIFY FOCUS OF THE SESSION

Whereas previous sessions have had an intrapersonal focus, in this session the treatment moves into the interpersonal domain. The therapist lets the client know that now that the client has learned (and, ideally, practiced) some useful emotion regulation skills, they will be able to use them to benefit their relationships. In this session, the focus shifts onto the client's relationships and relationship patterns. The therapist will be helping the client to understand how their models for relationships have developed and how these patterns continue to influence their interactions. The therapist will also help the client to identify how traumatic experiences have influenced their beliefs about themselves and their expectations of others. Along with changing the emotions that they bring to a situation, the client can also learn to change their expectations about an interaction or a relationship.

INTRODUCE CONCEPT OF RELATIONSHIP MODELS AND PATTERNS

In introducing the client to the concept of relationship models and patterns, the therapist can emphasize and elaborate on the points in Handout 15.1, Relationship Models: Instruction Manuals for Relationships. As a way of facilitating meaningful dialogue and to get the client thinking about how these concepts relate to their life, the therapist can ask the client the following questions: "What are your expectations about relationships now? Which do you view as healthy, and which do you view as not so healthy?" The therapist highlights for the client the role of feelings in their present-day interpersonal problems, and describes how intense emotions related to relationship models that were developed in the context of early relationships can at times interfere with current interpersonal goals. In a current interaction, strong feeling states from the past may be triggered and then drive a client's behavior, regardless of important ways in which the present situation may be different or may call for a different response.

Individuals with abuse histories in particular often experience such derailments in situations that elicit power and control—especially when there is a power differential or imbalance, as these are central dynamics of abuse.

EXPLORE AND IDENTIFY CLIENT'S RELATIONSHIP PATTERNS

If possible, the therapist will use an example from the client's life to illustrate the points made above. If none are forthcoming, however, the following example may be useful: A client may feel overworked at their job and taken advantage of by their boss, who has not given the client the raise they deserve. This scenario may remind the client of their childhood exploitation and may quickly give rise to intense feelings of anger and grief. This is a situation in which the client is vulnerable to acting on strong feelings that belong to the past, instead of responding to demands and aims of the current interpersonal situation. Clearly, the feeling of anger at their boss is legitimate and understandable, but the client's level of feeling and the way in which they handle these feelings are what will dictate the outcome. If the client's behavior is driven by their feelings and relationship models related to the past, it is unlikely that they will be able to meet their interpersonal goals in the current situation. In response to the boss's perceived exploitation and abuse, the client may withdraw and become passive, or may alternatively counterattack by expressing anger inappropriately to their boss in an effort at self-defense. Neither of these approaches is likely to result in meeting the client's goal of getting a raise and improving their status at work.

The therapist communicates to the client that a primary goal of this treatment is to help them identify the relationship models that are coming into play in their current relationships and causing problems in their interpersonal functioning. The client will first learn how to recognize when they are being influenced by expectations and strong feelings from the past, and then how to catch and manage these feelings before they interfere with present relationships. Becoming aware of these issues will ultimately give the client more control and choice in terms of how they respond and will make it more likely that their interpersonal goals will be met.

When addressing distinctions between strong feelings from the past and current interpersonal goals, the therapist needs to emphasize that choosing not to act on these strong emotions does *not* invalidate them or imply that they are inappropriate. Many individuals with histories of maltreatment are quick to feel ashamed, discounted, or invalidated. The goal is not to increase a client's sense of distrust in their own perceptions, but rather to help them become aware of ways in which feelings that belong to the past are being activated and are not working in their favor now. Although the client will still be vulnerable to having these feelings triggered in various interpersonal situations, ideally they will feel more aware and in control of them, and can make choices about the extent to which these reactions dictate current behavior.

REVIEW COMMON RELATIONSHIP BELIEFS AMONG SURVIVORS OF TRAUMA

Handout 15.2, Common Relationship Beliefs among Survivors of Trauma, specifies some common expectations that shape relationship patterns among survivors. The therapist directs the client to examine them, to see which expectations they recognize as ones they hold. After the client has checked off these beliefs on the list, the therapist asks the client some questions such as the following, to allow them to reflect on the answers:

> "Do your responses surprise you? How do these thoughts help or hinder your relationships? In what situations are these beliefs helpful or not helpful? How do the beliefs you checked influence your behavior with friends, family members, romantic partners, and acquaintances?"

INTRODUCE RELATIONSHIP PATTERNS WORKSHEET–1

Handout 15.3, Relationship Patterns Worksheet–1, is designed to help clients identify and understand their relationship patterns and the ways old relationship models (which represent assumptions about the self–other dyad) may come to bear on current interactions. This analysis is framed within a cognitive perspective, which includes two parts: beliefs about the self, and beliefs about others' perceptions of the self. With this intervention, the concepts described earlier can be concretized and personalized for each client. The initial goal is to help the client get in touch with experiencing themselves as a "self" with expectations, beliefs, and feelings. Next, the client needs to become aware that they bring a set of expectations, beliefs, and feelings about others into relationships. Given that this is likely to be the first time many clients have tried to articulate these complex concepts, it is critical for the therapist to describe this worksheet and its rationale thoroughly.

PRACTICE USING RELATIONSHIP PATTERNS WORKSHEET–1

The therapist uses time in the session to fill out a copy of Handout 15.3 with the client, and to answer any questions about how the client will proceed in using the form on their own. The purpose of this handout is to help the client articulate their key relationship models and to identify ways these models are negatively affecting current relationships. The therapist can begin by eliciting an example from the client of a recent challenging interpersonal situation. Preferably this situation will have taken place over the past week, so that the details and emotional relevance will be fresher in the client's mind. If the client cannot think of a recent example, the therapist can provide one, based on information discussed in previous sessions. The therapist prompts the client to respond to queries raised in each column of the form as follows, and records their answers:

"What happened in this situation? Who was involved? What did you feel and believe about yourself in this situation? What did you feel and believe the other person thought of you in this situation? How did you expect the other person would respond to you? What action did you take, and what was the result?"

In Session 7, an expanded version of this handout (Handout 16.1, Relationship Patterns Worksheet–2) is presented. It may be helpful to inform the client now that the goal of the next session will be to begin creating and testing alternative models—that is, alternative ways of thinking, feeling, and behaving in relationships, which will create new patterns of relating. However, it is not necessary (or even of much value) to move directly into the generation of alternative models. Initially, it is enough for the client to identify relationship models that are represented in specific interactions. As time goes by, the articulation of a model will become more refined and will become linked to a list of other relationship models.

CASE EXAMPLE: IDENTIFYING A RELATIONSHIP MODEL

Below, we provide a dialogue that took place between a client and therapist as they worked through completing Handout 15.3 (see Box 15.2 for the client's completed copy). The client, Maria, was in her late 20s, with a history of childhood sexual abuse by her stepfather and of military sexual trauma during her time in the Army. In her family there were many "secrets," and the clear message was that these should be kept quiet. Family members rarely discussed their feelings or problems openly, as this was seen as a sign of weakness or self-indulgent complaining. Maria's parents frequently responded to her with statements such as

BOX 15.2

Maria's Completed Relationship Patterns Worksheet–1

Interpersonal situation	What did I feel and think about myself?		What were my expectations about the other person?		My resulting behavior
What happened?	**My feelings**	**My thoughts**	**Their feelings**	**Their thoughts**	**What did I do?**
I had a fight with my sister. I thought about sharing it with Brian, but then decided I shouldn't, that he didn't seem too interested.	Upset. Stressed out. Alone. Worried about seeming Negative.	I am too emotional. I am weak. People can see I am messed up.	Annoyed. Stressed out with work. Frustrated.	She can't get along with anyone. She is always making a big deal about things. Why do I bother with her?	Didn't tell him about it, kept it to myself, shut him out.

Relationship model: "If <u>I share my feelings</u>, then I <u>will be abandoned</u>."

248

"Snap out of it," "Pull yourself together," or "A lot of people have it worse than you; there's nothing to complain about." These messages that she should not burden others with her problems were reinforced during her time in the military. When Maria reported her military sexual trauma, she was punished for doing so and sent away to a different unit.

In treatment, Maria shared that she was beginning a new relationship. Her past romantic relationships had been short-lived and disappointing. Previous boyfriends had told Maria that she was "hard to get close to." Despite Maria's wish to become more open and emotionally close, she found herself repeating the old pattern in this new relationship and came into the session upset about a specific situation. The therapist used this situation to demonstrate the use of Handout 15.3, Relationship Patterns Worksheet–1.

THERAPIST: In this session, we have been talking about relationship patterns—how they develop and are maintained in your current relationships. The situation you mentioned earlier with your boyfriend seems like a familiar one for you, and it caused you some distress. Let's use it as an example to break down the pattern, so we can understand more clearly what happens and how your relationship models may come into play. This is also a good way for us to practice using Relationship Patterns Worksheet–1, so I am going to record the information on a copy of this worksheet. Can you tell me a little more about what happened in this recent situation?

MARIA: Well, I was very upset about the fight I had just had with my sister. I was still really stressed out about it and in a bad mood by the time Brian came to pick me up, but I was trying not to show it. I guess he could tell something was bothering me, even though I was trying to act like it wasn't. He asked me what was wrong.

THERAPIST: How did you respond?

MARIA: I said that nothing was the matter, that I was just tired, and so he left me alone. But then that made me feel even worse, like he just asked to be polite. I figured since he didn't bring it up again that he didn't want to deal with any negativity.

THERAPIST: OK, so I'm going to write down in the "Interpersonal situation" column that you were upset and stressed out about your fight with your sister. Brian asked you what was going on, and you didn't tell him because you thought that he was not that interested. Is that right?

MARIA: Yeah, that's what happened. I considered telling him so I did not have to feel so alone, but then I started worrying that he would get annoyed and think I was being overly dramatic, especially compared to the stress that he is having at his job.

THERAPIST: OK, so let's work it through with the form. Identify the specific sequence. Now that we know what happened, let's think about the next column: What feelings and beliefs did you have about yourself in this situation?

MARIA: I felt like I was too emotional—that I shouldn't be so upset about the thing with my sister. I should be strong enough to handle it on my own and not burden anyone else with it.

THERAPIST: What did you think Brian thought or felt about you in this situation?

MARIA: I don't know. He probably thought I was being negative.

THERAPIST: How did you expect him to respond?

MARIA: Well, if he really wanted to know, he could have asked me more about it.

THERAPIST: What did you expect he would have done if you had told him what was the matter?

MARIA: I figured he would probably be nice about it—but he'd wonder what my problem is, why I can't get along with people, and why I have to make such a big deal out of things.

THERAPIST: So you had an expectation that he would feel annoyed or frustrated with you if you had actually told him.

MARIA: Yeah—that he would have found it a pain to have to deal with a girlfriend who was so emotional. He would see that I am messed up, can't handle things.

THERAPIST: So what did you do in the situation? How did you act?

MARIA: Like I said, I didn't tell him what was wrong, so we drove in silence the whole way to his house.

THERAPIST: And what was the result? How did you end up feeling, and what happened between the two of you?

MARIA: I ending up feeling even worse that there was awkwardness between us, and worried that he would decide he doesn't want to bother with me.

THERAPIST: Good job filling in the details. How did it feel going through this exercise?

MARIA: It was fine, but I don't always remember things in such detail.

THERAPIST: That's OK. Just do your best, and also the sooner you fill out the form after you have a situation like this or some other relationship situation, the easier it will be to remember details. Did you learn anything from what we just did?

MARIA: Basically, just that I tried to act in a way that I thought would be better for the relationship, and it ended up that I still felt bad, and then he felt bad.

THERAPIST: Right. Well, I think it is a good example that gives us useful information. We can start to really see how your feelings about yourself—that you are too emotional, and your belief that others will also see you this way and find you a burden—really dictate how you choose to act. Even in a situation where someone cares about you and wants to know what is going on, you keep them at a distance and maybe miss an opportunity to feel better and also closer.

After completing this exercise with a client, it is helpful for the therapist to ask how it felt and what was learned. The therapist can share their own observations about how the identified feelings, expectations, and beliefs of self and other may have contributed to the situation's outcome.

SUMMARIZE THE GOALS OF THE SESSION

The purpose of this session is to help the client describe interpersonal difficulties and identify potential trauma-generated relationship models that might be underlying these difficulties. Validation of relationship models based in actual experience is important, as is the awareness that trauma-generated relationship patterns were originally developed by the client during childhood as an adaptation to their toxic environment. The therapeutic goal is for the client to achieve better understanding or insight into why they behave and feel the way they do in their current relationships. The articulation of relevant relationship models is the first step in creating change in relationship patterns. Once the client has a clearer grasp of why they behave the way they do, then they are free to decide to do something differently. It may take a while for the therapist and client to identify the core relationship models. It is a process of identifying a possible model and assessing whether it "feels" right and whether the model helps explain behaviors in other relationships as well. The use of Relationship Patterns Worksheet–1 is intended to facilitate discovery of the models at work in the client's various interactions. At the end of the session, the therapist provides the client with the copy of Relationship Patterns Worksheet–1 that was completed during the session, along with blank copies of this handout to complete during the week. Handout 15.4, How to Complete Relationship Patterns Worksheet–1, provides support for the client in filling out this worksheet independently.

PLAN SKILLS PRACTICE

The therapist asks the client if they think they can try applying Relationship Patterns Worksheet–1 to specific interpersonal situations that may arise over the week. Ideally, they should try to complete a copy of this worksheet once daily. The therapist can remind the client again of the rationale and say something like this:

> "In addition to helping you with PTSD symptoms, another central way this treatment can be useful is by helping you improve the quality of your relationships. In order to do so, we need to begin with specifics as to what is actually happening in your day-to-day interactions with others."

The therapist will also want to discuss any potential problems or concerns that the client might encounter in trying to do this work between sessions. For example, the therapist will want to make sure that the client doesn't feel pressure to complete the form "correctly." Instead, the client is encouraged to view it as an experiment and to see how it feels to use on their own. In addition, the therapist will remind the client to continue to practice Focused Breathing, to identify and engage in at least one pleasurable activity, and to keep trying out other emotion regulation skills that feel applicable to situations that arise over the week.

Relationship Models: Instruction Manuals for Relationships

WHAT DOES YOUR RELATIONSHIP INSTRUCTION MANUAL LOOK LIKE?

- **What are relationship models?** These are models we develop of relationships that act as "blueprints" or "instruction manuals." They reflect our beliefs about ourselves, about others, and about how relationships work. They guide our expectations, feelings, and behaviors in relationships.

- **How are they created?** They are initially formed in our early environments, in the context of our relationships to caregivers and our experiences in our families. We learn to think, do, and feel *what allowed us to be successful or kept us safe* in those situations:
  - *We do what rewarded us then.* For example, being a nurturer led to love, or being distrustful/ keeping people at a distance led to safety.
  - *We don't do what led to punishment/negative consequences then.* For example, trusting others or relaxing your guard led to abuse, or asserting your needs led to aggression, criticism, or danger.

- **How are they influenced by trauma?** Abusive or neglectful environments, or other traumatic experiences, affect how these models are developed and often result in negative beliefs about ourselves and expectations that others will view and treat us poorly.
  - Example: "I can't trust others; other people will hurt me."

- **How do they affect us now?** The relationship models we developed earlier in life continue to play a central role in shaping thoughts, feelings, and behaviors in ways that we may not be aware of or notice. We bring them into adulthood and apply them to current situations.
  - Example: " I still can't trust others, even now."

- **How do they become relationship patterns?** Relationship models can act as self-fulfilling prophecies, because they lead us to behave in ways that prepare us for what we expect will happen in relationships. Over time the relationship models we rely on become more generalized and ingrained, and form our relationship patterns. We don't give ourselves opportunities for new experiences or look for evidence that might contradict our beliefs. Instead, we may continue to behave in ways we learned in early relationships, which may not be effective or helpful in current relationship situations.
  - Example: Shelby has a belief that no one will love him because he is unlovable. So he keeps others at a distance and isolates himself. Therefore, he misses opportunities for others to get to know him. He then uses the fact that he does not have close friends or a romantic partner as evidence that he must be unlovable.

- **The good news: Relationship patterns can be modified!** You can write a new instruction manual for yourself. This treatment will help you explore, identify, and change patterns to be more flexible and effective in your current and future relationships.

Common Relationship Beliefs among Survivors of Trauma

The first step to changing your relationship patterns is identifying them. Check the beliefs that you recognize in your life.

SAFETY

☐ If I let someone close to me, I may get hurt.

☐ The only way to stay safe is to keep others at a distance

☐ If I am alone, I can't take care of or protect myself.

TRUST/INTIMACY

☐ I can't trust my own judgment to stay safe, or I have bad judgment.

☐ No one can be trusted. I can't trust that others will keep me safe or have my best interests in mind.

☐ I can't trust anyone enough to share what happened to me.

   ☐ Others cannot handle hearing my experiences.

   ☐ They will judge/hate/disrespect me if they find out what has happened to me.

POWER/CONTROL

☐ I cannot control anything in my life. I am powerless to solve problems in my life.

☐ I cannot trust others to be in control.

☐ People who have power abuse it.

☐ Who has power is an either–or situation. Only one person can have power (either another person has it or I have it, but both of us cannot have power).

SELF-ESTEEM/NEEDS

☐ If I share my problems or disclose my feelings, I will not be respected or will be seen as weak.

☐ If I don't sacrifice my goals/needs in relationships, others will not love me.

☐ Others' needs are more important than my own.

☐ Asserting my needs will cause problems in my relationships.

☐ Only one person's needs can be met at a time.

☐ If I am not in a romantic relationship, something is wrong with me.

☐ I am broken/crazy/unlovable.

Relationship Patterns Worksheet–1

Interpersonal situation	What did I feel and think about myself?		What were my expectations about the other person?		My resulting behavior
What happened?	My feelings	My thoughts	Their feelings	Their thoughts	What did I do?

Relationship model: "If _____, then _____."

How to Complete Relationship Patterns Worksheet–1

- Take note when your interactions with others feel uncomfortable, confusing, or stressful, or lead to misunderstandings or conflicts.

- Notice your thoughts and emotions in these challenging interactions.

- Notice what your expectations of others are in these situations. Notice what you believe is going on for them (their thoughts, emotions, and behaviors) and your evidence for your expectations (is it "hard evidence," or could you be "mind reading"?).

- You will summarize this by using two new tools called the Relationship Patterns Worksheets. Today we will introduce the first of these sheets, Relationship Patterns Worksheet–1.

- You will note that Relationship Patterns Worksheet–1 is just like the Feelings Monitoring Form, in that you will focus on situations, thoughts, and feelings. The only difference is that now it involves two people, and you will also focus on your beliefs about the other person's feelings and thoughts about the situations.

- After you have completed describing the problematic situation, try to identify what relationship model or "blueprint" you may have been using in this situation.

Changing Relationship Patterns

Focus on Assertiveness

> In emotional life as in much of history, we are only doomed to repeat
> what has not been remembered, reflected upon and worked through.
> —ROBERT KAREN (1998, p. 408)

Session 6 has focused on educating the client about interpersonal patterns and working to identify them. The next step, which is the focus of Sessions 7–9, involves helping the client develop alternative, more flexible interpersonal patterns—ones that allow for positive expectations of others, and for the possibility of effectively and adaptively negotiating interpersonal needs and difficulties. These three sessions will involve attention to various types of interpersonal problems.

We begin in Session 7 with assertiveness, because exhibiting appropriate levels of assertiveness is a common problem among individuals who have experienced interpersonal trauma. Interpersonal trauma, especially chronic interpersonal violence, is a situation in which an individual has lost the capacity for autonomy and effective assertiveness. As a result, problems in being underassertive (passive), overassertive (aggressive), or both can emerge. To reach an effective and comfortable middle ground between submissive and controlling or aggressive behaviors, STAIR encourages the client to identify their assumptions about assertiveness, to learn about the potential benefits of behaving more assertively or less aggressively, and to create opportunities to learn and practice specific skills accordingly. During the session, the therapist and client will conduct role plays to try out different ways of relating, followed by feedback from the therapist. Second, the therapist and client will identify the alternative interpersonal expectations that support these new behaviors. The alternative beliefs, feelings, and actions will be registered on Relationship Patterns Worksheet–2, an expanded version of Relationship Patterns Worksheet–1, which the client can use as a tool to extend their range of possible responses in interpersonal situations. The therapist will want to predict for the client that making these changes can be quite challenging, because old interpersonal patterns are pervasive and powerful, but that change is possible. Box 16.1 outlines the content for this session.

256

Theme and Curriculum for Session 7
Changing Relationship Patterns: Focus on Assertiveness

Once the client's key relationship models have been identified, the next step is to begin generating alternative, more flexible ones. Though this is not an easy process, therapist and client develop aspirational relational models and then experiment with new ways of interacting with others that align with the models. These include making new assumptions, trying out alternative behaviors, and exploring different feelings. Role playing and covert modeling are useful ways to develop and practice new interpersonal skills. This session focuses on identifying and revising problematic patterns related to assertiveness.

PLANNING AND PREPARATION

Using material from past sessions, consider what type of assertiveness problems the client may have. Bring handouts for this session, including several copies of Handout 16.4 (see list below). The work in the session is estimated to take about 60 minutes; a flexible application is assumed (i.e., not every client will need all interventions).

AGENDA

- Check-in and review of skills practice.
- Identify focus of the session.
- Provide psychoeducation about assertiveness and basic personal rights.
- Clarify basis of client's assumptions about assertiveness (as relevant).
- Review and practice an "I Message" (the first role play).
- Complete Relationship Patterns Worksheet–2.
- Introduce additional assertiveness skills to practice.
- Summarize the goals of the session.
- Plan skills practice:
  - Complete two copies of Relationship Patterns Worksheet–2, with a focus on assertiveness.
  - Use skills from all channels as applicable to interpersonal events described in the copies of Relationship Patterns Worksheet–2.
  - Do something pleasurable.
  - Continue to practice Focused Breathing twice daily.

(continued)

SESSION HANDOUTS

Handout 16.1. Understanding Assertiveness

Handout 16.2. Basic Personal Rights

Handout 16.3. "I Messages"

Handout 16.4. Relationship Patterns Worksheet–2 (several copies)

Handout 16.5. Additional Assertiveness Skills

Handout 16.6. Practicing Assertiveness to Improve Relationship Patterns

---

CHECK-IN AND REVIEW OF SKILLS PRACTICE

Before the therapist begins this session's work on assertiveness, the therapist spends some time reviewing the Relationship Patterns Worksheet–1 entries brought in by the client. The therapist quickly confirms that the client has correctly completed the entries, particularly the expectations they have about the thoughts and feelings of others, since assessing these expectations is a new task. As the therapist reads through the entries, they can highlight emerging interpersonal themes that fall into the categories to be discussed in the next few weeks: assertiveness, power, and closeness/intimacy. The therapist can explicitly note that these themes will be discussed in future sessions, as long as the client can remain focused on the present discussion. It is possible that at least one issue relates at least indirectly to assertiveness, which will allow the therapist to segue to today's topic.

IDENTIFY FOCUS OF THE SESSION

The therapist begins the session by noting its focus on using newly discovered insights on the client's relationship patterns (from the previous session) to begin to make improvements aligned with the client's personal goals and values. This session starts the process of applying insights by exploring relationships and/or social situations that involve opportunities to practice effective assertiveness.

PROVIDE PSYCHOEDUCATION ABOUT ASSERTIVENESS AND BASIC PERSONAL RIGHTS

Discuss Concept of Assertiveness

Therapists should not assume that clients all have the same ideas about the meaning of the word "assertiveness." Instead, a therapist begins by asking a client what the client thinks being assertive means. This question will provide a jumping-off point for the session and will give the therapist information about the client's assertiveness beliefs, as well as any assumptions about assertiveness that may need to be challenged. There are numerous misconceptions about assertiveness: for example, "Being assertive means being impolite, demanding, or selfish," "To be assertive, I must be prepared for fights or confrontations," or "If I assert myself, I'll be disliked or punished." These misconceptions are especially true of individuals who have experienced chronic interpersonal violence—who have been actively discouraged from asserting their rights and needs, whose personal boundaries have been violated, and who may have been penalized for trying to stand up for themselves.

After the brief introductory conversation, the therapist gives the client Handout 16.1, Understanding Assertiveness, so the client can follow along during the review of the information summarized below. The therapist can begin this review by emphasizing that assertiveness entails standing up for one's rights and presenting one's needs or wants in a way that is respectful of both oneself and others. "Assertive" behavior must be distinguished from "nonassertive" and "aggressive" behavior, and brief general examples of each can clarify these distinctions. It may be helpful to ask the client to provide some brief examples of their own or of others' nonassertive, aggressive, and assertive behavior, to make these concepts more personally meaningful.

In nonassertive behavior, an individual disregards or does not directly express their own rights, needs, and desires. They often act passively or submissively and permit others to violate their rights. Nonassertive behavior may lead to feeling hurt, resentful, angry, frustrated, anxious, ignored, and/or disappointed in oneself.

In aggressive behavior, an individual acts upon their rights at the expense of others through intimidation and bullying. They may behave in ways that are manipulative, openly hostile, and/or demanding; at the extreme end, these behaviors can lead to threatening, inappropriate outbursts or even physical violence. Aggressive behavior may lead to feeling angry, out of control, frightened, and/or guilty.

The therapist explains that the same person may at different times display both nonassertive and aggressive behavior, and that these shifts often occur cyclically. For example, a person who typically has difficulty being direct and setting limits with others is likely to become more and more resentful and frustrated over time. This type of emotional buildup that comes with being consistently overcompliant makes the person more vulnerable to losing control at some point and reacting angrily or aggressively in a situation that does not necessarily merit such a strong response. This type of reaction in turn may elicit defensiveness and anger from others—the very things that the nonassertive individual was so desperately trying to avoid.

In assertive behavior, on the other hand, an individual consistently stands up for their rights in a way that neither infringes upon the rights of others nor evokes interpersonal hostility. Assertive behavior may lead to feeling more confident and powerful, is likely to open the door to more choices, and can also result in increased intimacy and honesty in relationships. These potential benefits provide the rationale for the focus of the exercises in this session—identifying specific problems and interpersonal patterns related to assertiveness, and developing appropriate assertiveness skills.

After defining assertiveness and differentiating it from other behaviors, the therapist discusses basic personal rights, before going on to identify more specifically the client's typical beliefs and interpersonal patterns with regard to assertiveness.

Discuss Basic Personal Rights

For a client to initiate assertive behavior in which they advocate for their own welfare, they must understand that they are entitled to basic personal rights. Unfortunately, survivors of interpersonal trauma are often taught the opposite—that they do not have personal rights. Thus it is important for the therapist to introduce this concept by exploring the list in Handout 16.2, Basic Personal Rights. The therapist reviews these rights briefly with the client, elicits the client's reactions, and then asks where they may expect any difficulties. The therapist keeps in mind that although these personal rights may seem straightforward and self-explanatory, many clients with a history of interpersonal trauma may see these rights as new ideas, and reviewing them can be a powerful and meaningful experience. After the session, the client will review and reflect on Handouts 16.1 and 16.2 more carefully at home.

CLARIFY BASIS FOR CLIENT'S ASSUMPTIONS ABOUT ASSERTIVENESS (AS RELEVANT)

If time permits and the topic is relevant to the client, the therapist can encourage the client to give examples of how needs and wants were communicated and responded to in their family of origin. The goal of this discussion is for the therapist and client to have a concrete understanding and clear examples of the client's typical thoughts, feelings, and behaviors centering around assertiveness and control. These examples also provide elaboration of the more subtle aspects of how the client's interpersonal patterns work; as such, they can help clarify to the client their own personal history, and can also provide detail for use in the role plays later in the session. Linking assertiveness difficulties to these experiences will help reduce any sense of blame that the client may feel about what are now maladaptive ways of acting and thinking.

The following questions can be helpful in generating specific links between the client's current difficulties with assertiveness and experiences they had with their family of origin:

> "How did people in your family model assertive, nonassertive, and aggressive behaviors?"
>
> "How did you generally communicate your needs and wants, and how did family members respond to these requests?"
>
> "How did family members respond to your attempts to be assertive?"

Frequently, survivors of childhood maltreatment come from families in which assertive behaviors were not a viable option for communicating needs and wants. In these families, needs were often met through violent and aggressive means (e.g., by an abusive parent) or were denied and downplayed (e.g., by a passive parent). For example, a child not only may be the target of a parent's aggressive style of getting their "needs" met, but also may witness the abusive parent behaving aggressively toward other family members. In such an abusive environment, a child may see the mother, for example, responding passively to the abusive father; or the mother may tell the child, "Don't bother your father with that, or he'll get angry." In addition, survivors have often experienced negative consequences of attempts at assertiveness. A child who does gather the courage to protest against any maltreatment often experiences additional maltreatment in response. Often only models of aggressive and nonassertive behavior are available in these families. There is typically neither any model of appropriate assertiveness nor any opportunity to learn that negotiation of needs is possible. Instead, children who grow up in this kind of family environment come to believe that getting needs met is an all-or-nothing process: One person gets what they want at another's expense.

REVIEW AND PRACTICE AN "I MESSAGE" (THE FIRST ROLE PLAY)

Now that the importance of being assertive and the specific difficulties in this area have been reviewed, the therapist can provide the client with information on how to develop more effective assertiveness skills. One of the most popular and universally helpful skills taught in STAIR is learning to communicate with "I Messages," as outlined in Handout 16.3, "I Messages."

Describe "I Messages"

"I Messages" are important assertiveness tools, because they promote communication with another person about the effects of the other's behavior. For the client, the purpose of "I Messages" is to focus on the negative impact of the other person's troubling behavior on the client, instead of blaming the other person's character or personality. As a result, the other person is less likely to feel attacked and to respond with defensiveness. An "I Message" has three parts: "behavior," "feeling," and "consequence." The following formula can be helpful:

> *Behavior:* "When I [state observed behavior] . . ."
> *Feeling:* "I feel [state the feeling] . . ."
> *Consequence:* "because I [state the consequence for the client]."

An example of an "I Message" is "When I wasn't picked up in time, I felt frustrated, because I missed my appointment." Another is "When I was yelled at, I felt hurt and upset, and it makes me not want to talk to you." The therapist models for the client how they might use an "I Message" in a recent interpersonal interaction, and then has the client practice using the skill.

Provide Rationale for Role Playing

Before conducting the first role play, the therapist communicates the rationale and potential benefits of role-playing exercises. Role playing provides an experiential basis for identifying the client's skills and comfort level with the new behaviors they are learning, and offers opportunities to demonstrate developing mastery. It also provides insight about what feelings and beliefs come up when the client tries to change their routinized behaviors and responses. A role play is not a test or evaluation, but instead an opportunity to practice and experiment with different ways of interacting in relationships. In this way, the therapy can serve as an "interpersonal laboratory" in which the client can practice difficult interactions "live" with the therapist and receive immediate feedback on the process in a safe environment. Role playing also gives the therapist and client a shared sense of what a particular situation is actually like—not just some theorized version of it. As a result, the therapist and client can talk more effectively about aspects of the client's approach that may hinder or derail them from reaching their interpersonal goals. The therapist can also highlight aspects that are particularly effective for getting a specific message across.

Role Play with an "I Message"

The first role play will be a practice of an "I Message." This basic skill is fairly well scripted and likely to be relatively comfortable for the client. The therapist asks the client to identify a situation in which they would like to share an uncomfortable feeling or message to someone. The therapist and client can refer to situations described in the client's filled-out copies of the Feelings Monitoring Form. The use of an "I Message" as a first role play is beneficial, because it provides a microcosm of many communication difficulties and problematic dynamics that are present in assertiveness situations more generally. An "I Message" includes the fundamental ingredients and building blocks for other forms of assertiveness, which may take the client more time to master.

The therapist can begin the role play by providing some general tips about communication, especially about how to express feelings without putting the other person on the defensive or getting caught up in side issues. For example, the therapist can explain that it is usually more effective to use an "I Message" and focus on one's own feelings than to focus on the other's behavior or potential motives. Emphasizing how any person's feelings cannot be "wrong" or "invalid" is also key, as is observing ways in which the client may undermine their own communication attempts. For instance, many clients will be overly apologetic or use disclaimers before even beginning, such as "I know this may seem like I'm making a big deal of this, but . . ." or "I don't mean to be picky, but . . ." Describing to such a client how this type of introduction is a "set-up" for them to be minimized can help them make important shifts. Alternatively, some clients will communicate with a more aggressive style. The therapist will want to make such a client aware that this type of approach could be off-putting and obscure their message.

Guidelines for Conducting Effective Role Plays

In our experience, role plays can be powerful tools in therapy, but they also require the therapist to have a deeper understanding of the process and alternative approaches. Box 16.2 outlines the general process and format. Below, we describe some key components of

BOX 16.2

Basic Steps of Role-Playing Exercises

1. The therapist provides the rationale for role playing.
   - It is a method for "trying on" and fine-tuning different ways of interacting in interpersonal situations.
     - It provides an opportunity to get immediate feedback from the therapist.
2. The client and therapist identify a relevant interpersonal situation.
   - If possible, they use an example client has recorded on Relationship Patterns Worksheet–1 between sessions.
     - Otherwise, the therapist asks the client to describe a recent relevant interpersonal situation.
     - Therapist and client choose a situation with a moderate distress level.
3. First role-play sequence: The client plays themselves, and the therapist plays the other person.
   - After initial sequence, the therapist obtains any needed clarification on the client's goals in the interaction, shares observations about the role play, provides feedback, and makes suggestions for improving the communication.
4. Second role-play sequence (with therapist modeling): The therapist role-plays behavior, language, and tone of voice that would align with the client's goals. The client imagines what the other person might feel and think on receiving the message as presented by the therapist.
   - Afterward, the therapist asks client for feedback on the approach. Does the client have any suggestions or observations? Can the client see themselves using this alternative approach?
5. Third role-play sequence: The client plays themselves, and the therapist plays the other person.
   - Afterward, the therapist asks the client to describe how the role play felt this time, as compared to when the client did it in the initial role play of the situation.
     - The therapist and client discuss how the client can continue to practice.

the exercise and one alternative for clients who are not ready for direct role plays with a therapist.

Setting the stage and sequencing the role play

To set the stage, the therapist and client must agree upon basic background information before beginning the exercise (e.g., the context for each specific interaction, the nature of the client's relationship with the other person involved, the client's main goal for the interaction). This clarification also allows the therapist to respond in a realistic and helpful way during the role play itself. Once the therapist has identified the interpersonal situation and has ensured that the client understands the rationale for the exercise, the role playing can begin.

In the first role play, the client acts as themselves and the therapist as the other person in the interaction. This initial role play will give the therapist an opportunity to see how the client has addressed (or plans to address) this situation, rather than relying solely on the client's description. After the first role play has been completed, the therapist can ask questions, share observations, provide feedback, and make suggestions for improving the communication (see the next subsection for tips for providing feedback).

In the second role play, the therapist can model how to implement the feedback in the same situation, with the therapist now playing the role of the client and the client taking the role of the other person. After this run-through, it is crucial to ask the client how it sounded to them and whether they could realistically picture themselves using the modeled approach. The goal is to help the client come up with a style of communication that remains genuine and fits their personality, rather than having the client adopt the therapist's particular wording of a response in a memorized, rote way. In this role play, the therapist's approach should be presented as just one alternative, rather than as "the right way." This attitude also demonstrates the key theme of flexibility, which is woven into STAIR's philosophy of emotional and relational well-being throughout the treatment protocol. In this spirit, the client should be encouraged to discuss what may or may not work about the way the therapist managed the situation in the role play. It is also helpful for the therapist to validate how challenging it can be to respond in certain situations, especially when emotions are strong and conflict is present. The therapist will be in a good position to comment on this complexity after having had the experience of playing the role of the client (e.g., "I can really see now how having your mother say those things would feel pretty intimidating").

In the third and usually final role play, the therapist and client reverse roles again, giving the client the opportunity to play themselves a second time. In this role play, the client is encouraged to try out the therapist's feedback and experiment with an alternative approach. Afterward, the therapist asks the client to describe how the role play felt this time, as compared to the first time they did it. Ideally, the client will notice some differences after incorporating the feedback. The client can practice the situation both within and outside the session until they feel a sense of mastery.

Giving feedback on interpersonal style

Giving feedback to any client on their interpersonal style can be a challenging task. Many individuals who have experienced sexual, physical, or emotional abuse have an enhanced sensitivity to perceived disapproval. If such clients feel they are being criticized, they may become defensive, shut down, and/or feel ashamed—none of which are conducive to practicing new interpersonal skills. Feedback is most effective if it follows a sequence in which the therapist provides positive feedback (what went well), followed by constructive feedback (what could be even better), and then ending with encouragement or reiteration of the positive feedback. To minimize the risk of a client's feeling judged or misunderstood, the therapist keeps the following guidelines in mind when providing feedback:

- Reiterate that interpersonal skills are learned—we are not born with them—and that learning any new skills takes practice. It is likely that the client did not have role models for effective communication or opportunities to practice these skills in their childhood environment. These factors probably make managing current interpersonal situations more challenging.
- Put the emphasis on generating alternatives, as opposed to rejecting the client's current approach. Communicate explicitly that there is no "right" or "wrong" way to express oneself, but rather a range of options the client can choose from, depending on the interpersonal message they would like to convey in a given interaction.
- Provide information about both strengths and weaknesses in discussing the client's style of communication, and be as specific as possible.
- When addressing problems or sticking points, provide the potential experience of the other person in the interaction, rather than directly using your own perceptions, as the latter might be overwhelming or confusing to the client. An example of such a comment is "A person in this situation might feel rejected by what you said about not really caring about their point of view."
- Ask the client how it felt for them to receive feedback, and whether there were things with which they agreed or disagreed.

Using covert modeling as an alternative

For some clients or in some situations, a technique called "covert modeling" may be more appropriate than explicit role playing. This approach is the same as role playing, except that the client is asked to imagine the situation and then describe and discuss it in detail with the therapist, rather than acting it out. The therapist can prompt the client by asking questions such as "What could you say to this person?", "How do you think you can best communicate your feelings to meet your goal in this situation?", or "How do you think you would handle it if they got angry?" The therapist can suggest that the client "try on for size" various approaches until they find one that fits their style.

This method is particularly useful for clients who are too self-conscious to engage in role playing, or for situations that do not lend themselves to effective role plays (e.g., sexual intimacy). If a therapist observes that a particular client is struggling with the role playing, or that it does not appear helpful for the client, covert modeling may be the preferred method of generating alternative scenarios. In fact, the therapist can bypass role playing altogether and start here instead if it appears that a role-play approach would not be maximally effective.

Another strength of covert modeling is that clients can use this method to work through future distressing or difficult situations without the therapist's presence. Between sessions, clients can practice talking themselves through situations by asking themselves, "What could I say in this situation?" or "How would it sound if I said it this way?" This exercise can be particularly effective if a client has the capacity to use it in combination with "positive visualization"—that is, actually imagining themselves in the situation and managing it successfully.

COMPLETE RELATIONSHIP PATTERNS WORKSHEET–2

The next step in the session is to introduce and complete Handout 16.4, Relationship Patterns Worksheet–2. This worksheet is new to the treatment, in that it includes space not only for a description of the old relationship pattern (as in Relationship Patterns Worksheet–1), but also for the formulation of a healthier alternative. The role-play experience of using an "I Message" can be used to help illuminate old beliefs, feelings, and behaviors, as well as the client's comfort level with the articulation of an alternative.

CASE EXAMPLE: AN "I MESSAGE" ROLE PLAY

Caroline, a client with a history of multiple sexual traumas, came to Session 7 acknowledging her need to practice assertiveness. When asked to give a recent example in which she had had difficulty with assertiveness, she shared her experience with Paul, a new man she had met during the course of the treatment. Caroline described being interested in Paul, but not ready to begin serious sexual involvement. Caroline felt that she had communicated this to Paul on their first two dates through her avoidance of situations in which they would be alone in private. On the third date, Caroline agreed to let Paul drive her home. When he asked to come in, she consented, even though she did not think it was a good idea. She became very uncomfortable when he told her that he was attracted to her and felt confused when he began to kiss her. She let it go on for several minutes and then told Paul that she did not feel well; she apologized and said she thought she should get some rest. After Caroline had shared the specifics of the situation, she and the therapist used a role play of an "I Message" to communicate her wishes. After they practiced, they discussed what underlying beliefs had made it so difficult for her to say what she meant, and explored alternative beliefs that could support new and healthier behaviors. These were worked through, using a copy of Relationship Patterns Worksheet–2 (see Box 16.3 for Caroline's completed example). The discussion began as follows:

THERAPIST: How did you feel about yourself in this situation?

CAROLINE: I felt silly—like "Why should this be such a big deal? I am a grown woman and should be able to handle a man kissing me." But the reality is that I was nervous and confused and just wanted him to go, so I could get my thoughts together.

THERAPIST: How did you expect him to respond to you asking him to leave?

CAROLINE: I didn't know how he would react—maybe get angry that I led him on by having him come up and then making him leave, or maybe just think I was nuts and never call me again.

THERAPIST: Neither of which were appealing outcomes. So what did you do?

CAROLINE: I was searching my mind for what to say without offending him or having

BOX 16.3

Caroline's Completed Relationship Patterns Worksheet–2

Interpersonal situation	What did I feel and think about myself?		What were my expectations about the other person?		My resulting behavior
What happened?	**My feelings**	**My thoughts**	**Their feelings**	**Their thoughts**	**What did I do?**
Allowed Paul to come in, but then wanted him to leave when he started kissing me.	I felt scared and nervous.	I should be able to handle this. I don't know what to say or do. Do I have a right?	He might get angry, feeling I led him on.	He will think that I should have stopped before and it is too late. He might think I am nuts and never call again.	I waited until I couldn't handle it any more and made up an excuse for why he should go. I felt relieved, but also bad and guilty.

Relationship model: "If I want to have a relationship _____, then I should not have opinions or make a fuss _____."

Interpersonal goals for situation	Alternative beliefs and feelings about myself: What else could I . . .		Alternative beliefs and feelings about the other person: What else could I expect the other person . . .		Alternative actions
What are my goals in this situation?	**. . . feel about myself?**	**. . . think about myself?**	**. . . to feel?**	**. . . to think?**	**What else could I do?**
Share my feelings about not wanting to be kissed, and continue to see Paul.	I could feel confident that I have the right to express my feelings and slow things down.	It is OK to begin a relationship without sex or even without kissing. I have a right to express this preference.	He could feel compassion and empathy for me.	He might be OK with this. He might like that I shared my discomfort and preferences.	I can tell him that when he kisses me, I feel nervous, because I am not ready for it. I can also say that I like him and want to see him again.
					What else might they do?

Alternative relationship model: "If I want to have a (real, true) relationship with someone _____, then it is important for me to share my preferences, beliefs, and feelings (kindly) _____."

to get into a whole thing about it. I waited until I couldn't handle it any more, and then I made up an excuse for why he needed to go.

THERAPIST: OK. What was the result of that action?

CAROLINE: Well, he did leave, so I felt relieved, but I also felt bad and guilty.

THERAPIST: What did you feel badly about?

CAROLINE: Everything—I didn't handle it right. He hasn't called me, and I feel like I blew a chance with someone I liked.

Caroline and the therapist spent time talking about how Caroline could have responded in this particular situation. While neither of them could say how the situation would have sorted itself out, Caroline could have been more assertive about her wishes and preferences to Paul, which could have led to clearer communication and plans for the future.

THERAPIST: It is clear that you were feeling overwhelmed and were having trouble putting your thoughts together. Why don't we try to formulate an "I Message" that identifies what you were feeling and why? That might make it easier for you to propose an action plan in this scenario if it comes up again, and for him to have a chance to know what you want and why.

CAROLINE: OK, here goes . . . When you kiss me, I feel nervous, because I am not ready for this (*said very softly and apologetically, with eyes downcast and an air of guilt*).

THERAPIST: You were really able to put the words together. So congratulations to you for stringing together all the words together and saying what you meant. But the tone of voice sounds like you have something to apologize for. This is your point of view, and you can say it more firmly, but also with kindness and compassion to him and for yourself. I am going to say your words, but in a different tone of voice. (*Does this, looking straight at Caroline, and using a soft but clear voice.*)

CAROLINE: That sounded so much more like a communication than an apology!

THERAPIST: Why don't you try it again? Say the same sentence, but with a sense that you are sharing something about yourself, and that you believe he will hear it and understand you.

CAROLINE: (*Completes role play with more energy and direct eye contact. Also adds at the end of the sentence:*) I'd like to end the night now. See you again another time.

THERAPIST: How did that feel?

CAROLINE: Very, very scary. But good. Once I said that I was nervous about kissing, the action plan to meet another time just tumbled out naturally.

THERAPIST: That is awesome. Not everyone would be able to make the transition from stating a feeling to making a plan, but you did it!

CAROLINE: Yes, I would really like to see him again. But I can see how much better I feel if I can share my feelings and thoughts with him first.

Caroline and the therapist spent some time talking about how, in this particular situation, Caroline's beliefs about herself and Paul were related to some of her core beliefs about assertiveness. Caroline was aware of her long-standing difficulties in being able to assert her needs, especially in the face of others' competing needs. In thinking about how assertiveness was typically managed in her family, Caroline noted that she and her siblings were "not allowed" to say if there was something they didn't like: "If my mother even thought she saw a sour look, she would threaten to smack it off our faces."

Caroline seemed to have coped with this environment by learning to distance herself from her feelings and needs. As she put it, "we just learned not to have opinions," which made going along with her parents' demands easier. What she also learned was that her needs were really not important and that it was best for her not to show them. Thus she did not have much experience with tuning in to her needs, let alone trying to express them effectively to other people. The sense that it was better to go along than to fight for what she wanted was further confirmed by the times she did try to assert herself: "People either don't listen—they act like they didn't even hear me—or I have been told that I am making things complicated."

The therapist then shifted to working with Caroline on the potential for other scenarios, despite the fact that it was hard for her to imagine any.

THERAPIST: Let's just experiment with the possibility of other options, starting with identifying what your goals were in this situation with Paul. What did you want in terms of the relationship in this interaction?

CAROLINE: I wanted him to like me, and I wanted him to ask me out again.

THERAPIST: All right, we've identified that you wanted to continue the relationship. That's important, because if you did not want continued contact, that would change your approach. What else, including what you did *not* want in this particular situation?

CAROLINE: What I did not want is exactly what happened. I didn't want to get in a situation where sex was a possibility. I wouldn't have minded a quick kiss, but I knew I wasn't ready for anything more.

THERAPIST: OK, so you wanted to maintain the connection, but didn't want it to get sexual.

CAROLINE: Yes—but I'm not sure if that's even possible with a man, if he would put up with that.

THERAPIST: Right. Well, it seems like that assumption is part of what made it hard to be direct. What else could you have felt or believed about yourself in this situation?

CAROLINE: That I wasn't crazy or ridiculous?

THERAPIST: Yes—that your wish to continue the relationship without getting sexual at this point was valid instead of shameful. What about your expectations of Paul? You feared he would get angry or reject you if you said something. What else could you have expected from him?

CAROLINE: I guess to not get mad or reject me, but I don't know if that would have worked.

THERAPIST: But you did a good job of saying what you wanted. And in the end, you seemed to feel better about yourself. We really don't know what Paul would have liked or not liked. You did signal that you wanted to maintain a connection with him. Just try to stretch your mind to let yourself think of other possibilities.

CAROLINE: OK, I could have expected him to be nice and understand—that's what I would have wanted.

THERAPIST: Now if you had these alternative beliefs and expectations that your feelings were valid and that Paul might understand them, what other belief might you be proposing?

CAROLINE: That I could share my feelings and still maintain a connection with him. Or that I could share my feelings and he might see them as legitimate.

THERAPIST: Right. At least if you believed that there was a possibility of him being understanding, you could have taken the risk and be more direct about what was really going on. Also, you might have been able to tell him right off the bat that you didn't want him to come up to your apartment, without being apologetic or guilty.

CAROLINE: Maybe, but even then I don't know if I could say it in the right way.

THERAPIST: Right. Well, that might take some practice, since these are new skills you are learning. That's why we are going to do more role playing.

The therapist and Caroline then completed a copy of Relationship Patterns Work-sheet–2, as shown in Box 16.3. It included a summary of what actually happened, as well as a formulation of an alternative scenario in which Caroline's beliefs, feelings, and actions differed, based on a change in a core interpersonal pattern. As indicated in Box 16.3, therapist and client jotted down what actually happened during the interaction in the top portion of the worksheet. They then spent some time discussing what belief was driving this interaction. As indicated above, Caroline was raised with a core interpersonal belief that "If I want to have a relationship, then I should not have opinions or make a fuss." This core belief had helped her get along in an abusive home environment, but this belief and the attendant feelings and behaviors were, at a minimum, leading to confused communications.

The alternative core belief that the therapist proposed during the session was "I can be connected and share my feelings and preferences," or "If I want to have a (real, true) relationship with someone, then it is important for me to share my preferences, beliefs, and feelings (kindly)." The therapist proposed the second wording of this alternative explicitly to the client. Then, assuming the alternative core belief, the therapist and client completed the concrete details of this particular scenario. Here the therapist and client articulated that Caroline's interpersonal goals in this situation were to share her feelings about not wanting to kiss *and* to continue seeing Paul. With this goal, the therapist and Caroline completed alternative feelings and beliefs that Caroline could have about herself. These included that she could feel confident about having the right to express her feelings and slow things down, that it was OK to begin a relationship without sex or kissing, and that she had a right to state her preferences. Regarding her expectations of Paul, she included the alternative beliefs that he could feel compassion for her, that he would be OK with her statements, and that he might even feel good about her sharing her preferences.

This case example illustrates the process by which survivors of trauma can begin developing new ways of expressing themselves and interacting with others. As the example shows, survivors may initially err by being too passive in expressing their needs. Caroline's difficulty in looking out for her own interests came up repeatedly during subsequent sessions, as Caroline continued to work on developing ways of feeling more confident and powerful. Typically, role plays will have to be practiced many times and with a variety of situations until the client feels natural, comfortable, and effective in enacting appropriate assertive behavior in a real-life situation.

INTRODUCE ADDITIONAL ASSERTIVENESS SKILLS TO PRACTICE

It is important to strike a balance in the session between teaching new skills and exploring/clarifying the underlying beliefs and patterns that are driving behaviors. Teaching "I Messages" is useful because it is a fairly simple skill, but learning it can be a powerful experience for the client. Below, we identify other skills that may be equally appropriate depending on a specific client's needs. These skills are Making Requests and Saying No. The therapist can introduce these skills as relevant to the client either in this session or in later sessions. A summary of these skills is found in Handout 16.5, Additional Assertiveness Skills.

Making Requests

Asking for something that a client needs or wants is an important assertiveness skill to master. Asking for something assertively does not guarantee that the client will get it, but it is highly unlikely that they will get what they want without asking. To make a request assertively, the therapist instructs the client to do the following:

- Make the request specific, and state it clearly and simply (e.g., "I would like you to come to the doctor's appointment with me").
- Couch the request as an "I Message" ("I would like . . ." vs. "You need to . . .").
- State the positive consequences of the other's compliance with the request (e.g., "If you take care of that errand for me, I will have more time to spend with you this evening") and/or the negative consequences of the other's noncompliance (e.g., "If you don't do that errand for me, I won't make it on time for our dinner date tonight").
- Avoid making excuses, downplaying or apologizing for the request, or blaming the other person (e.g., "I would like you to help me with my move" vs. "It's a shame that I'm going to have to move all alone," "I know you probably don't have time, but if you have nothing better to do, would you maybe be able to help me move?", or "You are so inconsiderate. You never do anything for me").

Another important assertiveness tool is to leave or temporarily put off the situation if the other person responds aggressively (e.g., "I can see that you're angry right now. Let's talk about this after lunch").

Saying No

For many individuals raised in abusive environments, it can be difficult to say no assertively. In cases when a client is dealing with a person with whom they do not want to foster or maintain a relationship, it is often sufficient to say, "No, thank you," in a firm and respectful tone. If the other person persists, the client should repeat herself while maintaining eye contact and slightly raising the tone of their voice.

A useful technique for dealing with someone who will not take no for an answer is the Broken Record. In this technique, the client simply repeats a concise sentence over and over, without backing down or getting sidetracked by other issues. For example, if a salesperson keeps badgering the client to buy something they do not want, they can keep repeating, "I understand what you are saying, but I'm not interested."

In situations involving a person with whom the client does want to maintain a relationship, it can be useful to begin by acknowledging the request by reflecting it back to the other person. Without apologizing, the client should give a brief explanation of the reason for turning them down and then say no. If possible, the client can end by suggesting an alternative plan in which both the client's and the other person's needs will be met. For example, in response to a friend's request to help with a move, the client could say, "I understand that you need help with your move. Unfortunately, I have other plans for that day, so I won't be able to help you. If it would be helpful to you, I'd be happy to help you pack boxes the day before." If Saying No is an especially difficult skill for a client, it can be useful to build in time before responding to a request. This can help counter the tendency to agree automatically to others' requests before the client has considered whether they are in their own best interests (e.g., "I need to check my availability and so will let you know tomorrow"). A final point for the therapist to make is that the client can practice low-level acts of assertiveness in a kind but firm way. Being assertive does not mean being hostile or rude. Additional ideas are found in Handout 16.5.

It is also important for the therapist to point out that behaving assertively does not guarantee that people will respond positively to a request or statement. Sometimes people will respond negatively, no matter how assertive or respectful the client is. The therapist explains to the client that they may still receive some negative or unhelpful responses to their assertive behaviors, but that they will be more generally successful in their interactions.

SUMMARIZE THE GOALS OF THE SESSION

This session has a lot of substance to it. It is the first session that explicitly articulates and discusses potential alternative relationship models for the client. It also introduces role plays as a way of realizing what acting in accord with an alternative relationship model might feel like and how hard or easy doing this might be for a particular client. The session introduces the topic of assertiveness because it is something that, in one form or another, is a challenge for individuals who have experienced intimidation and violation by persons in authority or with power over them. The use of "I Messages" is a simple and relatively flexible skill that can be applied in a variety of situations that support alternative relationship models where the client experiences themselves as being appropriate active agents in the expression of their beliefs, feelings, and preferences.

PLAN SKILLS PRACTICE

After the therapist and client have completed Relationship Patterns Worksheet–2 and reviewed assertiveness skills relevant to the client, the therapist asks the client how doing these exercises felt and whether they learned anything. The therapist then asks the client if they think they can try out using the new worksheet and skills over the week, as a way to build on the work they did outside of session last week and in session this week. The therapist provides the client with several blank copies of Relationship Patterns Worksheet–2 (Handout 16.4) in order to detail interpersonal situations that arise during the week. Guidelines for how to complete this worksheet are provided in the first section of Handout 16.6, Practicing Assertiveness to Improve Relationship Patterns. The therapist can recommend that the client complete this sheet twice during the week. If necessary, the therapist reminds the client again of the rationale for skills practice and discusses any possible things that could interfere with the client's being able to utilize the worksheet. The therapist also reminds the client to continue using emotion management skills from the three channels as they apply to the client's meeting their interpersonal goals, as well as to continue the twice-daily practice of Focused Breathing. Finally, the therapist and client should maintain the client's commitment to engage in at least one pleasurable activity per week.

Understanding Assertiveness

- "Assertive behavior" means standing up for your legitimate rights and presenting your needs/wants in a way that is respectful of both yourself and others. Assertive behavior may lead you to feel confident, self-respecting, and good about yourself.

- "Nonassertive behavior" means ignoring or not expressing your own rights, needs, and desires. Nonassertive behavior may lead you to feel hurt, resentful, anxious, disappointed, and/or angry.

- "Aggressive behavior" means expressing your own rights at the expense of others through inappropriate outbursts or hostility. Aggressive behavior may lead you to feel angry, indignant, out of control, and/or guilty.

Basic Personal Rights

1. I have the right to ask for what I want.

2. I have the right to say no.

3. I have the right to feel and express my feelings, both positive and negative.

4. I have the right to make mistakes.

5. I have the right to have my own opinions, convictions, and values.

6. I have the right to be treated with dignity and respect.

7. I have the right to change my mind or decide on a different course of action.

8. I have the right to protest unfair treatment or criticism.

9. I have the right to expect honesty from others.

10. I have the right to be angry at someone I love.

11. I have the right to say, "I don't know."

12. I have the right to negotiate for change.

13. I have the right to be in a nonabusive environment.

14. I have the right to ask for help or emotional support.

15. I have the right to my own needs for personal space and time, even if others would prefer my company.

16. I have the right not to have to justify myself to others.

17. I have the right not to take responsibility for someone else's behavior, feelings, or problems.

18. I have the right not to have to anticipate others' needs and wishes.

19. I have the right not to have to worry all the time about the goodwill of others.

20. I have the right to choose not to respond to a situation.

"I Messages"

- Goal: To express hurt feelings or distress, or to give feedback about another's behavior.
  - The key is to focus on the consequences you experience due to the other person's troubling behavior, rather than focusing on the person themselves. Focusing on the consequences their behavior causes you makes it less likely that the person will feel attacked or criticized.
- Format: Situation (or Behavior) → Feeling → Consequence.
- The following formula can be helpful: "When I [state observed behavior], I feel [state the feeling], because [state the consequence for you]." Example:
  - "When I had to wait longer to be picked up today, I was upset, because I did not have time to get all my errands done."
- Success in this exercise means stating your concerns clearly and respectfully, not necessarily having the other person agree with you.

An "I Message" has three parts: a situation, a feeling, and a result.

1. **Situation:** What is happening around you? What is the other person doing?

2. **Feeling:** How does the person's behavior make you feel?

3. **Consequence:** What happens as a result?

Use this structure for your sentence:

"When I _____ [situation],

I feel _____ [feeling],

because _____ [result]."

Relationship Patterns Worksheet–2

Interpersonal situation	What did I feel and think about myself?		What were my expectations about the other person?		My resulting behavior
What happened?	My feelings	My thoughts	Their feelings	Their thoughts	What did I do?

Relationship model: "If _____, then _____."

Interpersonal goals for situation	Alternative beliefs and feelings about myself: What else could I . . .		Alternative beliefs and feelings about the other person: What else could I expect the other person . . .		Alternative actions
What are my goals in this situation?	. . . feel about myself?	. . . think about myself?	. . . to feel?	. . . to think?	What else could I do? What else might they do?

Alternative relationship model: "If _____ ,

then _____ ."

Additional Assertiveness Skills

1. **Making Requests.** Be specific about what you want, and state it clearly and simply.
   - Couch your request as a sentence beginning with "I," such as "I would like . . ."
   - State the positive consequences of the other's following through with your request, and/or the negative consequences of the other's lack of follow-through (an "I Message" may be helpful in this case).
   - Avoid making excuses, downplaying your request, or blaming the other person.
   - Delay the situation if the other person responds angrily or aggressively. Use a coping skill, if useful, to help you calm down before deciding your next step.

2. **Saying No.** The approach you choose depends on the kind of relationship and your interest in maintaining the relationship.
   - If you *do* want to maintain the relationship:
     - Acknowledge the other person's request by repeating it (do this also to make sure you understand it).
     - Without apologizing, give a brief explanation of your reason for declining.
     - If appropriate, suggest an alternative plan in which both your needs and the other person's will be met.
     - If Saying No is especially difficult, give yourself some time before responding to a request. You can try coping skills you've learned to ease your distress!
   - If you *do not* want to maintain the relationship:
     - Say, "No, thank you," in a respectful but firm tone. You may still explain why if it will benefit you or ease the situation.
     - If the other person persists, repeat yourself while maintaining eye contact and slightly raising the tone of your voice.
     - Or use the Broken Record approach: Repeat a concise sentence over and over, without getting sidetracked by other issues.

Remember: Behaving assertively doesn't guarantee that people will respond positively. Though you may sometimes receive negative or unhelpful responses to your assertive behaviors, you will generally, in the long run, be more successful in your interactions with other people.

Practicing Assertiveness to Improve Relationship Patterns

GUIDELINES FOR COMPLETING BOTTOM HALF OF RELATIONSHIP PATTERNS WORKSHEET–2

1. Identify a positive goal for the relationship.
2. Identify a belief and feeling that supports the relationship goal. Ask your therapist or a friend for suggestions if you get stuck.
3. Imagine a response from the person that supports your goal. What could they be feeling and thinking? Ask for help if you get stuck.
4. Imagine actions that you can take to support the goal or maintain that goal if you reach it.
5. Try out the action you came up with, see if it works, and adjust your approach as needed.

OTHER ASSERTIVENESS PRACTICE SITUATIONS

- Ask a salesperson to help you find something.
- Call or text a friend you haven't seen in a while to schedule a time to catch up.
- Ask your therapist to explain a concept or skill again if you're having trouble understanding or remembering the details.
- Ask your therapist for additional copies of handouts if you need more or if you misplaced old ones.
- Ask the pharmacist for information on an over-the-counter drug.
- Ask for a substitution on the menu when ordering a meal.
- Ask coworkers or classmates to do a favor for you (for example, ask for them to get you a cup of coffee while they get their own).
- Disagree with someone's opinion politely but with confidence.
- Ask a friend for help in fixing something.
- Ask your landlord to fix a problem in your apartment.
- Ask a person to stop doing something that bothers you—a great opportunity to use an "I Message"!

Note. The majority of the other assertiveness practice situations are adapted from *DBT Skills Training Manual, Second Edition* (p. 255), by Marsha M. Linehan. Copyright © 2015 Marsha M. Linehan. Additional ideas come from authors of this book.

Changing Relationship Patterns
Managing Power

> I've learned that people will forget what you said,
> people will forget what you did, but people will
> never forget how you made them feel.
> —ATTRIBUTED TO SEVERAL AUTHORS

In Session 8 of STAIR, the work of identifying maladaptive interpersonal schemas and developing alternative ways of approaching and processing relationships continues. The focus, however, is narrowed to the specific difficulties individuals who have experienced interpersonal trauma have with managing power balances in relationships. Often people who have experienced such trauma equate power with abuse. The goals of this session are to help clients separate power dynamics from risk for abuse and other maltreatment. The session reviews different kinds of power balances—including circumstances when the client has the same amount of, less, or more power than the person with whom they are interacting. It describes ways in which trauma can adversely affect managing relationships with each of these dynamics. The psychoeducation component in this session presents the idea that regardless of the nature of the power balance, respect for oneself and for others is a constant in all relationships and is the solution for managing conflict and other difficulties. In this session, the therapist and client select the power balance with which the client has most difficulty. They then explore the interpersonal schemas associated with the dynamic, identify an alternative way to view the dynamic, and try out a skill called Respect Bookends to facilitate the development of respect for oneself and others. Copies of Relationship Patterns Worksheet–2 (Handout 16.4), introduced in Session 7, are used to organize and summarize the particular relationship problems that are being explored and for which solutions are being evaluated. Box 17.1 outlines the theme and curriculum for Session 8.

Theme and Curriculum for Session 8
Changing Relationship Patterns: Managing Power

This session addresses the effective negotiation of power dynamics in relationships. Individuals who have experienced violence or exploitation often feel uneasy in situations where they feel the pull of power in the interactions. The session introduces the inevitability of power dynamics in relationships—whether the client is in a situation where the power balance is equal, or whether the client feels they have more or less power than the other person. The therapist proposes that the solution to discomfort around power is to experience respect for oneself and for others in every interaction, regardless of the type of power balance. Respect for self and others is critical for good communication, effective partnerships, and social functioning. The session provides skills training in acknowledging and signaling respect for others with an attitude of respect for oneself. Copies of Relationship Patterns Worksheet–2 are used to organize and distill problematic relationship power dynamics, and to provide alternative models of relating that support skills practice in the expression of respect for oneself and others.

PLANNING AND PREPARATION

Consider what kinds of problems in power management the client has been experiencing to organize your discussion in the session. Bring the handouts for Session 8 (listed below), as well as multiple copies of Relationship Patterns Worksheet-–2. The work in the session is estimated to take about 60 minutes; a flexible application is assumed (i.e., not every client will need all interventions).

AGENDA

- Check-in and review of skills practice.
- Identify focus of the session.
- Review and discuss three types of power balances.
- Discuss respect and power: Respect is the constant.
- Introduce the Respect Bookends skill.
- Summarize the goals of the session.
- Plan skills practice:
  - Complete two copies of Relationship Patterns Worksheet–2, with a focus on power dynamics.
  - Practice Respect Bookends.

(continued)

○ Use emotion management skills from three channels to support interpersonal work.

○ Do something pleasurable.

○ Continue Focused Breathing twice daily.

SESSION HANDOUTS

Handout 17.1. Power Balances in Relationships

Handout 17.2. Impact of Trauma on Managing Power Balances

Handout 17.3. Managing Power Balances with Respect

Additional copies of Handout 16.4. Relationship Patterns Worksheet–2

CHECK-IN AND REVIEW OF SKILLS PRACTICE

Before the therapist begins the session work on managing power, the therapist spends some time reviewing the Relationship Patterns Worksheet–2 entries brought in by the client. The therapist briefly confirms that the client has correctly completed the entries, particularly their expectations about others' thoughts and feelings regarding the client's own efforts in behaving more assertively. The therapist also briefly discusses whether the client has completed any assertiveness exercises, particularly any "I Messages" that were role-played in the previous session, and praises any efforts made. If there were difficulties, the therapist elicits information about them. Often difficulties with effective assertiveness are associated with difficulties in managing the underlying power balance—the topic of this session. The therapist can plan with the client to return to these issues in the current session. Similarly, if there were any difficulties executing an "I Message" or if the client was unable to practice this skill during the week, the therapist can tell the client that today's session will include a new skill (focusing on expressing respect for self and others) that incorporates the "I Message," so that there will be time to practice the skill again and adapt it to the client's needs and situation. The topic of power flows fairly directly from that of assertiveness, so the relationships that are of concern to the client can remain the focus of discussion in this session as well.

IDENTIFY FOCUS OF THE SESSION

The therapist begins the session by noting its focus on managing power dynamics in relationships. The therapist can mention any difficulties the client has identified that may be the result of problematic power dynamics. The therapist elicits from the client examples of difficulties the client is experiencing, to set the focus of the session on the types of problems the client is interested in discussing and resolving.

REVIEW AND DISCUSS THREE TYPES OF POWER BALANCES

The therapist and client first review the information presented in Handout 17.1, Power Balances in Relationships. They walk through the three central kinds of power balances in relationships and identify people that the client has a relationship with that fit into each type of power balance. These are the three types of power balances presented:

- *Type I.* The client has the same amount of power as the other person in the interaction. Typical examples of people in this power balance are colleagues, friends, and siblings.
- *Type II.* The client has less power than the other person, as is typically the case when the person is an employee, student, or trainee.
- *Type III.* The client has more power than the other person, as is the case when the client is an employer, teacher, coach, or parent.

Discuss Trauma-Generated Barriers in Managing Each Type of Power Balance

Following the information in Handout 17.2, Impact of Trauma on Managing Power Balances, the therapist and client can explore the client's views on each type of power balance and identify which is the most difficult. Below are descriptions of ways in which trauma can affect each type of balance, along with some case examples.

- *Type I.* Although the power balance is equal in these relationships, individuals who have experienced childhood maltreatment or been in other situations of sustained exploitation (e.g., domestic violence) may be highly sensitive to the power dynamics of a situation and may see themselves as having more or less power than the other person. For example, they may relate to work colleagues as abusive parents and have difficulty seeing that their colleagues do not hold that kind of power over them. On the other hand, a survivor may act as if they hold more power in a relationship, for fear of being "victimized" or taken advantage of by the other person. The case examples below illustrate both of these types of problems in Type I relationships.

> At the beginning of treatment, Angie, a 20-year-old student, described tremendous anxiety in interactions with most of her friends. She constantly feared letting her friends down or making them angry with her. When there was any issue or conflict, she would become uncomfortable and distressed, which would lead her to call and smooth things over regardless of the situation. Despite the reality that Angie was (or should have been) on an equal footing with her friends, she certainly did not feel or act this way, which continued to fuel her anxiety and obsequious behavior.

> In contrast, Joanne came into treatment because she feared losing her boyfriend of several years. He had threatened to break up with her because of her "bossiness," saying that he could no longer stand her efforts to control him. When Joanne and her therapist

examined these relationship interactions, it became apparent that Joanne often treated her boyfriend as though he was a child. She would often tell him what to eat, pick out his clothing, and even make plans for him. Rather than being a girlfriend, Joanne had taken on the role of an intrusive mother. Although initially her boyfriend had felt taken care of, over time he began to feel resentful.

Type II. Type II relationships can be especially difficult for survivors of childhood abuse, because people in positions of power are often equated with abusive caregivers (or can behave in ways that are abusive and have special impact upon the survivors). This can leave survivors feeling angry, helpless, scared, and anxious in interactions with these people. The primary challenge of a relationship in which the client has less power is to try to achieve a balance between meeting the other person's demands or requests, while getting the client's rights recognized and needs met. The following case examples illustrate such problems in Type II relationships.

Beth had recently seen a doctor who had diagnosed her with a thyroid condition and had prescribed medication without giving much explanation or information. Shortly after she began taking the medication, she reported to her therapist that she felt fatigued and dizzy. Her therapist recommended she call the doctor to ask about possible side effects rather than waiting for her next appointment, which was scheduled for next month. Despite her discomfort, Beth felt hesitant to call the doctor, since it was not an emergency situation. She did not want to annoy or question the doctor, as she feared this might affect the quality of care he was willing to provide. Beth's therapist used this example to discuss ways Beth interacted with those she viewed as being in authority. She did not feel entitled to ask questions even when her own needs were being compromised. The therapist tried to provide a "reality check" and discussed with Beth that part of her doctor's job was to provide follow-up care and information.

Dawn worked as an assistant to a prestigious editor. Though she knew that her job would include long hours and little pay, she had taken it because she knew the experience could further her career. However, when Dawn's boss asked if she could come in on a weekend in order to meet a pressing deadline, Dawn felt that she was being taken advantage of and needed to stand up for herself. She told her boss in no uncertain terms that she would not be treated like a slave and walked out of the office. In treatment, Dawn identified that one of her major relationship models involved the assumption that those in positions of power would inevitably exploit her. In response to this expectation, she was always on the lookout for this possibility and likely to interpret others' behavior as fitting with this model, which at times caused her to take actions she later regretted. The therapist acknowledged the importance of Dawn's self-protective instincts, but also noted the need to develop other relationship models in which exploitation was not a given. The therapist also worked with Dawn on building skills (e.g., identifying relationship goals and considering pros and cons of continuing the relationship) that could help her assess current situations with authority figures more objectively before taking actions.

* *Type III.* Because of experiences in past relationships, survivors of childhood abuse or other maltreatment may not understand that they have more power in these types of relationships, or they may deny that they do for fear of what it means to be powerful (e.g., power may be equated with aggression). In contrast, some survivors find themselves taking on the perpetrator role in this power situation, becoming literally or figuratively abusive. Behaving abusively in these interactions can lead a survivor to feel frightened, anxious, guilty, and disgusted with herself. The case examples below illustrate both of these types of problems in Type III relationships.

> Jen, a high school teacher, was distressed by the fact that her students did not seem to respect her. She felt ineffective and embarrassed by her reputation as a "pushover." When her therapist asked her more about what was going on in her classroom, Jen described an atmosphere in which she gave her students tremendous freedom and imposed minimal limits. She was surprised and hurt when students disregarded assignments, but she had difficulty giving consequences. Though Jen appeared to be a skilled teacher, her discomfort in taking on the role of an authority figure was having a negative impact on her professional life and self-esteem.

> At the opposite end of the Type III spectrum, Becca, the eldest of three children, was named executor of her mother's will; this included overseeing the sale of her mother's properties and ensuring that each of the three children received an equal percentage of the profits. Rather than implementing her mother's plan and involving her siblings in the process, Becca became very secretive and manipulative. She delayed putting the properties on the market; she also made important decisions without talking to her sisters and refused to provide them with updates, saying that since she was the one chosen to handle things, she should not have to run things by her sisters for their approval. Becca acknowledged that she felt entitled to more than her two sisters because she was taking on more responsibility, noting that this had always been the case. In this way Becca was using this opportunity to fulfill her own agenda by unilaterally assuming power, instead of taking the lead while also acting collaboratively with her siblings, as her mother had intended.

DISCUSS RESPECT AND POWER: RESPECT IS THE CONSTANT

Those who have experienced interpersonal trauma, often at the hands of people who have more authority and power, may equate power with the risk of more trauma. Similarly, being the object of someone else's maltreatment is likely to be associated with a feeling of powerlessness. Victims are often treated like objects and told (explicitly or implicitly) that they "deserve what they get"; some victims, particularly children assaulted by caregivers, may internalize these messages and believe themselves to be worthless, deserving of abuse, or "failures" because they could not defend themselves. Maltreatment is indeed an act of disregard for a person's value and worth, but the blame for these behaviors falls squarely on the shoulders of the perpetrators of these acts.

Recovery from being a victim of interpersonal trauma includes recovery of self-worth. This session focuses on the client's inherent right to self-respect and their inherent obligation to treat others with respect. The rehabilitation of sense of respect for self and other can occur in a variety of ways. In this treatment, the therapist simply reminds the client of their inherent worth as a human being and points out ways that they have treated themselves in a respectful and appreciative manner. Discussing the impact of trauma on sense of self-respect is an important initial and eye-opening step. The client may be able to see that they were not born defective or a "loser," but that certain unfortunate experiences have led them to this belief. Current relationship patterns that appear to replay traumatizing power dynamics are explored to identify underlying relationship models that hold that one or the other person in the relationship is worthless. These beliefs are challenged, and alternative models of relating are proposed. Experiential exercises in the form of a skill called Respect Bookends are introduced in this session, so that the client can practice behaviors that express respect for others as well as the self and are intended to contribute to a revised and more positive respectful view of oneself and others.

INTRODUCE THE RESPECT BOOKENDS SKILL

Handout 17.3, Managing Power Balances with Respect, describes the skill of Respect Bookends. This skill adds to the "I Message" communication by bookending one's own opinions, concerns, and distress with recognition of the other person's perspective at both the beginning and ending of a statement. On a superficial level, the process of recognizing the preferences and opinions of another person is intended to help engage that person in conversation and facilitate resolution of conflicts or differences. On a deeper level, this type of interaction recognizes the presence of another person and awareness of that person as a human being in their particularity and with respect for their position, whatever it may be. The statement is intended to express the shared humanity of the two people, and respect for the other person's rights to their opinions as well as one's own.

As with the skills training for "I Messages," the therapist and client start by sketching out the current problematic situation in the top portion of Relationship Patterns Worksheet–2 and formulating a preferred alternative scenario in the bottom portion, along with a hypothesized alternative relationship model. The client and therapist formulate a three-part communication, which begins with a statement that recognizes the concerns and positive aspects or behaviors of the other person; is followed by a statement of the client's request, concern, decision, or point of view; and ends with a statement that again recognizes the other person's concerns and positive aspects or behaviors. The therapist and client then engage in a role play of the planned communication. As described in Chapter 16/Session 7, the role playing can serve to highlight more details about what is problematic about the current situation, and to refine the alternative relationship model and interpersonal goals associated with the situation. More details on this role playing are provided in the case example below.

CASE EXAMPLE: WORKING THROUGH A POWER PROBLEM

Using Relationship Patterns Worksheet–2

Julie identified a chronic problem with her boyfriend—that he did not listen to her opinions. Even though she viewed the relationship as having an equal power balance, she often ended up feeling as if she had less; as she expressed it, she felt that her opinions and preferences "don't count." The therapist asked Julie to describe recent experiences in her relationship; together, they then used the top portion of Relationship Patterns Worksheet–2 to describe a recent situation and identify what might be the underlying relationship model contributing to the dynamics and outcome of the situation (see the top portion of Box 17.2).

THERAPIST: You have described similar situations with your boyfriend. There are some real similarities in this and past examples. What do you notice?

JULIE: Well, I always end up feeling bad and feeling that everything I do is wrong.

THERAPIST: Yes, that does seem to be a theme. In this and previous situations, you seem to expect the worst from the other person. You anticipated that your boyfriend would not listen to you. Do you think these expectations affected your behavior in any way?

JULIE: Well, yeah. That's why I didn't try to talk to him about it.

THERAPIST: Which makes sense—if you expect no one will listen, then you are not likely to put yourself out there. Where do you think these expectations that you will not be heard come from?

JULIE: They come from people not listening to me.

THERAPIST: You have shared with me that this certainly was the case with your parents—that they would accuse you of something and not give you the chance to defend yourself.

JULIE: If I tried to explain, they would get mad and say I was being disrespectful. Usually I would get punished or even hit.

THERAPIST: In this context with your parents, it sounds like avoiding further discussion and leaving the situation before it escalated was an adaptive response and allowed you to avoid some negative consequences. However, in your current life, always expecting that you will be shut down and punished for trying to speak up has some potential negative consequences. Can you think of any?

JULIE: Well, yeah. I let people go on thinking whatever they want to think about me, even if it is wrong—but I would rather do that than try to convince them of something else.

THERAPIST: Yes, you are not inclined to try to clarify a misunderstanding or further discuss a situation, which leaves you unable to further discuss your intentions or understand the other person's perception of your behavior. Again, when you are dealing with someone who is toxic, this may be for the best; you avoid getting into

BOX 17.2

Julie's Completed Relationship Patterns Worksheet–2

Interpersonal situation	What did I feel and think about myself?		What were my expectations about the other person?		My resulting behavior
What happened? My boyfriend snapped at me because I lost the car keys. He called me irresponsible.	**My feelings** Stupid. Ashamed. Angry at myself.	**My thoughts** Why am I always losing things? I can never get it together. No point in explaining. He will just get more angry and insult me.	**Their feelings** Enraged. Tired of me.	**Their thoughts** Thinks I am worthless and can't get anything done. Wishes he had a better girlfriend. Wants to get rid of me.	**What did I do?** Went into the other room until he left for work. Was upset most of the day.

Relationship model: "If _I try to explain myself after an honest mistake has been made_, then _I will be punished, criticized, and insulted_."

Interpersonal goals for situation	Alternative beliefs and feelings about myself: What else could I . . .		Alternative beliefs and feelings about the other person: What else could I expect the other person . . .		Alternative actions
What are my goals in this situation? To apologize, but also to improve communication. I would like him to respect my feelings, and I don't like being snapped at.	**. . . feel about myself?** A little embarrassed. Compassion for myself. Hopeful he will listen to me.	**. . . think about myself?** I sometimes lose things, but I am not the only one. I can ask him to help develop a strategy to remember where the keys are.	**. . . to feel?** Irritated.	**. . . to think?** That he would hear my apology without being rude. That he might apologize for snapping at me if he knew that it hurt my feelings. That he might want to problem-solve around the key problem.	**What else could I do?** Talk to him about it. **What else might they do?** If he is a jerk, end the conversation.

Alternative relationship model: "If _I try to explain what happened after an honest mistake has been made_,
then _I will be given respect for my point of view and responded to without punishment (maybe even compassion)_."

a nonproductive interaction. But what about situations in which you are wrong in assuming the other person will respond negatively?

JULIE: Well, how do I know if this is going to be the case?

THERAPIST: True, you don't always know, so it involves some risk—but in certain cases it may be worth it. For example, there are likely to be situations in which others will not belittle or ignore your efforts to explain yourself. In these cases, you don't let the person know what's on your mind, and you miss out on the opportunity to have an important conversation that may improve things in the relationship. This is the main limitation of applying expectations across the board in your relationship. Although it is more nuanced and complicated, ultimately it is more adaptive to take each relationship on a case-by-case basis. This will help you to consider what approach you might want to take. In this example, you felt unheard by your boyfriend—but since this relationship is different from the one with your parents, you may want to approach him in a different way.

Using Julie's example, the therapist worked with her to identify interpersonal goals she had with her boyfriend and to construct an alternative relationship model she might apply to her interactions—a different model from the one generated by her traumatic past with her parents (see the bottom portion of Box 17.2). Julie's old relationship model based on her childhood was "If I try to explain myself after an honest mistake has been made, then I will be punished, criticized, and insulted."

With the help of her therapist, Julie was able to articulate an alternative relationship model: "If I try to explain what happened after an honest mistake has been made, then I will be given respect for my point of view and responded to without punishment (maybe even compassion)." She identified that a relationship goal with her boyfriend was to have him understand her feelings and to improve communication in the relationship. In addition, the therapist noted that Julie might want to work on being more assertive: Although she shared power in the relationship with her boyfriend, she often behaved submissively, as though he was more of a parent figure. If Julie believed that her boyfriend might not become more adversarial and would care about how she was feeling about their interaction, she might feel more confident about herself and be willing to share her feelings and ways she would like the relationship to improve.

Role Play Using Respect Bookends

After identifying the relationship model and specific interpersonal goals, Julie and the therapist walked through what she might say, using the Respect Bookends approach. They focused on an interaction with her boyfriend following her accidentally losing the car keys. In her typical fashion, Julie avoided her boyfriend and did not explain what happened for fear of his criticism and rejection. Her boyfriend misinterpreted her silence as lack of concern, which only made him angry, and then he snapped at her. The therapist pointed out that using Respect Bookends to explain what happened would be an effective way for Julie to express her feelings, while simultaneously validating her boyfriend's frustration and perspective.

This role play has three steps. In the first step, a client practices the planned communication, beginning and ending with the Respect Bookends. In the second step, the therapist shares observations and provides suggestions for improving the client's communication and clarifying the goals for the interaction. As always, it is important for the therapist to acknowledge both the client's strengths and weaknesses. When addressing problems, the therapist provides the potential experience of the other person in the interaction, rather than directly using their own perceptions. The therapist also role-plays what the client might say, incorporating any relevant modifications and improvements. While the therapist is speaking, the client imagines being the other person and evaluates how it might feel from their perspective. In the third step, the client practices aloud again, making any desired adjustments. Here is how Julie and her therapist role-played Respect Bookends:

> THERAPIST: Let's do a role play where you can try out the Respect Bookends approach. This role play will be a little different from the one we did last session, because when I repeat what you say, I would like you to really imagine what it might feel like to be your boyfriend. You can begin the conversation with your boyfriend by acknowledging his feelings and maybe even the impact losing the car keys has on him. Then tell him what happened and how you are feeling, and include your apology. Then end by recognizing what he may be feeling, and say something positive about him or the relationship.

> JULIE: Tim, I know you probably hate me and want to break up with me because I did something stupid again. I'm so sorry I lost the car keys! I was on my way into Safeway to buy groceries when I noticed this older lady trying to lift her heavy grocery bags and put them in her trunk. She looked so miserable, so I stopped to help her. You should have seen the smile on her face when I put the groceries in the car for her! It made my day. And then, after I finished shopping and I came out, I realized the keys must have fallen out of my pocket! I searched all over that parking lot, but couldn't find them. I think that maybe they fell out in the lady's trunk. Even though it was an accident, I am sorry that this happened. My relationship with you is very important, and I want you to know how much I appreciate everything you do for me.

> THERAPIST: That was great, Julie. That was very nice of you to help that lady; I am sure she really appreciated it. And I am glad you got a chance to tell what happened. One thing I am wondering about is in the beginning. You are very self-deprecating, and I am not sure about your assumptions that your boyfriend hates you and wants to break up with you. It is possible to validate and respect another person's beliefs and feelings without putting yourself down. I will repeat what you said, but I will try to be respectful of Tim without saying negative things about myself. And I would like you to imagine what it might be like to be Tim in this situation.

> JULIE: OK.

THERAPIST: (*As Julie*) It really means a lot to me that you helped me when I lost the car keys. I know how frustrating it is for you when things get lost. You were so sweet and kind to come bail me out. I would like to tell you what happened, so that you understand. I was on going into the store to buy groceries, when I noticed a lady who appeared to be very old and frail. She was trying to lift her heavy grocery bags and put them in her trunk. I stopped to help her. She was very appreciative. When I finished shopping and I came out, I realized the keys must have fallen out of my pocket! I searched all over that parking lot, but couldn't find them. I think that maybe they fell out in the lady's trunk. Even though it was an accident, I am sorry that this happened and that it distressed you. Our relationship is very important, and I appreciate everything you do for me.

THERAPIST: What do you think about what I said?

JULIE: I really liked how you said nice things to him and acknowledged his perspective, but never put yourself down. And when I heard the story as though I was listening to it for the first time, I thought it was a really nice thing to do. I'm pretty sure my boyfriend might think so too. Rather than being mad at me, he might even say, "Come here so I can give you a hug!"

THERAPIST: Terrific. Then let's do this one last time. Practice telling your boyfriend what happened, and use the Respect Bookends without putting yourself down.

JULIE: It really means a lot to me that you helped me when I lost the car keys. You were so sweet and kind to come bail me out, as I know how frustrating it is for you when things get lost. Let me tell you what happened so that you understand. I was on my way into Safeway to buy groceries, when I noticed this older lady trying to lift her heavy grocery bags and put them in her trunk. She looked so miserable, so I stopped to help her. You should have seen the smile on her face when I put the groceries in the car for her! It made my day. And then, after I finished shopping and I came out, I realized the keys must have fallen out of my pocket! I searched all over that parking lot, but couldn't find them. I think that maybe they fell out in the lady's trunk. I am embarrassed and sorry about all this, especially how frustrating it is for you, even though it was an accident. I appreciate all the things you do for me, and you really mean a lot to me.

Julie told the therapist how much better this way felt to her. She realized that telling her boyfriend what happened might lead to problem-solving the situation together, and thus that expressing her feelings could actually make them feel closer to each other. Julie was excited by this revelation and eager to try it out.

Use of Other Skills

Contextual information and awareness will also help clients determine the appropriate level of intimacy and assertiveness (e.g., avoiding the traps of not being sufficiently assertive and being overly assertive) in interactions. One way to do this is to help clients draw on the skills learned in the previous sessions and apply them to the various types of power relationships. For example, a therapist can tell a client:

"Remember to listen carefully."

"Slow down, and clarify what is being expected of you."

"Practice distress tolerance. Sit with your feelings, and realize that there will be opportunities to come back to the issue."

"Identify your goals and examine your Pros and Cons. What are you trying to accomplish? Is it worth it?"

"Get multiple perspectives before reacting."

"When you are confused, get more data. Ask for feedback about power dynamics. Make sure that this is the kind of person you can safely talk to."

"Remind yourself, 'This is part of my history.' Using this type of self-talk may help you contain your emotions and understand why you are reacting strongly in the moment."

SUMMARIZE THE GOALS OF THE SESSION

In this session, the therapist and client have practiced a new skill, Respect Bookends. The exercise prompts the client to think about another person's perspective, but in that process to develop an attitude of respect toward the self. The therapist and client also have identified how trauma can lead to an internalization of other people's negative attitudes, and accordingly to feelings of worthlessness and self-loathing. The client is encouraged to let go of these trauma-generated negative beliefs about themselves, as they tend to be self-fulfilling and lead to a vicious cycle of self-loathing. The client and therapist construct alternative, more positive relationship models that focus on respect for oneself and others. Practicing Respect Bookends provides corrective emotional experiences that provide evidence for the alternative relationship models.

PLAN SKILLS PRACTICE

The client's most important task for the week is to practice Respect Bookends with at least two people (ideally, in different types of power relationships) with whom they will interact during the week. The client can also complete two copies of Relationship Patterns Worksheet–2 (Handout 16.4) to track how these efforts at new interactions go. The sheets can also be used to record relevant emotion regulation skills used in response to each situation (e.g., Thought Shifting, Positive Self-Statements). The client should be encouraged to engage in one positive activity (preferably with someone they discuss in a copy of Relationship Patterns Worksheet–2) and continue to do Focused Breathing twice daily.

Power Balances in Relationships

There are three types of power balances in relationships:

Type I: You have equal power with a person (examples: someone who is your friend, sibling, coworker, partner, or team member).

Type II: You have less power than the other person (examples: someone who is your employer, supervisor, parent, teacher, or coach).

Type III: You have more power than the other person (examples: someone who is your child, employee, supervisee, student, or trainee).

Name people you interact with where each type of power balance exists:

I have equal power: _____

_____

_____

I have less power: _____

_____

_____

I have more power: _____

_____

_____

Impact of Trauma on Managing Power Balances

Type I: You have equal power (*examples:* friend, sibling, coworker, partner, team member).

Barriers: Although you are equal in power, there are problems. You may see yourself as having more or less power than you do.
Related thoughts:

- Your work colleagues, peers/friends, or family members are threats or enemies.
- They will be aggressive, will be competitive with you, or will exploit you.
- You need to be vigilant and aggressive.
- You need to act like you have more power and authority than you actually have to protect yourself.
- You need to keep a safe distance from them, not trust them.

Type II: You have less power (*examples:* employee, supervisee, child, student, trainee).

Barriers: You have less power than someone else, and you expect them to take advantage of you.
Related thoughts:

- The authority figure or boss is a threat or enemy.
- You feel anxious and worried that something bad will happen to you if they are displeased with you or they are in a bad mood.
- You may be too eager to please, may find it difficult to say no, or may not ask for the authority or resources you need or want, because you are afraid they will punish/hurt you.
- You become angry and accuse them of being exploitative when that might not be true, but you were too afraid to ask about things you were seeing going on and made your own interpretation.

Type III: You have more power (*examples:* parent, employer, supervisor, teacher, coach).

Barriers: You have more power than others, and this makes you very uncomfortable.
Related thoughts:

- You cannot execute your authority, so you do a bad job (as a boss, parent, or leader).
- You are afraid that you will be abusive when you use your power, so you don't exert it at all.
- You feel taken advantage of by those under your authority.
- Sometimes you do exert your power, but the results are unsatisfactory.
- You feel mean/abusive, so you are apologetic and sometimes take back what you say
- You actually act mean/abusive, and then you feel bad.

Managing Power Balances with Respect

MANAGING DIFFERENT POWER BALANCES: RESPECT IS A CONSTANT

While differences in power balances are a fact of life, respect for oneself and others should be a constant, no matter what a specific power balance is like. **When you have less power**, remember that you have a right to act in ways that respect yourself and your values (for example, politely express your point of view, but also remember also to express respect for those with more power, rather than mistrust or fear of abuse). When you interact with others with whom you have **more power**, remember to show respect for their personhood and express your power in a positive way, with confidence and warmth.

A SKILL FOR MANAGING POWER BALANCES: BEGIN AND END WITH RESPECT

Skill: Select the power balance that causes you the greatest difficulty. Select a situation that you can also describe in the top portion of Relationship Patterns Worksheet–2. Formulate the point of view you want to express in a way that is open, direct, and clear (for example, use an "I Message"). But now begin and end what you want to say in a manner that acknowledges positive aspects of the person or relationship. This skill is called Respect Bookends.

- Begin with a statement that recognizes positive aspects or behaviors of the person.
- State your request, concern, decision, or point of view.
- End with a statement that again recognizes the person's positive aspects or behaviors.

Example: Mother to child (mother has more power than child):

"I so enjoyed seeing you talk with your grandmom. She just lights up with you. I noticed she was in that hard-backed chair. What do you think of giving her the cushioned chair you usually sit on when she visits, as her back hurts and it's the only one that is comfortable for her? [Discuss.] She'll be coming by next week, and I am sure she will be much more comfortable with the cushy chair. Thanks so much for doing this. I know you want her to be happy by the way I see you pop up and get her the tea. This will definitely make her comfortable and happy as well."

Try out this practice:

- Say what you plan to say aloud, remembering to use Respect Bookends.
- Your coach/therapist repeats what you plan to say. Now imagine yourself as the other person.
- How does it feel? What are your thoughts and reactions?
- Practice again, to maximize the chances that you will get a good response. Make adjustments as desired.

CHAPTER 18

Changing Relationship Patterns
Increasing Closeness

> Loneliness does not come from having no people about one,
> but from being unable to communicate the things that seem
> important to oneself . . .
>
> —CARL JUNG (1963/1989, p. 356)

Although issues with intimacy and closeness are introduced toward the end of STAIR, they are fundamental to the experience of clients who have survived interpersonal trauma, particularly childhood abuse. Their problems with intimacy range from efforts to isolate and protect themselves from further betrayals, to efforts to keep loved ones so close that the survivors lose contact with the parts of themselves that are separate and distinct from the other persons. These problems can occur at either end of the spectrum of isolation to enmeshment, but some people can experience issues with both extremes. For example, an individual may have an unhealthy boundary with their romantic partner that reflects being too dependent on the loved one, while their boundaries with friends reflect the opposite problem—great distance and lack of any real kind of intimacy.

No matter what the specific problems in this domain may be, this session reviews the importance of healthy boundaries that allow real intimacy and closeness, but that also avoid the loss of the identity and healthy independence that mark mature, functioning adult relationships.

Several interpersonal skills and approaches can aid the client and therapist in exploring more optimal levels of intimacy with others. For some clients, the focus of the session can be on repairing existing relationships and conflicts that arise. This work follows from that in the two previous sessions in a stepwise fashion: First, the client has learned how to make their own feelings, beliefs, and thoughts clear (through using "I Messages"). Then the client has become more skilled in recognizing other people's feelings, beliefs, and thoughts (through using Respect Bookends). These skills often help resolve differences and bring people closer. However, sometimes conflict does erupt and results in increased distance in a relationship. Individuals who have experienced interpersonal trauma often feel fearful about and avoid dealing with conflict or relationship ruptures. They can be fearful of being overwhelmed by the other persons, bullied into doing something they do not want to do. Alternatively, they can be fearful of becoming too angry themselves. For these clients, the goal of this session is to provide additional skills in conflict resolution and repair while maintaining or moving toward healthy boundaries.

For other clients who are highly avoidant of relationships, the focus of the session may be starting new relationships and mindfully developing appropriate levels of intimacy over time. These alternative skills include the basics of how to say hello to strangers or acquaintances and how to deepen relationships over time. Although these interpersonal goals are long-term ones, the therapist can offer hope and encourage these clients to start making small steps to decrease their isolation and put themselves on a path toward healthy social engagement.

CHECK-IN AND REVIEW OF SKILLS PRACTICE

The therapist begins, as usual, with a brief check-in on the client's emotional state and then about the client's skills practice since the last session, as well as entries on copies of Relationship Patterns Worksheet–2. The therapist can note any entries or relationships the client has discussed that may be of importance in today's session. The therapist can also reinforce any movement toward the client's interpersonal goals related to assertiveness and/or managing difficult power balances. Some of the client's practiced emotion regulation and communication skills may be relevant to today's session on intimacy. When reviewing Relationship Patterns Worksheet–2 entries, the therapist can focus on (1) reinforcing any skills the client has used (from the three channels of emotion or from previous relationship-oriented sessions), and (2) acknowledging any insights or discoveries the client has made about their interpersonal beliefs and behavioral patterns. Even if a client has reported not successfully navigating an interpersonal situation, the therapist can emphasize that gaining insight is the first essential step in making healthy changes.

For clients who have had difficulties with completing any exercise, the therapist can problem-solve any practical barriers, while also ensuring that they have time to focus on this session's content, which will include applying familiar skills and further Relationship Patterns Worksheet–2 entries to the theme of intimacy and closeness. If the client has had ongoing difficulty with exploring and changing their relationship patterns (including completing worksheets and practice), the therapist can say something such as:

> "Working on relationships can be really hard. It can be hard for everyone, even people who haven't had traumatic experiences. But improving relationships requires skills, just like any other area of your life. We'll keep chipping away at the things that get in your way, and as long as you can keep making small steps, things will slowly but surely get better."

IDENTIFY FOCUS OF THE SESSION

This session continues the previous sessions' focus on adopting healthier relationship patterns by introducing and exploring ways to manage intimacy and closeness. This final major theme of the interpersonal sessions of STAIR is often incredibly relevant to the lives of survivors who have experienced interpersonal trauma particularly during the developmental years. The session introduces the concepts of relationship boundaries and emotional intimacy, and describes how to use these concepts to move toward the client's goals for their relationships. Some clients may learn how to set better boundaries with their loved ones, friends, family, and coworkers while others may focus on beginning and deepening new relationships with others. Box 18.1 outlines the session contents and major tasks.

PRESENT CONCEPTS OF BOUNDARIES AND EMOTIONAL DISTANCE

Many clients will have heard of the concept of boundaries. This session fleshes out the concept by introducing the client to three different types of boundaries, categorized by the amount of emotional distance. For the purposes of STAIR, the term "boundaries" broadly refers to the intrinsic and rightful ownership of a person's own body, thoughts, and feelings, and respectful recognition of this ownership by others. We use the phrase "healthy boundaries" to describe an individual's sense of comfort and safety in relationships resulting from respect for the needs, rights, and values of each person in the relationship or interaction. Handout 18.1, Healthy Relationships = Healthy Boundaries (to be filled out in session with the therapist), provides information about three common types of boundaries and the advantages and disadvantages of each type. The emphasis here is on the degrees of emotional distance resulting from these configurations.

IDENTIFY CLIENT'S RELATIONSHIP PATTERNS RELATED
TO CLOSENESS

Together in this session, the therapist and client discuss each type of boundary (and review its pros and cons), while also exploring which ones typically fit the client's relationships. Sometimes clients report that they engage in both "too close" and "not close enough" relationships, and there may even be a relationship pattern (of feelings, thoughts, and behaviors) associated with each of them. Going through each style can help a client see that there is no clear right or wrong; different boundaries may be more or less helpful, depending on the specific relationship or situation. The therapist may wish to refer back to the client's trauma history to identify ways in which their preferred style was protective to them. In fact, in the case of childhood trauma, negotiating some level of emotional distance with others was often quite protective and even necessary to remain as safe as possible in interactions with past perpetrators.

BOX 18.1

Theme and Curriculum for Session 9
Changing Relationship Patterns: Increasing Closeness

This session continues the work on interpersonal relationship skills by focusing on optimizing closeness in relationships. Survivors of trauma often have impairment in this domain, due to the effects of avoidance and emotional numbing and/or reactivity. Previous sessions have introduced a range of interpersonal skills, but this session serves to apply such skills directly to the goal of either repairing intimacy problems in current relationships or establishing new relationships that can grow over time. Clients with childhood trauma that adversely affected their development in relational capacities may have more severe impairments in this domain, so the therapist can focus on more foundational skills with such a client as relevant.

PLANNING AND PREPARATION

Review concept of emotional intimacy/closeness. Bring extra copies of the Relationship Patterns Worksheet–2 (Handout 16.4), plus a copy of each handout for this session. Prepare several examples of ways the client may address struggles with intimacy and boundaries. The work in the session is estimated to take about 60 minutes; a flexible application is assumed (i.e., not every client will need all interventions).

AGENDA

- Check-in and review of skills practice.
- Identify focus of the session.
- Present concepts of boundaries and emotional distance.
- Explore client's relationship patterns related to closeness.
- Review and select steps for developing new relationships or deepening existing ones.
- Complete Relationship Patterns Worksheet–2.
- Complete one role play on chosen skill.
- Explore additional skill domains (optional).
- Summarize the goals of the session.
- Plan skills practice:
  - Complete Relationship Patterns Worksheet–2 twice a week before next session (to record practice interacting in a situation with opportunity to increase closeness).
  - Use coping skills from all three channels to support interpersonal goals.

(continued)

○ Schedule at least one pleasurable activity for the week.

○ Continue practice of Focused Breathing twice a day.

SESSION HANDOUTS

Handout 18.1. Healthy Relationships = Healthy Boundaries

Handout 18.2. What Creates Emotional Distance and Ruptures in Relationships?

Handout 18.3. Relationship Guidelines to Enhance Intimacy and Closeness

Additional copies of Handout 16.4. Relationship Patterns Worksheet–2

To help bolster the client's understanding, the therapist can use Handout 18.2, What Creates Emotional Distance and Ruptures in Relationships? This handout may be helpful for all clients, because emotional avoidance and numbing are key phenomena of post-traumatic reactions and are often expressed and observed in relationships. This handout encourages the client to share their personal viewpoint about why distance can grow in relationships, and to specify behaviors that they have noticed lead to greater distance. The therapist can help the client if they are at a loss by providing some examples:

"I've noticed that some people push others away by getting angry and yelling. Other persons create distance by not sending texts or not calling their friends or loved ones. How do you handle situations where you want to avoid being physically or emotionally close to someone?"

Regardless of the client's specific avoidance patterns or the origins of these patterns, the therapist introduces the idea of optimal, healthy boundaries that maximize benefits while mitigating risk. If the client is unfamiliar with such boundaries, it may be useful and reassuring to identify the Cons of moving toward these healthier, balanced boundaries. For example, the client may report Cons such as these:

"I'll need to learn new things."

"Getting closer (or moving farther away) will increase my anxiety."

"It'll create change in my current relationship, and I won't know what to expect."

"My partner might not like this."

The therapist may acknowledge the client's fears and concerns as relevant, and note that the client can take their time in changing relationship patterns. Relationship changes take practice, communication, and patience—both with the other person and with oneself. To help manage any anxiety, the client can choose a specific relationship on which they would like to focus. The most important or difficult relationship might not necessarily be the best place to start. It is key for the client to experience and feel a sense of success as they work toward optimizing their boundaries and sense of intimacy with others.

REVIEW AND SELECT STEPS FOR DEVELOPING NEW RELATIONSHIPS OR DEEPENING EXISTING ONES

The therapist can then guide the conversation to identifying the interpersonal patterns associated with distancing or relationship avoidance, and determining which skills might help change the pattern. Different clients will benefit from different acquisition and practice of different skills. By this point in therapy, the therapist will have a reasonable sense of whether the client would benefit most from focusing on managing conflict and repairing current relationships, or from developing skills to enter into new relationships or greater socializing. Of course, these goals are not mutually exclusive; skills related to both of these goals are necessary throughout life. Nevertheless, choosing a focus for the session will support the client's ability to take smaller, mindful steps toward making important improvements in their life. The client's growing skills in distress tolerance and emotion regulation will likely be crucial to integrate into this discussion, and the therapist can remind the client as necessary that they can make more conscious choices in how to develop their relationships. Handout 18.3, Relationship Guidelines to Enhance Intimacy and Closeness, outlines the skills related to different goals and tasks for the remainder of the session.

Developing New Relationships

Some clients have avoided relationships and emotional intimacy for years. The resulting isolation is painful and dangerous to their well-being, but they often feel as if they have no choice and must continue being alone, even if deep down they want to connect with others. For these clients, the first two sections of Handout 18.3 can provide concrete ideas for starting the process of tackling their isolation through (1) increasing their general social engagement and (2) developing new relationships. The therapist and client may want to review both sections instead of choosing only one. The key factor in how to proceed is increasing the client's sense of hope and willingness, while minimizing the risk of overwhelming the client. Throughout the discussion, the therapist can check in with the client on how they are feeling (reinforcing the client's growing emotional awareness), and can encourage them to communicate what they may need if they experience distress in talking about developing new relationships (reinforcing appropriate assertiveness, distress tolerance, and active coping).

As an example, if the therapist notices that the client is not making eye contact when discussing the topic, the therapist may acknowledge this and say, "I see you looking down as we talk about the idea of developing new relationships. What's going on for you in the moment? How are you feeling?" This statement gives permission for a shy or anxious client to express their genuine reaction and collaborate with the therapist. Not only will this communication increase client engagement; it will also provide *in vivo* modeling (by the therapist) and direct experience of practicing new skills of emotional awareness (see Chapter 11/Session 2), as well as even newer skills of healthy communication and assertiveness (see Chapter 16/Session 7). The therapist and client can then engage in active problem solving as appropriate, and can connect agreed-upon solutions to the client's personal goals.

After introducing the topic of developing new relationships and ensuring the client's engagement, the therapist can delve into the specific skills listed in Handout 18.3. The first set of behaviors is geared toward increasing basic social engagement, while the second set focuses on starting new relationships. As mentioned earlier, the therapist and a socially isolated client can choose either or both of these options. Some clients may be significantly socially isolated and report that they have no one with whom to practice any of these skills. For such clients, it is necessary to highlight how the most basic of behaviors can start them on a path toward social engagement. No step is too small to matter. By slowly chipping away at their social distance, even with strangers, anyone can begin forming new relationships over time—whether that entails garnering new friends, activity partners, or potential romantic partners. The therapist can review each item on the list.

Deepening Existing Relationships

For clients who already have close relationships when they come to therapy, focusing on these relationships may be most sensible. Clients with trauma often have difficulties with intimacy, which may be manifested within existing long-term romantic relationships and/or relationships with family members or friends. Attachment theory provides one framework for understanding how individuals negotiate emotional distance in their close relationships. For example, even people in committed, long-term marriages can have well-developed patterns of emotional distance. One member of the relationship may prefer more independence and fewer verbal and nonverbal displays of affection (akin to a more dismissing style of attachment), while the other prefers greater closeness and emotional expressiveness (akin to either a secure attachment or a preoccupied one, depending on other factors). Though neither partner may be fully comfortable and satisfied, the marriage may "work," in that both members have found ways to compromise and accept the way things are.

In the case of childhood trauma, a survivor's pattern of emotional avoidance may be pronounced, but tolerated by a more securely attached partner. This situation is an ideal one for a client in STAIR, as the survivor can learn to open up more with the partner and then experience emotionally corrective responses that reinforce a sense of safety and intimacy. For other clients, romantic partners or family members may themselves be uncomfortable with growing intimacy and may require patience and time to adjust to it. Whatever the particular situation, the therapist normalizes any challenges and emphasizes that the client is only responsible for their own behavior, not for the reactions of others. With commitment and practice, new ways of relating can emerge.

The third and fourth sections of Handout 18.3 outline two general options for deepening current relationships: (3) increasing intimacy and reducing distance, and (4) repairing relationships after a fight or conflict. The therapist briefly introduces both options and lets the client choose one to focus on.

The third set of skills (increasing intimacy) may seem on the surface to be a "feel-good," all-positive one. However, increasing levels of intimacy can provoke a great deal of anxiety for some survivors of trauma. This reaction is especially likely for clients who experienced severe interpersonal trauma from a caregiver and/or close loved one (as in the case of intimate partner violence). In these examples, an attachment relationship was the vehicle through which the trauma and betrayal occurred. Thus learning to emotionally open oneself up again to trust another person can take ongoing effort.

The other (and, of course, complementary) option for deepening relationships is actually the most broadly applicable, and thus is often the "go-to" intervention for clients who can tolerate it—repairing relationship conflict. Navigating conflicts in relationships is a universal skill, regardless of trauma exposure or symptom presentation. Even the healthiest relationships involve occasional conflict. Acknowledging this shared human experience may help normalize some clients' concerns, reduce their sense of shame or feeling "broken," and put their minds at more ease. After the therapist and client go through each step of conflict resolution in Handout 18.3, the therapist tells the client that using these skills does not always have an immediate impact the first time around. The client may need to use emotion regulation skills to tolerate the process of conflict resolution. Sometimes the other individual needs time to absorb a message, and the client will need some level of patience. The therapist can highlight again that conflicts and their resolution are part of all relationships, so learning this skill is important and can be adapted for use in a variety of relationships and contexts.

COMPLETE RELATIONSHIP PATTERNS WORKSHEET–2

Before the therapist and client conduct the role play, the client can complete a copy of Relationship Patterns Worksheet–2, focusing on the scenario chosen for the exercise. The client can write down their initial concerns and feelings, as well as alternative, healthier thoughts, behaviors, and/or other skills identified and practiced to increase the likelihood of a positive experience. They will then do the same for the thoughts, feelings, and behaviors they expect from the other person. After the role play is completed, the therapist and client may wish to go back to the worksheet and refine the client's interpersonal goals or clarify what a new relationship model might be. The worksheet serves to document the approach the client takes in the role play, so that they may reference it when they get ready to do the real work outside of session.

COMPLETE ONE ROLE PLAY ON CHOSEN SKILL

The therapist and client's collaborative discussion in session will have set the foundation for practicing a role play with a chosen skill. Ideally, this role play can be a standard one, with the client playing themselves and the therapist taking on the role of the relevant communication partner (e.g., parent, romantic partner, or even child). Alternatively, the role play can be completed via covert modeling, where the client and therapist explore what would happen in such an interaction, as outlined in Chapter 16/Session 7. This approach may be most appropriate for more complex, lengthy scenarios. In general, the interaction is likely to look like the following:

1. The client tries out the message they want to communicate (where the client plays themselves and the therapist plays the other person).
2. The therapist then gives feedback—first identifying what went well, and then, in a supportive and positive manner, identifies what might help improve the chances of a positive outcome even more. The therapist checks in with the client, and the two come to a collaborative conclusion about how the client can revise the communication approach (verbally and nonverbally).
3. The therapist provides modeling by playing the client.
4. The client then completes the message for the second time, incorporating the suggestions presented by the therapist (with the client playing themselves and the therapist playing the other).

The therapist can adapt these steps as needed to tailor the interaction to the client and the chosen focus. What follow are examples and suggestions for completing these role plays by domain.

Role-Playing How to Develop New Relationships

Clients with a history of trauma vary greatly in their social isolation, but a subset may be so isolated that they rarely even leave their own homes. For these clients (or similarly isolated ones), the role play may be most effective if it focuses on very basic rules of social engagement and pleasantries. Although such rules may seem simple on the surface, highly traumatized individuals may be so preoccupied with their efforts to manage their symptoms and avoid triggers that they have little energy or attention left for acknowledging others. The first two sections of Handout 18.3 provide suggestions for such clients to begin opening the door, so to speak, to other people for social engagement. A therapist can encourage a client to list upcoming plans to leave their home and go to some public venue, even if the visit is routine and brief. This information may provide opportunities to highlight specific, real-world scenarios for a role play. For some clients, just saying hello to their local grocery store clerk is a big step. Others may be ready to share a simple, appropriate compliment with an acquaintance they see in passing. Regardless of the specifics, the therapist helps underscore the nonverbal elements of social interaction—especially making eye contact and using appropriate body posture and interpersonal distance—to make the situation as comfortable as possible for all people involved.

A more advanced option for the goal of developing new relationships is role-playing how to broaden a conversation from a smile or saying hello to practicing small talk or sharing an introductory conversation. Starting a relationship of any kind requires first that the involved people make a choice to interact. Then the two can make further choices to spend time together and deepen their new relationship over time. The therapist can acknowledge that sometimes, for example, an individual may want to start a friendship with another person, but for whatever reason, the other person may not follow through. It does not have to be a personal or explicit rejection, but instead may perhaps be due to the other person's limited time or priorities. This point may be important for some clients who are particularly sensitive to rejection. Thought channel skills from Session 4 (see Chapter 13) may be help-ful to review before doing this kind of role play or planning for similar practice between sessions.

We find that practicing small talk can be an especially useful topic for a role play. The label "small talk" is a misnomer for a social interaction that can perplex many clients with a history of social isolation (or may even be challenging for therapists, who are used to having deep conversations as part of their job!). The therapist keeps a positive attitude and even encourages having fun in finding ways to practice small talk. The therapist tells the client that the content of small talk is not important (that's why it is called "small talk"!). Rather, the goal is finding a way to engage in a process where people are simply acknowledging each other's presence or possibly "warming up" to become more comfortable in each oth-er's presence. The classic example of small talk is discussing the weather. Of course, other options exist, and the client can benefit from having a range of options to choose from when the situation arises. Using some humor in this exercise can help ease any sense of anxiety. It can also model the positive, upbeat quality shared by most forms of small talk.

For either type of role play for establishing new relationships, the therapist can share any relevant information about local organizations, interest groups, or meetings that an isolated client might be willing to explore. Completing an online search for events related to the client's interests may be an appropriate between-session task in this regard. As men-tioned previously, the role play ends with a discussion about the client's reactions to the exercise and plan.

Role-Playing How to Deepen Existing Relationships

The client who chooses to work on increasing intimacy in relationships may generally feel connected to select individuals, but still recognize that they (and/or the other individuals) maintain certain emotional walls. Going through a role play tied to a specific relationship can be very helpful in providing concrete options for how to move forward. The correspond-ing list in Handout 18.3 (the third one) offers several options to practice. The therapist and client can choose from this list one or more approaches to try out together. For example, a survivor of interpersonal trauma may find it challenging to express positive feelings for even their romantic partner. This hesitancy can develop from several angles, such as the fear that expressing positive feelings will make others uncomfortable or push them away, or it can result from general anhedonia or emotional numbness associated with some posttraumatic reactions. Fortunately, many of the options provided in Handout 18.3 correspond well with STAIR's broader focus on increasing positive emotions and enjoyable activities—a focus already familiar to the client by this point in therapy. The conversations and activities pro-moting closeness with others vary in depth, so the role play can be tailored to the client's specific circumstances. They may choose, for example, to role-play asking an old friend to dinner and a movie to catch up, or talking to their partner about hopes and dreams for the future.

For clients in ongoing relationships, the last five points in this section of Handout 18.3 may be most relevant. Some clients may still need to start small, so the therapist can highlight that even doing very simple things can increase one's sense of closeness, even if it is just talking about the ordinary events of the day. Socially avoidant clients may not be aware of the importance or strength of these relatively simple activities, even if they have maintained ongoing relationships of some kind over the years.

Role-Playing How to Repair After Conflicts

Alternatively, the client and therapist may choose to focus on repairing after conflicts in relationships. For this exercise, they can use the fourth and last section of Handout 18.3 to guide their practice. Because the provided guidelines in Handout 18.3 are long and sequential, we suggest in most cases that rather than doing an actual, complete role play, the therapist and client can walk through an imaginal role play and identify places where the client feels they might get stuck. Combining discussion about the approach in a specific scenario with some circumscribed role playing of the more difficult moments that may occur can be highly effective and efficient. As with other interpersonal skills learned throughout this treatment, the therapist can note that a key part of conflict resolution includes many other skills already learned (respect for the other person, clarity of one's own message, managing one's emotional reactions, etc.). Using "I Messages" is especially important to review and practice for effective conflict resolution. While checking in on the client's reactions throughout the exercise, the therapist keeps the focus on using the steps outlined in the fourth section of Handout 18.3.

No matter what the focus of the practice is, the therapist asks the client afterward about their reactions to the exercise. The client can identify where they feel more comfortable after the practice (which the therapist reinforces) and areas where they acknowledge needing additional practice. The therapist can encourage the client to take time between sessions to practice any particularly difficult statements or adjust them to fit the client's own style and language.

EXPLORE ADDITIONAL SKILL DOMAINS (OPTIONAL)

Although the therapist has referred to and used Handout 18.3 in relation to the client's specific interpersonal scenario and relationship goals, the two may also choose to explore additional components of the handout's relationship guidelines to preview further approaches to improve relationship communication and intimacy. The therapist only does so if the client is feeling comfortable, engaged, and ready to explore more options to consider for the future. If the client displays any signs of hesitancy or anxiety, it is best to keep the focus only on the agreed-upon skill domain or behaviors already explored.

Because this additional work is optional, it is expressly guided by the client's voiced wishes and interests. The therapist and client may choose to apply guidelines to a different relationship from the one already covered in the session (e.g., a relationship with a close friend or a potential new partner in the early stages of dating). Exploring how to apply these guidelines to different kinds of relationships has the added benefit of reinforcing the concept of healthy flexibility introduced in Session 8 (see Chapter 17).

All clients can continue reading the handout at their own pace outside of their sessions with the therapist. Later in treatment (or outside of treatment), clients may feel more prepared to deepen their practice and set out to meet more advanced goals after experiencing initial successes with earlier, smaller ones.

CASE EXAMPLE: MOVING TOWARD HEALTHY LEVELS OF CLOSENESS

Samantha was a 39-year-old transgender woman who came to therapy a year after successfully undergoing two gender-confirming surgeries. For the first time in her life, she felt equipped to deal with the impact of her childhood traumas. Samantha had experienced sexual abuse from the ages of 6 to 9 perpetrated by a female babysitter, as well as severe emotional abuse from her father. Her mother had died when Samantha was 3 years old, and her father, often overwhelmed by the burdens of being a single parent, frequently lashed out and demanded that Samantha "buck up and handle things like a man." She was berated and deemed weak if she expressed any feeling other than anger. Samantha learned not to express emotions or opinions in any of her relationships, and she never shared her turmoil about her personal gender identity not matching her assigned gender. Sadly, when Samantha finally told her father about her decision to pursue gender transition, he disowned her and had not spoken to her since. To protect herself from further heartbreak, she decided to preemptively sever all ties with the few friends she had with whom she had not come out.

Samantha had been working over the past few sessions to learn to express her feelings and opinions. She had gained some newfound confidence in asserting basic requests, such as asking for help in a store and asking for a menu substitution in a restaurant. Her therapist was thrilled that she brought in a copy of Relationship Patterns Worksheet–2 (see Box 18.2) related to an old friend of hers who wanted to get together. The therapist guided the discussion to the topic of getting closer to people.

THERAPIST: I see from your worksheet that your friend Bob reached out to you.

SAMANTHA: Yes, I was shocked that he did. I didn't return any of his calls or texts last month. He's always been a really good guy, but it's just a lot easier to avoid everyone. I don't know how people are going to react.

THERAPIST: So it's easier just to avoid people altogether?

SAMANTHA: Oh, yeah, way easier!

THERAPIST: And I see on your worksheet that this potential meeting with Bob brings up one of your key relationship patterns that we've been discussing—that if people really get to know you, then they will reject or punish you. This belief makes total sense in the context of the messages you received while growing up and from your father after coming out to him, but I wonder if you might be making a lot of

BOX 18.2

Samantha's Completed Relationship Patterns Worksheet–2

Interpersonal situation	What did I feel and think about myself?		What were my expectations about the other person?		My resulting behavior
What happened?	**My feelings**	**My thoughts**	**Their feelings**	**Their thoughts**	**What did I do?**
My friend Bob called and invited me to come to the diner for lunch next Thursday, like we always used to do.	Scared. Ashamed.	I am defective. No one would want to be friends with me now.	Disgust. Pity. Anger.	What a freak! He can't believe he was friends with this creep.	Didn't call him back.

Relationship model: "If _I share my true self_ , then _I am rejected and punished_ ."

Interpersonal goals for situation	Alternative beliefs and feelings about myself: What else could I . . .		Alternative beliefs and feelings about the other person: What else could I expect the other person . . .		Alternative actions
What are my goals in this situation?	**. . . feel about myself?**	**. . . think about myself?**	**. . . to feel?**	**. . . to think?**	**What else could I do?** **What else might they do?**
I want to be me and have relationships. I just want to be accepted for who I am.	Proud.	I am who I am, and I do try to be a good person.	Curious.	He may still want to be friends.	Call him and meet him for lunch. Maybe he will still want to be my friend.

Alternative relationship model: "If _I share my true self_ ,

then _someone might still like me_ ."

assumptions here about Bob's possible reaction. You said yourself that you don't actually know how Bob will react.

SAMANTHA: Well, that's true. It's just so risky and probably painful! I don't want to have to deal with more rejection. That's what makes relationships so hard. I wish I had some guarantee that people would accept me for who I am.

THERAPIST: I agree! Wouldn't it be nice if they did? Unfortunately, establishing, building, and maintaining relationships do require a little bit of vulnerability on your part. But, the key here, as we discussed earlier in our session today, is to open up slowly over time, in gradual ways, so that you can evaluate how you feel and how the other person treats you. If you don't open up at all, then it's preventing the possibility that Bob could be understanding and your friendship could even deepen. Rather than taking a gradual approach to opening up, though, often people who have experienced trauma behave in ways that are all-or-nothing: putting everything out there when they first meet someone, or cutting people off entirely.

SAMANTHA: Yes, that sounds familiar.

THERAPIST: Looking at your entry, you did a great job filling out the bottom line! You stated that your goal is to be accepted for who you are.

SAMANTHA: That's right. When I thought a lot about it, I realized that this *is* the bottom line. I'm not going to pretend any more. And I know from the Basic Personal Rights handout [Handout 16.2] that I have the right to my feelings, too! I'm still scared to act on it, though.

THERAPIST: Have you called Bob back yet?

SAMANTHA: No. I have no idea what to say. I even attended a few classes on "how to come out," but I still just kind of freeze up.

THERAPIST: Well, it seems like the first and simplest thing you want to tell him is that you would like to have lunch with him. I know you used to do that every week. And maybe, if it feels appropriate, apologize for being out of touch? Do you want to tell him over the phone about your becoming Samantha, or do you want to wait and tell him in person?

SAMANTHA: I definitely want to tell him over the phone. I look so different now. I think it would be good to tell him first, so he is not so shocked when he sees me. *If* he wants to see me.

THERAPIST: Sure, that sounds very reasonable. I think it's wonderful that you're going to give him a chance, and not assume everyone falls into the same relationship pattern. How will you tell him?

SAMANTHA: I can call him back and say something like "I'm sorry for not returning your calls sooner. I've been going through a lot lately, and I've been nervous to tell you about it. But I've missed hanging out with you, and I hope we can stay friends." Then I'd tell him that for my whole life I have struggled with understanding and expressing my true gender, and I finally built up the courage to do something about it. I would tell him I have changed my name to Samantha. Then I'd say I value his friendship and still want to see him for lunch if he wants to.

THERAPIST: That sounds great. You are very clearly telling him your feelings and explaining why you've been so out of touch. And you are clearly letting him know that you would still like to be friends. So can we plan that you will call him before our next session, and then we can talk about how it goes? If you get anxious thinking about what you plan to say, take a look over the Relationship Guidelines handout [Handout 18.3]. The section on repairing relationships will help remind you of things you might want to say to him.

SAMANTHA: Yes, I can do that.

THERAPIST: I'm happy to hear that. Know that, regardless of his response, you're doing something very healthy for yourself. It may be hard, but I'm so pleased that you're choosing to take what you deem an acceptable risk to protect a relationship you value. Your doing that is also a great example of choosing to tolerate distress. Know that I'll be here to support you, no matter how the conversation goes.

SUMMARIZE THE GOALS OF THE SESSION

At the end of the session, the therapist briefly summarizes the goals of the session and indicates how these fit within the larger framework of improving the client's relationships. The therapist can check in with the client to see how they are feeling about improving their levels of intimacy in their relationships (or starting new ones). The therapist praises the client for the work done in this session and beforehand. They also instill some level of hope that the client can develop their relationships in ways they find most helpful, while also highlighting the necessity of continuing to practice both new and old skills to make such changes happen.

PLAN SKILLS PRACTICE

In keeping with the conversation about the importance of continued practice, the therapist ends the session by discussing with the client which skills to practice before the next session. If these choices have not already been made earlier in the session, the therapist can spend some time helping the client identify a specific relationship and skill for practicing efforts to optimize intimacy and closeness. As with all skills practice, the therapist can provide encouragement to the client and suggest that accepting and listening to their feelings, while keeping in mind their larger goals, can help them navigate changes in their relationships. The therapist reminds the client that creating positive changes in relationships takes practice, just like the practice needed to learn emotion regulation skills. The therapist may say something like: "You can use copies of Relationship Patterns Worksheet–2 as a personal diary to jot down important things that happen as your move toward healthier levels of closeness with others. We'll use what happens during the week as the basis of our continued work together."

Before the next session, the client will complete Relationship Patterns Worksheet–2 at least twice and focus on situations related to increasing intimacy and closeness with others. Entries can include the client's planned efforts to improve levels of closeness in their relationships (or other specific relationship goals the client has chosen in this or previous sessions). Continuing to practice coping skills from the three channels of emotion remains important as the client focuses more on interpersonal goals. The therapist encourages continued practice of these skills, including the ongoing twice-daily practice of Focused Breathing. Finally, the therapist and client confirm the client's commitment to engage in at least one pleasurable activity per week.

Healthy Relationships = Healthy Boundaries

COMMON BOUNDARIES IN RELATIONSHIPS

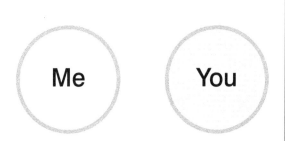

NOT CLOSE ENOUGH
Holding others at a distance

Pros:
- Feel protected and safe
- Less or no conflict

Cons:
- Not connected
- Lonely
- Lack of support
- Too much self-reliance

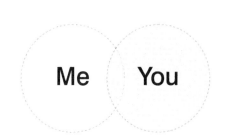

TOO CLOSE
Being "codependent"

Pros:
- Feel connected and "in sync"
- May feel support sometimes

Cons:
- Lack of support for your own priorities
- Lose sense of unique identity
- Not getting your needs and/or goals met
- Not enough self-reliance

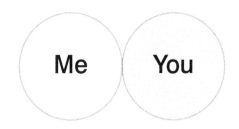

OPTIMAL
Healthy boundaries

Pros:
- Feel connected
- Feel support
- Strong sense of individual identity
- Support of each other's goals and needs

What Creates Emotional Distance and Ruptures in Relationships?

What leads people to create emotional distance in relationships?

What specific behaviors create emotional distance?

> **Remember, no matter where your relationships are now,
> you can work to improve them and grow closer to people.
> Just take it one step at a time!**

Relationship Guidelines to Enhance Intimacy and Closeness

How to increase social engagement:

1. Smile kindly at stomeone (a grocery clerk, a pharmacist, a neighbor walking down the street, etc.).
2. Say hello to someone.
3. Compliment someone on doing good work or being kind.
4. Make eye contact during these exchanges or other interactions.

How to start new relationships:

1. Initiate contact with small talk.
2. Get to know the other person, and identify common interests and/or values.
3. Make a point of acting respectfully and expressing positive emotions.
4. Initiate spending time together in low-effort ways (for example, coffee).
5. If things go well, start spending more time together (movies, hikes, etc.).

How to increase intimacy and reduce distance:

1. Ask about the other person's life, values, and interests.
2. Be willing to support them in their interests and activities.
3. Share your interests and opinions or recent life events.
4. Express positive emotions.
5. Address unresolved conflicts and issues respectfully.
6. Spend time together in enjoyable ways.
7. Express caring and respect.
8. Invite them to weigh in on your decision-making processes.
9. Be genuine and sincere.
10. Offer to help and/or ask for help and support when needed.

How to repair relationships after a fight or conflict:

1. Ask if the other person is willing to talk about what happened.
2. Acknowledge that the last contact did not go well.
3. Convey your respect and caring for the other person.
4. Acknowledge mistakes that you may have made and the hurt/damage that you think you caused.
5. Share your feelings and thoughts about your behavior and about the other person's behavior in a way that is respectful and minimizes the risk of the other person's feeling defensive. In other words, use "I Messages."
6. Ask how the other person felt about what happened.
7. Ask questions for clarification, and invite the other person to ask such questions.
8. Ask if you can make amends, or ask the other person to make amends, if appropriate.
9. Discuss how you can avoid similar situations in the future.

CHAPTER 19

Self-Compassion and Summary of Skills Training

If you want others to be happy, practice compassion.
If you want to be happy, practice compassion.
—THE 14TH DALAI LAMA (quoted in Schaef, 2000, p. 11)

This session marks the ending of one phase of treatment and a transition to another—either to more independent growth or to more advanced trauma work. For all clients, though, this session includes a new overarching theme to help shape their continued efforts at growth and psychological well-being. That theme is compassion. The word "compassion" may evoke many different feelings from clients and therapists alike. Some people may immediately latch on to the concept of caring for oneself and others in a deep, open-hearted way. Others may feel resistant to a word that may be associated with religious, political, or otherwise personal baggage. What we mean by "compassion," for the sake of this treatment, is an attitude of open, nonjudgmental kindness and recognition of the challenges one faces.

The capacity for feeling compassion for oneself and others is inherent for most of humankind. For survivors of trauma, particularly those who have experienced sustained violence (especially in childhood), there may be many blocks to experiencing compassion. These blocks can stem from a lack of foundational experiences with caregivers or intimate partners who themselves were blocked in developing their own sense of compassion. Clients who have experienced abuse during childhood or sustained violence by a partner have often internalized both explicit and implicit messages that they "deserved" the abuse/violence and are not worthy of care or respect. Such messages can lead to sustained self-loathing. Sometimes clients also feel guilt for acts of omission—for example, not helping others when they felt they should have—or for acting in ways inconsistent with their beliefs and values, such as can occur during war (i.e., "moral injury").

Still other barriers to compassion arise from experiencing interpersonal harm when trying to help other people. For example, one client came to therapy with a history of boundary violations tied to her efforts to reach out to men who were in financial and emotional need. After repeated betrayals, including a sexual assault, this client decided to wall herself off not only from these men, but also from other loved ones. Through therapy, she learned to soften these edges again so she could live her value of compassion while being mindful of appropriate boundaries and emotional warning signs.

For all these reasons, survivors of trauma can find it difficult to reconnect with a sense of compassion. By this time in treatment, at the end of STAIR, they likely have acquired enough skills to be more open to reawakening their inner capacity for compassion for themselves as well as for others. The timing of the explicit introduction to compassion also corresponds nicely with the other component of this session—transitions. This session marks a key transition to either ending therapy or moving on to the second, trauma-focused component of treatment (Narrative Therapy). The therapist's modeling of a hopeful and compassionate attitude in the session sets an important tone for this transition. As throughout this treatment, the therapist holds a compassionate attitude toward the client, which in turn can allow the client to experience this compassion and internalize it. This session concretizes this process by explicitly focusing on the role of self-compassion in the client's continued efforts to recover from trauma.

The other major task of this session is planning for the transition to the client's next step. Because not all clients will move on to Narrative Therapy, we have structured this chapter to acknowledge two pathways forward. Although all clients will explore self-compassion and review the progress they have made thus far in treatment, the paths diverge roughly halfway through the session, when the focus moves to the future. Box 19.1 outlines the content of the session. It also corresponds to the organization of this chapter by including the two branching paths, the choice of which will depend on the client's treatment plan.

CHECK-IN AND REVIEW OF SKILLS PRACTICE

Although Session 10 is the final session of the STAIR module, it begins as the others do—with the therapist conducting a brief check-in on the client's current emotional state, followed by a review of the client's skills practice. The therapist begins by reviewing the client's Relationship Patterns Worksheet–2 entries and then identifying and praising successes while acknowledging any challenges. Particularly because this session is the last one focused entirely on skills training, the therapist provides necessary guidance while recognizing that change takes time, along with continued commitment and practice. For example, the therapist may say something like:

"I see you had some challenges with your efforts to get closer to other people in the last week. That's hard to experience, but I know with time and practice, you can grow your relationships as you'd like. Nothing is radically changed in a day or a week. But I think you're going in the right direction. We'll talk today about how to keep yourself on this healthier path."

BOX 19.1

Theme and Curriculum for Session 10
Self-Compassion and Summary of Skills Training

This session marks the ending of one phase of treatment and a transition to another—either to more independent growth or to more advanced trauma work (such as Narrative Therapy). For all clients, though, this session includes the new overarching theme of compassion to help shape continued efforts at growth and psychological well-being. Although the capacity for feeling compassion is inherent for most of humankind, survivors of trauma can find it difficult to reconnect with a sense of compassion for themselves. Clients who have experienced childhood maltreatment or sustained domestic violence have internalized the explicit and implicit messages that communicate they "deserved" the abuse/violence and are not worthy of care or respect. By this time in treatment, clients ideally will have enough skills to develop an emerging sense of compassion for themselves and what they have been through. The timing of the explicit introduction of self-compassion also corresponds nicely with the other component of this session—transitions. Self-compassion is important for a client moving on to Narrative Therapy, where they will be reviewing and appraising the meaning of past traumas. However, not all clients will move on to Narrative Therapy; they will pursue life without therapy or explore other options. Here too, self-compassion is important in recognizing that important recovery tasks remain, in planning for potential relapses, and in understanding that recovery in its entirety will take time and that patience is needed. The material for this session is organized so that guidance for a client following either pathway is provided: moving to Narrative Therapy, or ending this particular treatment.

PLANNING AND PREPARATION

Review concept of self-compassion (and consider client's potential barriers to living more compassionately). Review changes in symptoms and problems over the course of skills training to aid reflection on progress. Bring extra copies of forms relevant to client's treatment plans, such as the Feelings Monitoring Form (Handout 11.3) or Relationship Patterns Worksheet–2 (Handout 17.4). The work in the session is estimated to take about 60 minutes; a flexible application is assumed (i.e., not every client will need all interventions).

AGENDA

Check-in and review of skills practice.

Identify focus of the session.

(continued)

Introduce concept of compassion.

Practice Self-Compassion Meditation.

Summarize accomplishments in skills training.

Prepare client for next step: Select Option 1 or 2.

Option 1: Moving to Narrative Therapy

- Prepare client for move to Narrative Therapy.
- Summarize the goals of the session.
- Plan skills practice:
  - Complete Relationship Patterns Worksheet–2 twice a week before next session, with a focus on situations related to increasing compassion.
  - Practice interacting in a situation where there is an opportunity to feel and express compassion for oneself and for another person (ideally as related to client's goals).
  - Use coping skills from all three channels to support treatment goals (including Focused Breathing twice daily, if preferred).
  - Practice Self-Compassion Meditation once a day.
  - Make a list of questions and concerns about the transition to Narrative Therapy.
  - Schedule at least one pleasurable activity per week.

Option 2: Completing Treatment—The Final Session

- Review and summarize the treatment as a whole.
- Prepare client for independent skills practice.
- Plan for independent skills practice.
- Present completion certificate.

SESSION HANDOUTS

Handout 19.1. Compassion: Recovery Is a Journey

Handout 19.2. Summary of Accomplishments (So Far)

Handout 19.3. STAIR Skills for Continued Practice

Additional copies of Handout 16.4. Relationship Patterns Worksheet–2

Additional copies of Handout 11.3. Feelings Monitoring Form (optional)

IDENTIFY FOCUS OF THE SESSION

Because this session is the final session of STAIR, it integrates all previous skills training sessions while introducing an organizing attitude of self-compassion for whichever next steps the client choses. The main goal of the session is to share and enjoy reviewing the client's accomplishments so far and to prepare for their continued work—whether that will be continuing to practice skills independently after ending treatment, or moving on to Narrative Therapy.

INTRODUCE CONCEPT OF COMPASSION

Rationale for Compassion

As noted at the beginning of this chapter, the concept of compassion can be loaded with personal and cultural meaning. For this reason, we recommend introducing the concept as in this example:

> THERAPIST: As I mentioned earlier, today we're going to start by talking about the idea of compassion, specifically self-compassion. What comes to mind as you hear the word "compassion"?
>
> CLIENT: To be honest, I think about people who are too "touchy-feely." The people who haven't experienced the dark side of people, like I have.
>
> THERAPIST: That's a good point. Sometimes when people talk about compassion, it can sound like they're ignoring the ugly side of the world. What if I were to say that feeling compassion actually requires recognizing that bad things happen?
>
> CLIENT: I guess that sounds more honest. How does that work?
>
> THERAPIST: At its core, compassion is simply an attitude of kindness in the face of suffering. It's being open and nonjudgmental to yourself and to others, while recognizing the challenges we all face by just being human while living in an imperfect world.
>
> CLIENT: OK, I can get on board with that. But how do I do that?
>
> THERAPIST: Good question! Luckily, there are many options. We'll explore some today, including a meditation we'll do together in a few minutes.

After a brief introduction like the preceding example, the therapist can expand on any especially important aspects of compassion relevant to the particular client. For most clients, we recommend focusing on self-compassion, as it is foundational for appropriately feeling compassion for others. It also addresses a common boundary issue for survivors of early trauma—prioritizing others' needs over one's own basic rights (see Chapter 16/Session 7). For other clients, the therapist can discuss how compassion can be expressed both for oneself and for others.

Compassion for self

Feeling compassion for oneself provides the groundwork for experiences of compassion directed outside of oneself. Saying that it provides the groundwork, however, does not mean that it is basic or easy. In fact, for many people, consciously spending time in developing self-compassion is quite challenging and may even be belittled as self-indulgent! Certainly some people can "wallow in their own self-pity," but in our experience, what may look like wallowing is actually withdrawal and depression involving high levels of self-judgment and shame. What is different about self-compassion is that it involves a higher aspect of self-awareness—the observing self. The observing self recognizes, validates, and cares for the parts of the self that are suffering, all without any level of judgment, prescription, or invalidation.

The good news is that by this point in treatment, the client has already experienced this part of the self. Any time the client has completed a Feelings Monitoring Form or a Relationship Patterns Worksheet–2, they have been observing their own behavioral and emotional patterns. By examining what has and has not worked in their efforts to change unhelpful patterns, they have had at least fleeting moments of observing without experiencing undue levels of self-judgment and shame. Fully experiencing self-compassion involves mindfully expanding these nascent moments of self-observation and awareness, while caring for the part of the self that is in pain.

Compassion for others

Developing greater compassion for others can be complicated for a variety of reasons. It can be difficult for many people to maintain a sense of compassion for others who do not share their personally held values and/or who are vastly different on various dimensions of identity. Nevertheless, when people are able to get in touch with a sense of shared humanity and the resultant compassion for other people, really important changes can and do occur.

At an individual level, fostering greater compassion for others can help transform relationships. Compassion for self and compassion for others are highly complementary. Indeed, it is nearly impossible to have one without the other. Having compassion for others does not mean giving up one's own needs and rights, but it does mean considering the needs, rights, and perspective of other persons while communicating interpersonally and making decisions. All of these characteristics are consistent with the interpersonal relationship skills previously introduced in this treatment.

Discuss Barriers to Compassion

If compassion was easy in the modern world, then everyone would be practicing it. Unfortunately, people experience many barriers to compassion, whether or not they have a history of trauma. Box 19.2 lists some possible barriers clients may face, along with corresponding responses the therapist can adapt to address these client-specific attitudes. By this time in treatment, the therapist and client will have established a strong therapeutic alliance; we

BOX 19.2

Addressing Barriers to Compassion

Possible Barrier and Client Response	Potential Therapist Response
Limited time "I don't have time to be compassionate to myself or others."	"Even small movements toward compassion can open the door more and more over time. You just need a few seconds to start down that path. If you take one step at a time, you'll begin to feel some changes, and the compassion will become easier to experience."
Shame or worthlessness "I have too much guilt and shame to care for myself in that way." "I'm worthless. How can I feel like I even deserve self-compassion?"	"I know we've explored ways, in this treatment, for you to start moving beyond these deep feelings of shame. What's really important to know is that everyone deserves compassion. I can say, too, after getting to know you over these several sessions, that you really do deserve compassion—I feel it for you, and that's not just because it's my job! I hope over time you begin to see this and even feel it deep down. I know it'll take practice and time, just like everything else we've done."
Lack of reciprocation "But if I'm more compassionate, I still won't receive more compassion from other people."	"You're right that you're only in control of your own behavior and attitude. But if you continue to be compassionate, eventually others can begin trusting that the feeling is genuine and eventually responding in kind. It's like when you smile at someone, it's hard for them not to smile back."
Not leading to action "Yeah, I may be able to feel more compassion, but that means nothing if I can't do anything with the feeling."	"Good point! As you've learned in this treatment, though, feelings do matter and do affect how we behave. How you live your growing feelings of compassion is up to you, but with time and self-reflection, I'm confident you'll see it show in how you act toward yourself and others."
Mismatch with persona, identity, or culture "That's too 'touchy-feely' for me." "That sounds like something only women are good at. I don't want to be a pushover or soft."	"There are a lot of stereotypes about who can and should feel compassion. But if we buy into those, then we're all limited in our choices in life! Compassion can seem 'touchy-feely,' but at its core, it's just knowing that we and other people experience pain in life. You don't have to go around hugging everyone or passing out flowers to show that you know and care. Sometimes a simple smile and nodding of the head can be what's helpful."
Anger/irritability "I'm just too worked up these days. Everyone and everything annoy me. My anger is too great right now for me to feel compassion."	"Yes, life can be frustrating sometimes! Especially from what you've told me, many things were getting under your skin before you started treatment. I think some of the skills you've been using to slow down, breathe, and make choices that help you meet your goals might be especially helpful to continue. As you do so, it will create space for other feelings beyond anger and frustration. I think that compassion for yourself and other people just might be one of those feelings you can start having again."

recommend using this alliance in discussing compassion. There are many ways to do so, and Box 19.2 gives a few examples. The therapist has been modeling a compassionate attitude toward the client throughout the treatment, without having to point it out explicitly. Nevertheless, expressing compassion for the client in a more direct way and using it as an example of how to feel and act compassionately may be especially helpful for clients who communicate reluctance to do so, or a lack of confidence that it is even possible.

Some themes in Box 19.2 are important for us to unpack, as they highlight important elements of compassion that the therapist may not have covered by this point in treatment. The first is the concern about lack of reciprocity for expressing compassion. This concern is most relevant for people who are interested in feeling more compassion for others. A central expectation for most people is social reciprocity. Regrettably, we cannot ensure that other people will reciprocate positive feelings and behaviors, including that of compassion. The therapy directly acknowledges this reality. What the therapist can also do, though, is reassure the client that the act of feeling and being compassionate is in and of itself a positive, healing experience—no matter what the responses from others may be. In fact, because of social reciprocity, it is very difficult to resist an honestly expressed attitude of compassion. The therapist can note that long-term relationships not characterized by mutual expressions of compassion will take time to change, but that it may be possible with continued effort and practice. Regardless of how others respond, though, if the client values having a compassionate attitude, then they are living that personal value every time they practice compassion. This alone is inherently meaningful and important.

Another significant barrier is related to cultural expectations of who can and should feel compassion. Even the word itself may be off-putting to some clients—ones who, for example, identify as particularly masculine, old-fashioned, or reserved. Still, as experienced professionals in the Department of Veterans Affairs, we know that even people embedded in a more masculine subculture, such as that of the military, are more than capable of experiencing and expressing compassion in ways congruent with their personalities and culture. As an example, one of us saw an African American Army veteran with traditional military values from a southern state, who was struggling with PTSD after combat exposure in Afghanistan. Through treatment, he began to tackle his symptoms of numbness and irritability by first expressing his caring for his dog, and then (with work) toward his young children and his wife. He had to acknowledge his own suffering and that of his family for experiencing his emotional absence over the years. His political beliefs and fundamental personality did not need to change for him to open up to increasing levels of compassion for himself and his family.

For some clients, experiencing compassion is not something they seem even willing or ready to do. For survivors of trauma, this reluctance can come from several different places. One common source of reluctance to practice self-compassion can be trauma-informed themes of inappropriate or excessive guilt and shame. By this time in treatment, the theme of guilt and shame will be familiar to therapist and client; ideally, it will have already been explored through use of the Feelings Monitoring Form and, if relevant to the client's current relationships, the two Relationship Patterns Worksheets. When reviewing possible barriers to self-compassion in this session, the therapist can explicitly make ties to any previous conversations about the client's pattern of self-blame. For a client continuing to Narrative

Therapy, the work will help address shame in more depth, so the therapist can preview how working on this barrier to self-compassion will be an ongoing process as the therapist and client continue to work together.

PRACTICE SELF-COMPASSION MEDITATION

Now that the therapist has introduced the concept of self-compassion and primed the client to develop this attitude, the therapist invites the client to participate in an exercise aimed at increasing self-compassion. The therapist can begin by acknowledging that recovery from trauma is a journey. At this point, the client has practiced many skills that will continue to be helpful in reaching their goals. Inevitably, though, there will be challenges and relapses into old behaviors. In response, the client can choose to refresh skills, begin again, or learn new skills. With any choice, having compassion for oneself will support the client in this process and make recovery from missteps easier and more successful. Compassion is a great emotion regulation intervention! After a brief introduction to the exercise, the therapist can read aloud to the client the meditation script from Handout 19.1, Compassion: Recovery Is a Journey, with appropriate pauses to let the client conduct the meditation mindfully and experience each step of the exercise fully.

Afterward, the therapist elicits and discusses the client's reaction. The therapist then encourages the client to practice the exercise over time, and to regard the Self-Compassion Meditation as a skill aimed at fostering a more compassionate attitude. If the client is going on to Narrative Therapy or some other type of trauma processing, the use of the Self-Compassion Meditation may be especially valuable as the client recalls things that provoke feelings of shame, guilt, and worthlessness. If the therapist feels that the client is ready to experience compassion for themselves, they can say something like:

> "Your being able to practice the Self-Compassion Meditation today is very encouraging. It's something that will serve you well as you move forward, especially when you think about very hard memories from your life. We want you to have compassion for the child [or person] who went through the trauma[s] you experienced. Maybe this skill can help center you. Then, from a more compassionate state of mind, you can make better choices about how to respond to a trigger, live your values, and meet your personal goals."

After the discussion on compassion ends, the therapist provides the client a copy of Handout 19.1, so that the client can use the Self-Compassion Meditation in their independent practice.

CASE EXAMPLE: FOSTERING COMPASSION IN A HARSH WORLD

Jazmin and her two sisters grew up with a mother diagnosed with paranoid schizophrenia. From birth, she experienced extreme emotional, physical, and verbal abuse. Her mother tortured her in the context of routine caregiving (e.g., injuring her during feeding). Later, Jasmin was prohibited from engaging in basic self-care, such as showering or brushing her teeth. As a young child, she spent many nights contemplating suicide, and even tried to kill herself on a few occasions from the ages of 7 to 11.

Entering therapy in her mid-20s, Jazmin built a strong bond with her therapist over the course of their work together, and she made considerable gains in her capacity to manage her emotions and advocate skillfully for herself. Although she was quite successful in her career, she worked in an abusive setting that in some ways was a repetition of her childhood home. She was now considering leaving her position for a more supportive and collegial environment—something she had never prioritized before. In spite of her significant treatment gains, Jazmin was approaching the end of the STAIR module with a sense of despondency. She described still feeling damaged to her core and could not believe that this feeling would ever change.

She could tell that her therapist had a very high regard for her and for all her accomplishments, but she dismissed it as just a routine part of the therapist's job. She had a very difficult time absorbing and believing any positive feedback, and even though intellectually she could challenge her negative beliefs about herself, she struggled to accept or even acknowledge her own self-worth. Her therapist turned to the theme of the session, compassion, as an important and possibly critical idea and experience for Jazmin to explore as she continued on the path of recovery from trauma. When the therapist presented the concept of compassion, she responded that compassion was great for other people, but not for her because she was too damaged.

> JAZMIN: I like the idea of self-compassion, but it's so abstract and not really for me.
>
> THERAPIST: It's a good thing for all of us that compassion doesn't discriminate. It may not seem like it at first, but it's for everyone. At its core, it means being kind to yourself as you navigate the ups and downs of life.
>
> JAZMIN: I just don't see how I'm supposed to have compassion for myself when I've made so many mistakes. I was constantly punished for even being alive. It's not that I'm not grateful for this program—I've learned so much about myself and gotten so much better at dealing with all kinds of things, and I even feel a lot better. But feeling compassion for myself? I just don't see it.
>
> THERAPIST: I wonder if you can tell when others have compassion for you. In fact, I have a great deal of respect and compassion for you and what you've been through. The reality is, when I hear a little about the things you've been through and the obstacles you've overcome, I'm amazed at how resilient you are. You are still alive, and you are a fighter.
>
> JAZMIN: I don't know . . .
>
> THERAPIST: Well, I firmly believe that. Remember, it was your mother's disorder that affected her thinking and behavior. The abuse didn't happen because there is something wrong with you or because you're a bad person. It was truly because of your mother's altered sense of reality.

JAZMIN: I know. Thank you for telling me this again. It really puts a whole new perspective on what happened. I had never really thought of it that way before therapy, and it's so easy to go back to blaming myself. Of course, I always took it personally, like I deserved it.

THERAPIST: Let's take a step back here. You mentioned that you've been thinking about finding another job. Tell me again why.

JAZMIN: Because I just can't stand it there any more. I am treated as less than human.

THERAPIST: This is a really big deal. For the first time in your life, you're setting healthy boundaries, dealing in a skillful way with emotions, and establishing a safe and supportive environment for yourself. Keep doing these empowering things, even if they feel small and even though they are hard to do. You know they are right to do. Recognizing that you're doing something hard but right is a wonderful way to cultivate a sense of compassion for yourself. Remember, like everyone else, you deserve to be treated with respect.

JAZMIN: I guess you're right. I was just a kid.

THERAPIST: Exactly, Jazmin. I know self-compassion will take practice. If in the future you find you are having difficulty with this, you can ask yourself how you would treat a friend. A lot of times, people who had early trauma like you find it easier to have compassion for others rather than for themselves, but in reality self-compassion and compassion for others go hand in hand. So even though our skills training sessions are ending, your own work—including creating space to acknowledge and respect your feelings, advocating for yourself, and nurturing compassion for both yourself and others—will continue to evolve.

Jazmin thanked her therapist for believing in her and for all the help she had received. The realization that her abuse was due to her mother's illness, and not due to her own inherent inferiority, was transformative for her. Although she needed to continue reminding herself of her own need for self-compassion, she felt inspired to keep making positive changes in her life, and wanted to allow herself to be open to the idea of experiencing more compassion as she moved forward in her recovery journey.

SUMMARIZE ACCOMPLISHMENTS IN SKILLS TRAINING

Prepare before Session

The therapist reviews their notes and the client's completed forms in preparation for this session, so they can identify problems and goals the client brought to the initial assessment and early sessions, and can summarize (mentally or on paper) the changes they have seen in the client. Creating a summary of accomplishments is especially important, because clients with a history of trauma tend to diminish their gains and to focus on their shortcomings and limitations. The therapist may organize the summary of accomplishments to highlight where the client first started and how far they have come. The therapist can refresh the client's memories of change that has occurred over time, and can add observations about changes that the client may have forgotten or overlooked. Using results from assessments collected along the way can be especially helpful in letting the data speak for themselves. If time allows, graphing the scores across treatment can provide a nice visual summary to use in session with the client.

Reflect on Work So Far

The therapist and client review and complete Handout 19.2, Summary of Accomplishments (So Far), to structure their reflections on the progress the client has made. Whether the client moves to Narrative Therapy or ends treatment at this session, this handout emphasizes the continuing role of the skills learned thus far in the client's ongoing health and recovery. The process of reviewing the handout will clarify and affirm the most important things that have happened in the treatment from the client's perspective. The therapist can reflect or elaborate on the client's observations with their own, keeping in mind that the conversation is still primarily led by the client. This stance reinforces again the role of the client as their own agent of change and primary source of knowledge as they gain increasing levels of psychological health.

To guide the discussion, Handout 19.2 lists reflection questions in the order of primary treatment targets: emotional awareness, emotional coping, and relationship patterns/communication skills. How does the client experience and express emotions differently from before treatment? In what ways are they approaching relationships differently? This reflection will help consolidate these lessons before the client moves on to the next step in their recovery journey.

Congratulate the Client on Progress

The therapist ends this discussion by congratulating the client on their hard work and accomplishments as reflected through both changes in their scores and positive experiences outside of sessions. The therapist can include any observations of change that they have wanted to share but might not have had the opportunity to do so up to this point. The therapist can also highlight specific successes and situations from any point of the skills training component of treatment, even if they have already provided positive feedback on the example in previous sessions.

PREPARE CLIENT FOR NEXT STEP: SELECT OPTION 1 OR 2

We designed this treatment with flexibility to allow therapists and clients to decide whether to combine the STAIR (skills training) and Narrative Therapy modules of the treatment protocol. Given this choice (which ideally is made before the beginning of treatment or in earlier sessions), the rest of this session/chapter is separated into two branching paths.

Depending on what the client and therapist decide, the therapist chooses Option 1: Moving to Narrative Therapy, or Option 2: Completing Treatment—The Final Session. To aid the discussion of ongoing skills practice, Handout 19.3, STAIR Skills for Continued Practice, is a component of both options and includes the new concept of compassion and its associated Self-Compassion Meditation skill in the thought channel of emotion. This handout also provides a summary for the interpersonal themes explored in the latter half of STAIR.

Option 1: Moving to Narrative Therapy

For clients continuing to Narrative Therapy, the following provides a structure for the rest of this session.

PREPARE CLIENT FOR MOVE TO NARRATIVE THERAPY

The next session and subsequent ones mark a shift in focus from skill acquisition to direct processing of the client's trauma history and memories in the context of their broader life. The next session will introduce the nature of this treatment approach (Narrative Therapy) more completely, but in this session, the client is given a "broad-strokes" understanding of this new approach in the context of the work they have already completed. Some key points for the therapist to share (and incorporate throughout the remainder of this session) include the following:

- Reviewing briefly with the client the work that they have done in building emotion regulation and interpersonal skills, and discussing how these skills support the second component of the program (Narrative Therapy).
- Asking the client to share their own thoughts about their progress, ways the treatment has been helpful, and areas that need further attention (which can be part of the next module of treatment).
- Congratulating the client on their hard work and progress during this first module of the treatment, and emphasizing the strengths the therapist has observed up until this point.
- Discussing together the areas in which the client is continuing to grow and improve, and letting them know that work will continue on these areas during the next component of treatment.

Review Format and Session Changes for Narrative Therapy

The therapist can remind the client that in Narrative Therapy, their work together will shift toward helping them to process and integrate their traumatic memories. This goal will be accomplished by going through their traumatic memories repeatedly and coming to a broader understanding of their meaning for the client now. The therapist can tell the client that during the Narrative Therapy sessions, the first part of each session will be spent reviewing the traumatic experiences and evaluating their meaning; the remaining time will be spent focusing on current issues and the effective use of emotion regulation and relationship skills.

Elicit Client's Questions and Concerns about Transition to Narrative Therapy

The therapist then asks the client whether they have any questions or concerns about the transition to Narrative Therapy. Is the format of this new approach clear to the client? Do they understand the rationale and procedure for Narrative Therapy? What are their concerns and fears about starting to do the narrative work? The therapist encourages the client to be frank about their concerns, but also indicates that there will be more time to discuss questions and more general information about the narrative approach in the next session. In fact, one of the activities the client will complete before the next session is to make a list of questions, concerns, or other thoughts they have about entering the next series of sessions.

Select Skills to Support Narrative Work

The therapist and client openly discuss how the skills the client have learned so far will still play a vital role moving forward, despite the shift in the treatment's focus. Handout 19.3 provides an overview of the emotion regulation and interpersonal skills they have learned, and a checklist for the therapist and client to complete in selecting the most crucial coping skills to bring to the next series of sessions. This conversation will parallel the one in Session 5 about distress tolerance (see Chapter 14), but will also incorporate newer skills and concepts related to self-compassion and healthier relationship patterns.

SUMMARIZE THE GOALS OF THE SESSION

As in previous sessions, the therapist provides a brief review and summary at the end of the session. For clients continuing to Narrative Therapy, the therapist can summarize similarly as they have done with previous sessions. That is, they review the major points of the session: reflecting on progress made in skill acquisition and symptom change; developing more compassion for themselves (and others, if explored); and planning for the transition to Narrative Therapy.

PLAN SKILLS PRACTICE

To support a client continuing to the Narrative Therapy module of this treatment, the therapist and client plan for ongoing skills practice aimed at (1) enhancing and maintaining skills learned in STAIR (to continue growth in emotion regulation and relationship skills), and (2) preparing for the more advanced narrative and trauma-focused aspects of Narrative Therapy. The client will continue completing Relationship Patterns Worksheet–2 twice a week with situations relevant to the client's broader treatment goals (including ones related to emotional triggers that may occur more spontaneously). If needed, the therapist can provide additional copies of Handout 16.4 for these new entries. The therapist can also confirm that the client has a copy of Handout 19.3 with the skills marked for continued practice, which the client will continue to do throughout the Narrative Therapy module to support their treatment goals.

As for new skills practice, the client can plan to (1) make a list of questions and concerns they may have about moving to Narrative Therapy, and (2) practice experiencing and showing compassion in two ways. First, they may use Handout 19.2 to practice the Self-Compassion Meditation completed earlier in the session once a day, to help keep the concept in mind. Second, they can practice interacting in a situation where they may express a feeling of compassion for either themselves or for another person. Ideally, this situation will relate to one of the client's goals. The client can also schedule at least one pleasurable activity in the next week, if this has not already been part of one of the activities planned thus far.

Option 2: Completing Treatment—The Final Session

For clients who end treatment after the completion of the STAIR module, the rest of the final session can follow the structure outlined below.

SUMMARIZE THE TREATMENT AS A WHOLE

For a client who is ending therapy, the review/summary serves as a broader one overviewing the course of treatment (summarizing key aspects of earlier sessions) and the client's commitments to continued practice and growth outside of therapy. Incorporating the conversation about compassion may be especially helpful in encouraging the client's continued growth and flexibility as they learn more about themselves and their relationships independent of therapy.

PREPARE CLIENT FOR INDEPENDENT SKILLS PRACTICE

Some clients may have entered this treatment expecting therapy to be something done to them, then completed, and finally left in the past. STAIR, however, has introduced these clients to a more active and collaborative role in therapy and in making changes in their lives. This sense of engagement, personal motivation, and responsibility is crucial to maintain for continued success in sustaining and expanding gains made in therapy. A therapist and client will both benefit from explicitly discussing how the client can continue to grow without the presence of the therapist or the sessions that provided structure for their initial skill acquisition. The client may share some concerns about how to maintain the progress they made, and the therapist can normalize some of this anxiety, while also eliciting the client's sense of ownership for what they have accomplished. The therapist can remind the client of specific instances when the client used skills during difficult moments, and/or of successes that occurred because of what the client did outside of the therapy room.

PLAN INDEPENDENT SKILLS PRACTICE

Which skills are practiced independently after treatment will vary from person to person. The client is ultimately the primary determinant of the plan, with guidance as needed from the therapist. In many cases, continuing to practice emotion regulation and communication skills will be a core component of the client's plan. Handout 19.3 provides the best framework for selecting skills across the three channels of emotion and reviewing interpersonal themes. Some clients may also prefer to use the structure of the Feelings Monitoring Form or Relationship Patterns Worksheet–2 to reflect on their ongoing experience. For these clients, the therapist can provide extra copies of the relevant worksheets. Any additional informational handouts or copies of worksheets provided by the therapist to the client also serve to reinforce the idea that the work is not over. That is, this transition marks primarily the move to independent practice, and not the leaving behind of lessons learned with the help of the therapist.

PRESENT COMPLETION CERTIFICATE

In the last moments of the session, the therapist can provide a certificate of completion acknowledging all of the client's hard work, achievements, and commitment to healing from their trauma. This moment is the final opportunity for the therapist to congratulate the client. The therapist can keep in mind that while some clients may like the idea of "graduating" from treatment, many others will prefer to view this transition as the beginning of the second stage of treatment—treatment as their own therapists. Even so, for most clients, having a formal certificate of completion can be a special indicator and reminder of the lessons they learned and want to continue to bring forward in their lives.

Compassion: Recovery Is a Journey

Having compassion for yourself can be challenging, given the messages you may have gotten from others and the negative beliefs you may still hold about yourself. There are several benefits to self-compassion, however, including:

1. Compassion for yourself goes hand in hand with compassion for others. So self-compassion may lead to having more compassion for others and improving your relationships.
2. Having compassion for yourself also allows you to change and experiment with new ways of behaving and feeling, such as asking for help or being more assertive. You'll be able to practice your new skills without fear if you just have compassion for yourself as a person who is learning, growing, and changing.
3. Finally, compassion for yourself allows success in the journey of recovery. There will be lapses and challenges. But the more accepting you are of your shortcomings, the easier it will be for you to focus your efforts on change. The energy you used up criticizing or defending yourself before you started treatment can be channeled into the work needed to reach your goals.

Consider your successes in this work and accept them. Consider your challenges and limitations and accept them too. Continue to work toward your goals with compassion for your past and your continuing struggles.

SELF-COMPASSION MEDITATION EXERCISE

Take a moment to focus on your breathing. If it feels comfortable, close your eyes.

Now take a slow, deep breath. Exhale slowly, allowing all of the air to leave your lungs. Inhale. And exhale slowly.

Continue to breathe at this pace.

Now imagine yourself. See all the parts of yourself.

View the parts that represent some of the positive aspects of yourself, such as happiness, joy, pleasurable feelings, positive beliefs, and loving memories. What do you notice?

Now, take a moment to view the painful parts of yourself—those that represent your distressing emotions, fears, negative beliefs, and painful life experiences. What do you notice?

Now imagine that these different parts of yourself are struggling with each other. It's a long struggle that has been going on for many years. The painful parts are trying to find an advantage over the positive parts, while the positive parts desperately respond with all of their might to avoid being taken over and ignored. What do you notice?

(continued)

Now imagine that instead of allowing the positive and painful parts of yourself to fight against each other, you allow them to exist together without needing to struggle. Rather than allowing the painful pieces to win and viewing yourself as all bad, worthless, or unlovable, allow yourself to hold all of these parts together with compassion. Imagine seeing yourself as a person with strengths and weaknesses, just like others, and at the same time seeing yourself as deserving love, respect, and compassion.

Focus on what this experience feels like. View all the parts of yourself as a whole, without judgment.

Now, return your focus to just noticing your breath . . . taking slow, deep breaths. And when you're ready, open your eyes, and slowly return your focus to the room around you.

Summary of Accomplishments (So Far)

Let's review all the things you've learned and accomplished during this treatment!

- We discussed how trauma affects emotion and how it affected you.

Before STAIR, how did you experience your emotions?

- We then explored skills that could change how you coped with your emotions. Later today, we'll select the skills from the three channels of emotion (body, thought, behavior) that you want to continue practicing. For now, consider:

What are ways you're experiencing your emotions differently from before starting treatment?

- We also explored how trauma affects relationships, and we identified different ways to approach and manage relationships—with flexibility, assertiveness, power, intimacy, and compassion.

What are ways you're approaching relationships differently in what you believe, feel, and do?

(continued)

Summary of Accomplishments (So Far) *(page 2 of 2)*

- As you prepare to move on, let's reflect on the progress you've made.

What are the most important lessons you've learned?	
What lessons felt most helpful?	
How have your thoughts, emotions, and behaviors changed?	
How will you continue to build on the progress you've made so far?	

STAIR Skills for Continued Practice

EMOTIONAL COPING

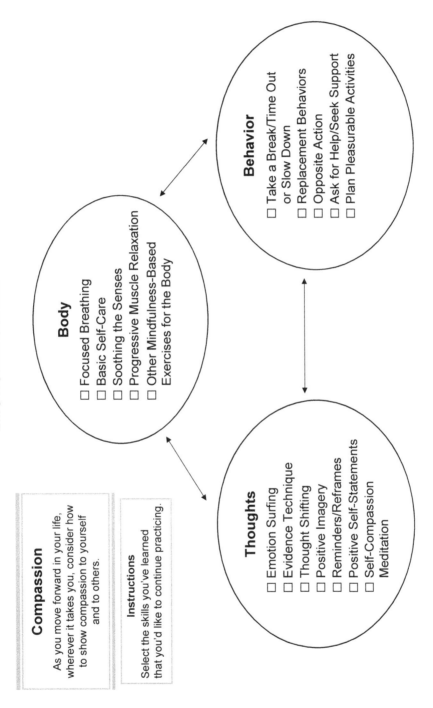

Body
- ☐ Focused Breathing
- ☐ Basic Self-Care
- ☐ Soothing the Senses
- ☐ Progressive Muscle Relaxation
- ☐ Other Mindfulness-Based Exercises for the Body

Behavior
- ☐ Take a Break/Time Out or Slow Down
- ☐ Replacement Behaviors
- ☐ Opposite Action
- ☐ Ask for Help/Seek Support
- ☐ Plan Pleasurable Activities

Thoughts
- ☐ Emotion Surfing
- ☐ Evidence Technique
- ☐ Thought Shifting
- ☐ Positive Imagery
- ☐ Reminders/Reframes
- ☐ Positive Self-Statements
- ☐ Self-Compassion Meditation

Compassion

As you move forward in your life, wherever it takes you, consider how to show compassion to yourself and to others.

Instructions

Select the skills you've learned that you'd like to continue practicing.

(continued)

From *Treating Survivors of Childhood Abuse and Interpersonal Trauma, Second Edition: STAIR Narrative Therapy* by Marylene Cloitre, Lisa R. Cohen, Kile M. Ortigo, Christie Jackson, and Karestan C. Koenen. Copyright © 2020 The Guilford Press. Permission to photocopy this material is granted to purchasers of this book for personal use or use with clients (see copyright page for details). Purchasers can download additional copies of this material (see the box at the end of the table of contents).

STAIR Skills for Continued Practice *(page 2 of 2)*

Compassion

Just as it's important for your own emotional coping, compassion is a key part of creating the relationships you want in your life. Compassion for yourself and for other people will help you thrive. Make sure you don't neglect one for the other—everyone deserves compassion, especially you!

RELATIONSHIP SKILLS

Instructions: Below is a summary of the relationship skills you've learned about, organized by theme. Jot down some relationship goals you still want to work toward, and list the skills you think would be most helpful in meeting those goals.

Assertiveness	Power	Closeness and Intimacy	Flexibility
"I Messages"	Understanding Power Balances	Increasing Social Engagement	Self-Compassion Meditation
Making Requests	Respect Bookends	Starting New Relationships	Compassion for Others
Saying No		Reducing Emotional Distance	Distress Tolerance to Meet Goals
		Repairing Relationships after Conflict	Pros and Cons

Your Relationship Goals	Skills Useful to Meet Your Goals

Narrative Therapy
Facing the Past and Imagining the Future

CHAPTER 20

Moving from Skills Training to Narrative Therapy

How Do You Know Your Client Is Ready?

My silences have not protected me.
Your silence will not protect you.
—AUDRE LORDE (1984, p. 40)

The transition to focused attention on trauma memories is often associated with increased anxiety and discomfort for a client, and sometimes for a therapist as well. Therapists often fear that their clients will get worse, suffer symptom exacerbation, or flee from the therapy when confronting painful memories. If not fearful of the task itself, therapists often uneasily inquire, "How will I know that my client is ready for narrative work?"

Both a therapist and a client need to keep in mind that some amount of increased anxiety in the anticipation of the task and in the initial efforts of confronting the memories is inevitable. It is frightening to face what one fears. However, it is our experience that narrative work is more difficult to think about than to do. The anticipatory anxiety resulting from imagining the next steps often requires more emotion management than the actual effort involved when therapist and client structure, agree upon, and begin the task. The skills training sessions have prepared the client and therapist for this work: The two of them have an established working relationship; the client has developed sufficient skills and self-confidence to face difficult emotions; and they have some amount of trust in the therapist to guide them safely and effectively through the process. The STAIR module enhances two therapeutic features that are important to successful narrative work.

Therapist's Knowledge of the Client

First, the therapist is by now thoroughly familiar with the client's trauma history, symptoms, and coping skills. The therapist is aware of the severity of the client's fear and emotional reactivity; has a working knowledge of the client's general coping style and distress tolerance; and has been able to evaluate, facilitate, and observe the client's skills strengths and areas of vulnerability. All of this information helps the therapist proceed effectively in the therapeutic task during the narrative work, which is to modulate the client's emotional experience. This task includes both encouraging the client to provide more specific and extended articulation of feelings and beliefs than they otherwise would have, and helping the client ease up on or move away from material that is overwhelming.

Shared Understanding and Commitment

The STAIR sessions also provide the template for the working relationship between therapist and client. The therapist's knowledge of the client is the result of a process in which the therapist identifies and characterizes the client's problems and skills, so that the client can confirm, correct, adjust, or extend the developing picture. This process engenders in the client a sense of being recognized and understood. The client develops confidence in the therapist's growing knowledge of their strengths and weaknesses. In addition, both client and therapist develop a specific language for referring to and describing internal emotional states and the traumatic memories. Lastly, the treatment goals and the means to reach these goals are repeatedly reviewed and take concrete shape through the emergence of the client's specific vulnerabilities, emotional reactivity, and strengths. Ideally, the therapist and client will be in agreement toward the end of the skills training work that the next task is the narrative work, and will have a good sense of how this task will go. Agreement on goals and the means to reach these goals, based on solid knowledge of the client's symptoms, needs, and strengths, secures the therapeutic foundation and provides confidence in both therapist and client for successful narrative work.

GUIDELINES FOR REVIEWING READINESS
FOR NARRATIVE THERAPY

There are no hard and fast rules about when to begin narrative work. Some clients may be ready in the second session, while others may not be prepared to do so for many months. The more important questions are whether an individual client is ready and whether the treatment relationship meets the criteria described above. This is a clinical judgment that therapists make on a case-by-case basis. The following basic questions may be helpful in assessing whether moving to the narrative component is indicated and appropriate for a certain client at a particular time in treatment. The assessment of readiness is helped if both therapist and client keep in mind the core features of narrative processing of the trauma (see Box 20.1).

Is the Client Committed to the Treatment?

Before embarking on narrative work, the therapist must have a sense of the client's motivation, ability, and willingness. Psychotherapy in general, and trauma treatment in particular, are challenging processes that require considerable investment and effort on the part of the

BOX 20.1

The Purpose and Nature of Narrative Therapy

The goal of trauma narration is for the client to experience trauma-related feelings in depth, but while safe and with control. Understood in this way, trauma narration is not a direct reexperiencing of the past. Rather, trauma narration allows the client to visit the past with the tools of the present, in the safety of the present, and with the companionship of an ally from the present.

Through the use of emotion management skills and awareness of the safety features of their current environment, the client reexperiences fear, but in a safe environment and without being overwhelmed by it. The client comes into contact with the feeling that there is no escape from traumatic events and memories, but that they have survived their past and the past cannot harm them. The client feels the anger and sadness of being betrayed, abandoned, and hurt by important people in their life, but with the therapist's presence, they need not feel obliterated by this knowledge. The client reveals the shame they feel about their trauma, and feels comforted by the compassion of an empathetic therapist.

client (as well as the therapist) to be fruitful. Even with a high level of motivation, facing often distressing and painful issues to the extent required to make changes is difficult for a client; without such motivation, a therapist is fighting an uphill battle. This is not to say that the client cannot express hesitation, ambivalence, or even resentment about having these problems as a consequence of traumatic experiences. The client does not necessarily have to feel positive about or enjoy being in treatment. In addition, a client may go through periods during the treatment when it feels particularly difficult to sustain involvement (for any number of reasons). These and other potential obstacles are manageable if they can be raised and addressed in the context of the therapy, and if they do not interfere with a basic level of compliance in treatment.

If the therapist doubts a client's level of commitment or ability to participate fully in the narrative work, then the treatment direction and goals need to be reevaluated in a nonjudgmental and realistic way. The following considerations about past experience in working with a given client may be helpful in this regard: Up to this point, has the client demonstrated interest and motivation in the treatment? If not, has the client been able to tolerate and participate in examining obstacles? Has the client made the treatment a priority, or does therapy tend to take a back seat? Has the client behaved in ways indicating a belief that the treatment is valuable (e.g., keeping most appointments, being generally on time, not putting other activities before treatment, doing between-session work, being actively engaged during sessions)?

Is the Client Relatively Stable at the Present Time?

The therapist evaluates the client's mental status and symptom severity continually throughout the therapy, as these will affect the treatment's direction and focus session by session. However, at this juncture when the therapist is considering whether to begin the narrative module, particular attention to assessing the client's current level of stability and current strengths and weaknesses is indicated.

"Stability" is a relative and hard-to-define term, especially given that so many survivors of trauma deal with a host of ongoing psychological, physical, and social problems on a daily basis. Many of our clients have chaotic and overwhelming lives; indeed, this has become the norm rather than the exception. Also, feeling consistently overwhelmed, "edgy," and easily emotionally triggered are hallmarks of the PTSD and CPTSD diagnoses for which many clients qualify (see Chapter 9). These factors make an accurate appraisal of a particular client's current level of stress, capabilities, and limitations challenging. It is important to keep in mind that for most of these clients there is no "optimal" time to begin narrative work, as there is typically some kind of disruption or crisis happening in their lives. Waiting until things are "calm" is unrealistic, as much of the chaos is perpetuated by the ongoing PTSD/CPTSD symptoms. If a therapist continues to move from crisis to crisis with such a client, it is the equivalent of continually putting out small fires rather than locating the main source of the primary fire, which will continue to rage. In fact, many of our clients have already had this type of experience in previous therapies, which did not systematically address the trauma memories and associated feelings at the root of their troubling symptoms.

However, if a therapist feels that a client is in a particularly vulnerable or precarious psychological state in which any additional stress may be intolerable or lead to decompensation, then engaging in narrative work (even in a modified format) is not indicated, as the potential risks outweigh the benefits. This type of situation most often arises when there are sudden major stressors or transitions in a client's life (e.g., unexpected death or loss of family member/friend, recent diagnosis of serious medical condition, loss of job or housing), or when for some reason the client has a particularly pressing situation that requires immediate attention and a high level of functioning (e.g., work situation that may jeopardize employment status, acute family emergency). In these cases, delaying narrative work makes sense, as it requires substantial effort and energy that may be in especially short supply. This is particularly relevant for clients who have a history of addictive or self-injurious behaviors.

Has the Client Demonstrated Some Capacity for a Therapeutic Alliance?

Addressing the client's capacity for a therapeutic alliance involves taking stock of how the client has worked with and related to the therapist up until this point. Specific key issues relevant to survivors of trauma, especially childhood interpersonal trauma, must be considered. Specifically, most of our clients struggle with building and maintaining healthy interpersonal relationships, and often this particular problem is what has brought them into treatment. A history of repeated violations by caregivers and others understandably has a negative impact on a person's ability to develop closeness and trust in relationships, particularly with those (such as therapists) who may be perceived as authority figures. Thus if a client demonstrates guardedness, suspiciousness, anxiety, hostility, or fear at times with the therapist, this is not surprising and is not in itself an indication that the client cannot develop an effective working relationship. In fact, these difficult feelings in the therapy relationship can be used in a beneficial manner if the client can directly express them or tolerate discussion of them.

However, if the client has not developed some level of trust with the therapist, has not been able to take in feedback constructively, or cannot communicate their reservations, there is cause for concern about moving into narrative work. The client needs to have some belief, even if it is tenuous, that the therapist is competent and motivated to help rather than to violate them. If not, it is unlikely that the client will be willing to engage in narrative processing, during which the therapist will be encouraging them to take risks by stepping outside their comfort zone. Or the client may agree to proceed with exposure, but may feel coerced and victimized by the therapist rather than feel that they are actively participating by their own choice. It is not uncommon in work with survivors of trauma for the therapist and client to find themselves in respective "perpetrator–victim" roles in the treatment. This dynamic does not have to be destructive if it can be processed in such a way that allows the client to recognize how this old relationship pattern related to past trauma is being generalized to the current situation. However, if the client continues to feel predominantly controlled, manipulated, or coerced by the therapist, narrative work is likely to be untherapeutic at best and retraumatizing at worst. One option is to continue trying to process these issues, with the hope of developing a more collaborative relationship before reconsidering narrative work. Alternatively, if this type of dialogue is not possible and the relationship continues in a similar vein over time, the therapist discusses the option of maintaining the treatment with a sole focus on further developing STAIR skills or of referring the client to a different therapist or treatment.

Has the Client Been Able to Learn and Use Skills Presented in the STAIR Module?

The STAIR Narrative Therapy program is designed so that before beginning intensive and emotionally demanding narrative work, the client has had the opportunity to learn skills to manage affective and interpersonal difficulties. We have typically found in our research that a 2-month (approximately 10-session) module of skill-based interventions is an adequate period of time for most clients to develop a basic repertoire of skills that they can experiment with in stressful situations. Of course, there are important individual differences—depending on how much time clients have devoted to practicing the skills both within and outside sessions, as well as their pretreatment level of coping skills.

It is not necessary or realistic to wait until clients demonstrate complete mastery over the skills they have been introduced to before making the transition to narrative work, especially given that continued work on skill building is integral to the Narrative Therapy module. Rather, it is important that the clients have been able to learn basics and have begun to use them outside sessions to cope with difficult feelings or situations. If a client is not exhibiting some degree of competence and confidence in using skills, then the STAIR module of treatment may need to be prolonged before narrative work begins. Questions to consider include the following: Has the client been interested in or found some value in learning the skills? Has the client practiced skill-building exercises regularly between sessions? Has the client made any modifications to skills that indicate an effort to integrate them into the client's own life? Has the client used skills independently both within and outside sessions with some success? Since narrative work will require the client to draw on some of the skills the client has learned in managing overwhelming emotions, it is important to review with the client which particular skills feel most beneficial and which skills need continued practice.

Might the Client Be Interested in Participating in "Conjoint Treatment"?

An alternative that we have found useful for clients who want to do narrative work but also want to continue intensive skills training is "conjoint treatment." In this arrangement, the client continues STAIR with the current therapist, but goes to another for the narrative work. The costs and time commitment for this type of approach need to be considered, but we have found this to work well: A client is able to maintain a useful treatment and good relationship with one therapist while engaging with another for more short-term and intensive work. This is also a good solution for situations where the primary therapist is trained in STAIR but not in Narrative Therapy.

To conclude, there is no perfect time to begin narrative work. The decision to make the transition from STAIR to Narrative Therapy is made by the therapist and client together, and is informed by the therapist's clinical judgment. Critical for this transition is that both the therapist and the client *believe* the client is ready for narrative work and can be successful. This belief, especially for the client, may be tentative. As we state above, most clients and therapists have some anxiety in anticipating this component of the treatment, but this anxiety tends to dissipate once the narrative processing has begun.

Introduction to Narrative Therapy

> I know this story well, because I have been stuck inside it. I have lived
> with its causes and effects, its details and indelible lessons my entire
> life. . . . And if I ever hope to leave this place, I must tell what I know.
> So let me begin.
>
> —MIKAL GILMORE (1994, pp. x–xi)

The goal of Session 11 is to orient the client to the narrative work that will begin in Session 12. The therapist provides a clear description and rationale for the use of Narrative Therapy. The therapist and client also review coping skills learned in previous sessions and identify ways in which these skills will support the goal of completing narrative work. Lastly, the therapist and client identify specific trauma memories that will be narrated, organizing them by the level of distress each of these memories causes, so that the narrative work can be planned with sensitivity to distress management.

Interwoven into these preparatory activities are the repeated reflections that, while painful, the task of revisiting and making sense of the traumatic past will allow the client to be freed of it. In telling about it, the client will confront, understand, and eventually master the trauma. By critically examining its causes and harmful consequences, the client will summon the reasons and the will to change their beliefs and behaviors.

Lastly, because Narrative Therapy is explicitly a *narrative* process, it conveys the message that a life story is composed of a past, present, and future. The client's retelling of the trauma both establishes and reinforces its "pastness." Moreover, narration assumes a chronological structure that not only allows the trauma to be located placed firmly in the past, but prompts the client to consider the present and imagine a future. Through narration, clients create important links between their past and present, as well as potential relationships among the past, present, and an imagined future. Through Narrative Therapy, clients express themselves and become the owner of their life stories. Box 21.1 outlines the theme and curriculum for this session.

Theme and Curriculum for Session 11
Introduction to Narrative Therapy

Narrative Therapy involves a client's repeated telling of specific traumatic memories, organizing these memories into coherent life events, critically evaluating their meaning, and deliberating about their place in the client's life history. Confronting the memories leads to the realization that the traumatic images and thoughts are simply memories that have no real power over the client. In addition, telling about the trauma allows the client to organize the traumatic events in a way that helps them understand what happened and explore their meaning. The client identifies beliefs about the self and others (relationship models) that emerged from the narratives, with the goal of understanding that these beliefs belong to a particular life context—namely, a traumatic past. The circumstances of the client's life have changed, and therefore these old beliefs and guidelines for living, which were once adaptive, are no longer necessary or even valuable. The client is free to choose alternative strategies for living.

PLANNING AND PREPARATION

Bring a copy each of Handouts 21.1 and 21.2, as well as several copies of Relationship Patterns Worksheet–2 (Handout 16.4). This session is 60 minutes in duration.

AGENDA

- Check-in and review of skills practice.
- Identify focus of the current session.
- Provide overview of Narrative Therapy.
- Review application of emotion regulation skills.
- Confirm client's commitment to narrative work.
- Create memory hierarchy.
- Summarize the goals of the session.
- Plan skills practice:
  - Read Overview of Narrative Therapy handout.
  - Complete distress tolerance exercise (Pros and Cons) for engaging in narrative work.
  - Complete Relationship Patterns Worksheet–2 twice during week.
  - Practice Focused Breathing twice a day, and other emotion regulation skills as relevant.

(continued)

SESSION HANDOUTS

Handout 21.1. Overview of Narrative Therapy

Handout 21.2. Memory Hierarchy

Additional copies of Handout 16.4. Relationship Patterns Worksheet–2

CHECK-IN AND REVIEW OF SKILLS PRACTICE

At the end of the last session of STAIR (Session 10), the client has been asked to make a list of questions they might have about Narrative Therapy. The therapist and client now review these questions. The therapist has prompted the client to consider issues such as whether the format of this new approach is clear, whether they understand the rationale and procedure for Narrative Therapy, and what concerns and fears they may have about starting Narrative Therapy. Often the client's questions will be answered during the course of this session. But the therapist now takes the time to answer each question, directly and briefly, and to state that more details about the process will be reviewed in this session. The therapist also reviews the Relationship Patterns Worksheet–2 copies completed by the client, and checks in regarding whether the client has maintained emotion regulation skills practice during the week. Clients sometimes experience increased stress in anticipation of the narrative work, and mentioning this might be helpful. The therapist can remind the client that maintaining regular practice of emotion regulation skills will contribute to emotional well-being.

IDENTIFY FOCUS OF THE SESSION

The goal of this session is to prepare the client for Narrative Therapy. After checking in with the client about their feelings of anticipation about this next step, the therapist begins by communicating that the purpose of this session is to introduce and orient them to the narrative work, so that they will know what to expect *before* beginning the process. Providing this structure is critical in giving the client the message that this work will be approached gradually, at a pace that will allow them to raise questions and concerns. This is particularly important for survivors of trauma, who commonly feel taken off guard and not in control of what is happening to them. It is also important that the therapist convey a sense of reassurance and empathy, because the client is likely to feel unprepared for narrative work. This is often the case no matter how much work clients have done on developing coping skills, or how clearly they have articulated alternative models for living in the here and now. The past is essentially uncharted territory. A critical part of the narrative process is that the client comes to feel strongly anchored in the present, and with the attitude that the resources they have within the context of the treatment are more powerful than any they had in the past. This feeling can be set in motion through a review of their coping skills, reassurance that the therapist is aware of their strengths and vulnerabilities, and promises that the therapist will be there to support and guide them in the process.

PROVIDE OVERVIEW OF NARRATIVE THERAPY

The therapist lets the client know that they will begin the narrative work in the next session. Although the client has been given the rationale for the narrative process at the beginning of treatment (Session 1), the therapist now reviews it in detail and describes the specific procedures involved in Narrative Therapy. The therapist delivers the information as though they are providing it for the first time, because many clients may not have retained important parts of the information they were initially given. The therapist also tells the client that they will be given a written version of this information at the end of the session, in the form of a take-home sheet on Narrative Therapy for review (see Handout 21.1, Overview of Narrative Therapy). A description of the purpose and implementation of each aspect of Narrative Therapy is provided below. Narrative Therapy has three goals: (1) to reduce the client's fear and PTSD symptoms; (2) to enable the client to organize the trauma memories in a coherent and meaningful way; and (3) to help the client develop a coherent life story by understanding how past trauma influences current feelings, beliefs, and behaviors.

First Goal of Narrative Therapy: Reduce Fear and PTSD Symptoms

Narrative work begins with repeated telling of trauma memories until they are no longer frightening. The therapist reviews the rationale both for this repeated telling of the trauma, as a skill to reduce fear, and for the process by which it is accomplished, based in the logic of prolonged exposure (see Foa & Rothbaum, 1998; Rothbaum & Foa, 1999). Talking about the memories is not identical to reliving them, as the client is in reality safe. This knowledge allows the task to be conducted with greater ease. The therapist starts by succinctly describing what the first step in narrative work will entail:

> "What we will be doing in the narrative sessions is revisiting your traumatic experiences—the ones that continue to cause distress and disruption in your life. I use the word 'revisiting' rather than 'reliving,' because during this process the aim is not to submerge yourself completely in the past, but rather to have one foot in the past and the other grounded in the present. The ultimate goal is to help you make sense of these disturbing memories, so that you will no longer feel so controlled and overwhelmed by them. During the narrative sessions, you will be describing narratives of your traumatic experiences and repeating them as many times as needed, in order to diminish the level of anxiety and fear associated with them. I will be there to provide support and to remind you that no matter how intense it may feel, you are not in the traumatic experience, but are instead in a safe environment.
>
> "You will see that with repeated telling, your fear reactions to the event will diminish. This process is called 'habituation.' The more often you tell the story, the less

frightened you will become, and the better this treatment will work. You will eventually experience the memories of the past as being in the past. That is, they are only
memories and cannot harm you."

Provide rationale for recording narratives

The narratives will be recorded during these sessions. The client will take each recording
home, with the goal of listening to it at least once a day. The recording contains not only a
narrative of the event, but also the discussion between client and therapist about the meaning of the trauma, the client's explanation of who they felt themselves to be in that story, an
exploration of the possible trauma-related relationship models embedded in the narrative,
and a consideration of how current relationship models developed during STAIR might differ. Listening to the recording will contribute to the client's habituation to the fear-eliciting
aspects of the narrative. It will also provide an opportunity for the client to reflect on their
reactions to the story and its meaning to them, both when it happened and now. The therapist describes the recording of each narrative in the first session, but a reminder of the
rationale for recording will help clients orient themselves to the work and elicit any specific
concerns they might have.

> "Each time you narrate your trauma memories, we will record them. Listen to the
> recording every day, and make sure you make time to do this. You will learn that a
> memory is just that—a memory—and that you have nothing to fear from recalling
> these past events, although doing so is painful. You will also listen to the discussion
> we will have about the meaning of the trauma. You will come to see that some of the
> negative beliefs you hold about yourself and others have their roots in these traumatic
> experiences. Recognizing their source will allow you to make sense of why you have
> the beliefs and behaviors you do. This is an important step in freeing yourself from
> them. The conditions of your life are different now, and the old beliefs do not need to
> hold power over you any more."

Respond to client's concerns

The client is likely to have a range of reactions to hearing the descriptions above, such as
anxiety, disbelief, confusion, and curiosity. It is important to recognize and address these
feelings and concerns. When presenting the rationale for repeated narration of the trauma,
the therapist explains the basis for recommending the procedure to this particular client at
this particular time. This involves reviewing how methods the client has used in the past,
such as avoidance, have not worked and indeed may have exacerbated the client's symptoms. In addition, the past trauma has invaded the present, so that the trauma continues to
shape the client's current behaviors in negative ways.

The therapist is mindful that the client may have some strong reactions to hearing that
their ways of dealing with trauma may in fact have resulted in an *increase* of symptoms and
problems. The therapist will want to "normalize" this way of managing painful experiences

and provide a sense that the client has been coping as best they could. Doing so minimizes the possibility that the client will feel criticized or judged for using avoidance or other unsuccessful skills. Instead, the therapist emphasizes to the client that their efforts have been attempts to cope with very stressful life circumstances while having limited resources or options available to them. The therapist reminds the client that they have developed skills in treatment that will enable them to engage in effective ways of coping, including the narrative process they are about to use.

In the service of building the client's willingness to trust the therapist during this new module of treatment, the therapist acknowledges that processing the memories connected with the trauma may be frightening at first. At the same time, the therapist provides assurance and belief in the narrative process by communicating that it will get easier, and that the client is likely to see not only a decrease in the fear and distress related to the traumatic memories, but positive changes in their attitudes toward themselves and their relationships.

Second Goal of Narrative Therapy: Organize Memories in a Coherent and Meaningful Way

In addition to reducing anxiety and fear, narrative work helps organize the trauma memories and allows discussion of their meaning and impact on the client. The therapist describes the narration of the trauma as a skill for making sense of traumatic memories. This point has already been discussed in Session 1, but the therapist reintroduces and expands on the topic.

Specifically, the therapist highlights the contribution of developmental stage to the impact of trauma. The therapist reminds the client about the particularly disorganizing force of trauma occurring during childhood, when cognitive and emotional resources to respond to trauma are developmentally limited. In addition, the survivor probably lacked social resources in terms of parental or other social support in understanding or making sense of the trauma when it happened, or even later in their lives. Survivors of abuse and other traumatic experiences often report they experienced negative reactions from others, such as disbelief, blame, and minimization, when they attempted to disclose their experiences. Thus many survivors have never had the opportunity to tell their stories in a supportive context that will help them organize and make sense of their memories.

The therapist can say something like this, for example, to a client who experienced abuse in childhood:

"Childhood abuse, like all traumas, is an event that overwhelms a person's senses. In times of extreme stress or danger, the typical mechanisms we have in place to interpret and process experiences become overwhelmed. We are particularly vulnerable to this type of disruption if we are faced with traumatic events during childhood, when these capacities for handling incoming information have not yet been fully developed. As a result, the memory of the trauma is often a disorganized, fragmented mess—parts of a puzzle in a heap. Many symptoms of PTSD, such as nightmares and intrusive images, reflect the disorganized nature of a trauma in the person's memory. The process of putting the pieces of the puzzle together includes organizing the images into a coherent memory. We will be doing this by organizing the events chronologically and putting words to the experience."

Individuals who experience trauma in childhood may have difficulty in putting the pieces of their memories together, as the experiences may have been mislabeled, or the attributed contexts in which the trauma happened may have been described in misleading ways by the perpetrators. Furthermore, children rely heavily on parents as interpreters of experience and as the central sources of names for things. In cases where children's parents are the perpetrators, the parents themselves rarely have the motivation or ability to label their experiences correctly or to discuss them coherently. Lastly, reliance on other adults may have been of little value. Childhood maltreatment is frequently stigmatized; it is an event (or set of events) that is not typically part of mainstream conversation in many educational and social environments. As a result, the event or events do not get named or understood. Children who have been maltreated often cannot even describe what has happened, let alone make sense of what has happened and why. The reason, purpose, and impact of the experience remain mysterious. It is essentially "unreal" and incoherent—often disregarded by the individual, but influential all the same. The therapist can describe the situation to a survivor of abuse in childhood as follows:

"Meaning is often made by putting words to our experiences. This capacity is disturbed during traumatic events, leading some to describe trauma as a 'wordless horror.' The process of organizing memories with words may be particularly difficult for survivors of childhood abuse. Children learn and understand life experiences through communication and discussion with their parents. If their parents were the abusers, the children are at a particular disadvantage in making sense of their experience, as their parents may mislabel or deny the experience. In addition, opportunities to make sense of the event (such as disclosing or fully describing the experience to others) are often not options, since abuse is often a stigmatized experience that adults may feel uncomfortable discussing. As a result, the impact of these experiences on the children's beliefs and feelings remain unexamined and disconnected from the rest of life. Still, they continue to influence thoughts, feelings, and behaviors, in ways that are often outside of awareness or control."

The therapist can also highlight the importance of telling what happened as an opportunity for the client to label and define their experience appropriately. The therapist characterizes this notion by reference to the often-used "file cabinet" analogy for memory organization. The analogy can be described to a survivor of childhood abuse as follows:

"The mind can be viewed as a kind of 'file cabinet' in which experiences are organized and stored. When something has its place in the file cabinet, the information in the file and the feelings that go along with it are more manageable, and new experiences can be integrated in the future.

"For example, we have files for things like 'school,' where we store information about how to act in school, things other people have told us about school, and our memories of school-related experiences. Over the years, a child accumulates knowledge of what school is like, how one is supposed to behave, what is expected at school, and so on. Parents, siblings, peers, and others help the child label and process these experiences by communicating about school.

"In contrast, there are no clear or accurate labels or organizing systems in which childhood abuse experiences can be meaningfully filed. There may be no label on the file, or perhaps one that is vague ('Special Times with Dad') or inaccurate ('Things That Everyone Does with a Drama Coach'). The files are placed in some separate drawer, or, if they are mislabeled, exist as part of another set of experiences in which they truly do not fit. As a result, these experiences do not become integrated with all other information about one's childhood. Rather, they remain apart from it, or they create an inaccurate and distorted sense of some of life's themes."

Third Goal of Narrative Therapy: Create a Coherent Life Story

As the discussion above suggests, if an individual's memories of trauma are not organized or appropriately labeled, they remain disconnected from the rest of the person's life experience and meaning system. Narrative work helps integrate the trauma into the context of the individual's life experience, particularly the impact that it has had on beliefs and life themes.

Relationship models connect past with present

The identification of problematic relationship patterns and of the relationship models driving them has been an integral component of the therapeutic work in STAIR. Narrative Therapy takes a next important step by identifying the particular ways in which problematic relationship models have their source in the client's past trauma. While the type of analysis conducted during STAIR acknowledges that current relationship models represent adaptations to past events, Narrative Therapy involves a detailed review and organization of the trauma that allows the client to make clearer and more specific connections between their particular past traumas and problems they experience in the here and now. Exploration of the client's traumatic experiences helps resolve the mystery of their current behavior. The past is connected to the present through the identification of trauma-generated relationship models that have a negative impact on daily living. Their current behavior no longer appears frighteningly irrational and nonsensical. The client now understands the motivation for their behavior.

The circumstances of the trauma articulated in the narrative allow the client to understand the logic of their models and the source of these models in traumatic experiences. This often enables the survivor to develop sympathy for their past self and understanding of the power of the models to intrude into their current life. The therapist can provide an explanation like this one:

"The belief system you now live with is one of the ways your trauma continues to influence you. Often you will recognize the relationship models from the work we have done in STAIR. Others will be new but will make sense, given the particulars of your trauma as you talk about what happened. One of the most valuable aspects of relationship model identification is that it will help you make sense of your current behaviors. Often survivors of trauma feel themselves to be crazy because they do not understand why they behave the way they do, particularly when the behaviors seem at odds with their desired goals. These behaviors are often driven by models formulated in the context of your trauma and are accurate reflections of your trauma circumstances. The identification of relationship models often solves the mystery of what appears to be nonsensical or irrational behaviors. You have a reason for acting the way you do."

The therapist notes that the models from the traumatic past will be critically examined and directly contrasted with the models that have been generated and tested in STAIR. This direct comparison will help the client distinguish beliefs based in the past from beliefs adaptive for the present. This comparison will help the client separate the traumatic past from the present. It is intended to give the client a sense of freedom from the past and a sense of choice about how they may live in the present.

Possibility of change supported by recognizing differences between past and present

Contrasting the internal and external resources of the traumatic past with those of the present will provide good examples of the fit between an environment and an appropriate model. For example, trauma narratives will often include themes of powerlessness, vulnerability, incompetence, and dependence, and these themes will be reflected in the client's relationship models. However, the current life circumstances of clients in this treatment are often far improved, and the therapist reminds such a client of essential differences as they pertain to their particular situation. Examples may include such differences as these: A client no longer lives in close proximity to the perpetrator; they do not rely on the perpetrator for food or shelter, but have some (even if limited) resources of their own; they are much stronger both physically and mentally than they were during the trauma; they are able to fend for themselves in work and sleep through the night without expectation of intrusion or retraumatization; they can come and go out of their dwelling as they please.

As the client recognizes the difference between the context of their present and their past, the client will gain additional motivation and confidence in adopting new models and expectations. Awareness of the distinction between the past and the present will reduce automatic repetition of trauma-based behaviors and functioning. When clients recognize that many of their current maladaptive feelings and beliefs have their origins in the trauma, they will find it easier to develop awareness of the anachronistic and generally counterproductive nature of these feelings and beliefs in their present environment, and to become motivated to develop present-focused feelings, beliefs, and behaviors.

Validating the past by understanding it rather than living it

Many survivors of childhood maltreatment have difficulty giving up certain trauma-generated behaviors, because they are among the few (or the only) forms of validation that the traumatic past actually happened. These survivors were often in circumstances where telling about what happened led to threats, punishment, or denial. Thus the survivors may experience their trauma-generated behaviors as evidence of their own experiences. For some such survivors, giving up these behaviors would mean "betraying" their own past and their former selves.

The development and articulation of trauma-related relationship models constitute a healthy and powerful alternative means by which to acknowledge and respect the past trauma. The client's awareness of changes in their circumstances allows them, with the help of their therapist, to develop and test new models. As clients identify models generated by their trauma and develop alternative models for their life in the present, these two sets of models can be placed side by side and examined for how they mark the evolution of change in clients' sense of self and opportunities for engagement with life. A therapist may explain narrative analysis to a client in the following way:

> "Narrative analysis is the experience of going back to the past, with the final goal of creating an alternative assessment and understanding of that experience for living in the present. During the narrative, you will experience many emotions and perceptions from the past as you felt them as a child, but will simultaneously be viewing the experience from your position as an adult. An adult is a person with additional life experiences and an experientially based understanding of the differences between the needs and abilities of children and those of adults. Given this additional perspective, the meaning of the traumatic event as it was formed during the trauma is available to you for reassessment.
>
> "This process is not intended to distort or minimize the trauma, or to diminish its importance. The goal is for you to have respect for your past, but an emerging awareness that you are not the same person as you were in childhood and need not have the same feelings or beliefs about your trauma as you did then."

REVIEW APPLICATION OF EMOTION REGULATION SKILLS

The therapist refers to skills the client has learned over the course of treatment to cope with anxiety, as a way to remind the client that they are actually more equipped to do the narrative work than they may feel they are. The therapist encourages the continued use and practice of coping skills, especially Focused Breathing, which will be called on during the narrative process. This is an opportune time to revisit the concepts presented in Session 5 about distress tolerance (see Chapter 14). During this session, the idea of making the *choice* to tolerate distress in the service of trying to reach an identified higher-level goal has been introduced. Having the client apply these skills to the narrative (identifying the goal as well as the Pros and Cons of tolerating associated distress) before beginning is another powerful way to provide inspiration for the work ahead. The therapist may suggest that the client do the Pros and Cons exercise on paper before the next session, so that it can be referred to when sustained motivation is needed throughout the process. Also, by anticipating potential obstacles and distress, both client and therapist can begin to think of ways the client might approach these challenges before they arise.

The therapist mentions again that the client will set the pace of the narrative work, and that the therapist will follow, support, and encourage the client. The therapist may also enumerate the client's strengths and convey a sense of their vulnerabilities, so that the client feels that the therapist truly understands them. The therapist then inquires whether either the client or the therapist may have overlooked any other aspects of the client's strengths or vulnerabilities.

Finally, it is important for the client to keep in mind that narrative sessions include continued commitment to maintaining good functioning in the here and now. The therapist reminds the client that throughout all the narrative sessions, the work on further developing and refining interpersonal skills will continue. This work will be particularly highlighted as the interpersonal themes picked up in the narrative work are further characterized and refined. Experientially based alternative models will be explored and contrasted with these old beliefs associated with traumatic events. The therapist reassures the client that all interpersonal tasks will be based on the resources available to support the client's success.

CONFIRM CLIENT'S COMMITMENT TO NARRATIVE WORK

Review Client's Understanding of Rationale for Narrative Therapy

After presenting all of the information described above, the therapist checks in with the client to see if they have understood the main points, and encourages them to share their reactions and questions. It is expected that the client will still have some anxiety and uncertainty about beginning the narrative; ideally, however, at this point they are clear about its purpose and goals. The narrative work does not proceed until the client generally understands and accepts the rationale for it, because otherwise ongoing and active collaboration between the therapist and client is not possible. Both the rationale and the therapeutic alliance need to be established before this work begins, as these are essential skills in sustaining the client's motivation and participation in this challenging yet potentially powerful process.

Plan Number of Sessions and Timeline

Once the client expresses an adequate understanding and acceptance of the process and goals of Narrative Therapy, it is recommended that the therapist discuss "making a commitment" before turning to the specifics of trauma memories. This entails a verbal contract in which the client and therapist agree to use the narrative for a set number of sessions (at least three or four). The duration and intensity of the narrative during these sessions remain flexible and will depend on the individual client's needs and reactions, but the minimum number of narrative sessions is clearly established before beginning. The impetus for this intervention is to put a structure in place that will encourage both the therapist and client to give the narrative work an adequate trial. The initial narrative sessions in particular tend to be the most challenging. It is not uncommon for client and/or therapist to want to retreat after an emotionally intense and difficult narrative session. This could, however, lead the client and therapist to abandon the treatment too early, based on the erroneous conclusion that the client is not actually ready to proceed.

In our experience, it is not only ineffective but can in fact be detrimental to start the narrative and then end it prematurely within a session or within the treatment. The process of starting and then abruptly stopping the narrative may significantly raise the client's anxiety level, because not enough time has elapsed to allow habituation to occur. This type of experience could inadvertently confirm the client's belief that approaching the traumatic memories is dangerous, and that they are incapable of managing the emotions associated with them. This could in turn result in an increase of symptoms, particularly phobic avoidance of trauma-related cues, as well as fear of engaging in future treatment.

CREATE MEMORY HIERARCHY

Generate List of Trauma Memories

During the pretreatment assessment, the client has probably reported the general nature of their traumatic experiences, but has not provided a series of specific memories. At this point, the therapist will need to assist the client in identifying several memories for use in the narrative work. The client does not need to go into extensive detail at this time, as the present goal is to identify the most critical memories for later work, not (yet) to conduct a narration of the event. The development of a hierarchy of distress is a common cognitive-behavioral skill; its application to trauma memories has been developed and nicely described by Foa and colleagues (see Foa & Rothbaum, 1998; Rothbaum & Foa, 1999). The procedure has three steps. First, the therapist elicits several traumatic memories from the client (the number of these typically ranges from 4 to 10), taking brief notes so that each memory can be referred to later. Once this list is complete, the client assigns a number that reflects the level of distress provoked by each memory, using a scale from 0 (no distress) to 100 (highest possible distress). The units on this scale are typically referred to as "subjective units of distress" (SUDs). The memory hierarchy is completed when the memories are rank-ordered, with revision as necessary following the SUDs ratings provided by the client. This process usually takes about 20–30 minutes. The therapist can complete two organized and clean copies (one for the client and one for the therapist) of Handout 21.2, the Memory Hierarchy sheet, after the session. Before the client and therapist start to develop the hierarchy, the therapist explains to the client:

> "Before beginning the narrative work, we need to decide which memories it makes
> the most sense for us to focus on. In order to do so, I am going to ask you to identify

your most important trauma memories and describe how they continue to affect you emotionally. In addition, you may want to identify additional memories of traumatic experiences that occurred later in life. The goal here is not to go into extensive detail about your memories at this point, but rather to identify and generally describe what you believe are the most significant trauma memories, so we can have a road map for future narrative sessions. So I would like you to think and tell me about the particular memories that are most disturbing and disruptive to you in your current life."

The therapist must encourage the client to discuss trauma memories in enough detail that they can be briefly recorded and referred to individually (e.g., "the time my father locked me in the closet"), but not in so much detail that the client feels overwhelmed. Achieving this balance requires the therapist to be active in containing the client during the session, so that the client does not open up without having time to process traumatic memories within the session.

The therapist is encouraged to keep probing to a minimum in the process of developing the memory hierarchy. If a client is having trouble, the therapist may want to ask some simple and specific questions about the perpetrator, the client's age when each traumatic event occurred, and/or the client's emotional reaction, in order to help the client articulate basics that they remember. Through the narrative process, the client may or may not be able to remember more details. The communication to the client is that whatever they remember is a good starting point, and that specific details about content are not likely to be as important as their emotional experience of the event(s).

Dealing with Challenges in Creating the Memory Hierarchy

Lengthy or overly elaborated reporting of memories

If the client is having trouble containing their description of an important memory, the therapist sensitively redirects the client to talking more briefly and generally about what happened and moving on to another memory, by saying something like this:

> "The information you are sharing with me is very important, and I appreciate your willingness to do so. We will have the opportunity to process it in our narrative sessions. However, right now we need to focus on identifying and briefly describing relevant memories, so that we have a sense of the big picture before getting into the specific details."

Few and fragmented memories

Some clients may have the opposite problem with this task: They have difficulty spontaneously providing specific information about their memories, and only relay brief and vague snippets. This may be because the details of the events were never encoded due to dissociation at the time of the trauma, or because they have strenuously avoided thinking about the distressing memories for so long. Whatever the reason, it is important to assure the client that having incomplete or fragmented memories of traumatic experiences is common and will not prevent the client from doing and benefiting from narrative work.

Abundant and diverse trauma memories

Many clients will have long and complicated trauma histories, which makes developing a hierarchy of memories particularly challenging. It is important for the therapist to be aware that this could be overwhelming; in such a case, the therapist explains to the client that they are not being asked to specify every memory, but rather to identify the ones that feel the most significant in the present. Some clients ask for more guidance on what memories are most important to focus on. Such memories include those that are the focus of a client's current reexperiencing symptoms (such as flashbacks or nightmares), or those where the related feelings and beliefs are most clearly interfering with the client's current life. By reminding the client to focus on the most significant memories, the therapist decreases the likelihood of the client's being flooded with anxiety or becoming detached in the face of intense emotion. However, the therapist still needs to check in repeatedly on how the client is feeling during this process.

Clients who have been repeatedly maltreated over a long period of time may describe a composite or confluence of many different episodes. This is to be expected. Again, the therapist encourages such clients to report what they do remember, rather than worrying about teasing apart the specificity or sequence of the memories at this point. If it is clear, however, that in the process of relaying one specific traumatic memory the client moves into talking about another specific memory, the therapist sensitively asks the client to stay focused on the first memory; after completing that description, the client can return to talking about the second memory. It is reassuring for clients who have numerous traumas to be aware that often work on one memory will carry over to other memories—ones that involve similar types of trauma and/or similar emotional responses to the trauma.

Explain the SUDs Rating Scale

The therapist tells the client that the SUDs ratings will be used in making decisions about which memories to focus on during narrative sessions and in what sequence. Before the SUDs scores are used to rate memories, the therapist operationalizes the meaning of these scores with each client, to ensure that the ratings can be used meaningfully and consistently. This is done by generating anchor points with the client, using the client's own words and descriptions as a guide. For example, 0 might be "no distress whatsoever" or "a totally neutral state in recalling this memory"; 50 might be "moderate distress" or "very aware of feeling distress, but definitely manageable"; and 100 might be "severe distress and discomfort" or "I can't manage." Using the analogy of a thermometer can be helpful. The therapist explains: "The SUDs scale is used to get a quick read on your current level of distress and anxiety, in much the way that a thermometer is used to gauge temperature." A SUDS score identifies the level of anxiety/distress the client is *currently* feeling about a memory, rather than what they may have experienced at the time of the traumatic event.

Finalize Memory Hierarchy

After obtaining the SUDs ratings for all identified memories, the therapist completes the hierarchy by using Handout 21.2, Memory Hierarchy, to create a list of memories in which the first entry is the memory with the highest score and the last entry is the memory with the lowest score. Both the memory and its SUDs score are noted. The therapist will want to check in with the client to be sure that the memories rated with the highest scores are in fact the most distressing. In cases where more than one memory is given the highest rating, the therapist and client will want to think further about which of these memories is the most disruptive in the client's current life. The therapist keeps the in-session copy of the Memory Hierarchy form and will make a copy to give to the client in the next session, plus another copy for the therapist's own use.

Describe Use of SUDs Ratings during Narratives

The therapist discusses with the client that the SUDs ratings will also be used during the narrative work itself, as a way for the client to indicate how they are feeling immediately before they begin, during the telling of the story, and immediately after the narrative is complete. During each session in which the SUDs scores are used, the therapist reminds the client that the scores are based on how the client is feeling in the present, rather than how the client felt in the past.

SUMMARIZE THE GOALS OF THE SESSION

The therapist can take this time to review what has been accomplished in the session. The rationale for conducting Narrative Therapy has been provided; the number of the sessions and duration of this module has been identified; and the Memory Hierarchy sheet has been completed. The therapist now congratulates the client for their good work in this session. The process of memory elucidation, in particular, although not part of the formal narrative processing, can be quite demanding in its own right—particularly if the client has many trauma memories to describe. Though it can cause distress, creating a list of significant trauma memories and having to view them as a whole can also be quite powerful, especially for those clients who lack compassion for themselves and/or minimize the extent of their traumatization. It is critical to allow some time at the end of the session to check in with the client about how it has felt to complete this session. If the client is still aroused or anxious, the therapist uses this as an opportunity to practice coping skills (e.g., Focused Breathing or Thought Shifting) before ending the session. It is also important to give the client feedback and encouragement about the fact that they have been able to complete an important first step in the narrative work. The therapist reminds the client that it would not be surprising if between now and the next session, they find themselves thinking more about their traumatic experiences than usual. This will subside. The therapist encourages the client to use their emotion regulation skills during the week (e.g., Focused Breathing and Soothing the Senses) to keep a good balance and to remind them that they are safe now and the memories are only memories. The narrative work will help the client put the memories into the past, where they belong and where they cannot harm the client.

PLAN SKILLS PRACTICE

The therapist asks the client to read Handout 21.1, Overview of Narrative Therapy, as it will be useful in future sessions. The therapist also assigns the distress tolerance exercise (i.e., evaluating Pros and Cons) in relation to beginning the narrative work. Finally, the client continues completing copies of Relationship Patterns Worksheet–2, practicing Focused Breathing, and engaging in other relevant emotion regulation skills (e.g., Plan Pleasurable Activities, Thought Shifting, and Positive Self-Statements).

Overview of Narrative Therapy

Beginning in the next session, you will carry out narrative exercises in sessions and every day at home for the duration of the treatment program. This is very likely to be one of the most difficult parts of your treatment. However, it will help to bring about long-term relief from your distress and to facilitate positive changes in the way you think about yourself and relate to others. It is important, therefore, that you do your best to do the narrative work and resist urges to avoid doing it. To assist you, this handout reviews the rationale and instructions for Narrative Therapy.

RATIONALE

The purpose of narrating the trauma is to have you revisit and organize your trauma memories. It is not easy to understand and make sense of traumatic experiences. When you are reminded of your trauma, you may experience extreme anxiety or other negative feelings. So you may tend to push away or avoid these painful memories. You may tell yourself, "Don't think about it," or "I just have to forget about it."

But as you have discussed in therapy, no matter how hard you try to push away thoughts about the trauma, the experiences come back to haunt you through nightmares, flashbacks, fears/phobias, and negative beliefs about yourself and others. These symptoms serve as signals that the trauma is still "unfinished business." This is because avoidance prevents you from processing the thoughts and feelings that go along with the memories.

After a traumatic event, your mind begins the work of organizing the experience. When various aspects of the experience are organized into a story, this process is completed. Additionally, your feelings are organized within the context of the story and as a result become more manageable. The meaning of the event—particularly beliefs about yourself and the world—is evaluated and placed in the larger context of other life experiences. If, however, the process is interrupted, the story never gets organized, and the emotions remain intense and unmanageable. Powerful and emotionally charged fragments of a story never settle into a sensible or coherent account of what happened or how it affects you. The unanchored memories dominate your internal experience, leaving you feeling fragmented, disorganized, hostile, out of control, and fearful. Relationships are equally fragmented and undermined by strong and unexpected emotions. These reactions are often intrusions of unsettled feelings from the past. They may have little to do with the present.

The goal of Narrative Therapy is to help you process the memories connected with your traumas and create a life story that (1) helps you understand the trauma's impact on your feelings and relationships, and (2) allows you to put the past in its place. As you confront the memories and experience the intense emotions that go with them, the emotions will become less distressing. This process is called "deconditioning" or "habituation." In addition, the process of narrating the trauma will help you distinguish the feelings and beliefs that are results of the trauma from your current desires, wishes, and plans for yourself—in other words, to separate the past from the present. By identifying the relationship models in your narrative after you finish it or finish listening to a recording, you can explore how those beliefs influence your functioning in the present, whether they are helpful to you, and how relevant they are to your current goals. Although these relationship models were consistent with and adaptive to your traumatic environment, they are not likely to help you now that you are out of this environment and have goals other than avoiding, escaping, or confronting threat. Awareness of these

(continued)

models and their lack of relevance to your current life will help you recognize when you are using them and help you disengage from them. Practice and success with the alternative relationship models that you have developed in the STAIR treatment module will gradually replace behaviors generated from the trauma-related models.

PROCEDURE FOR BETWEEN-SESSION NARRATIVE REVIEW
AND ANALYSIS

To help you carry out the narrative work you will do between sessions, your therapist will have you record the narratives you have completed in your treatment sessions. Listen to the recordings of the narrative conducted with your therapist in the session, and use the material from the session to guide you through the narrative analysis (relationship patterns work) again. When you listen to the recording, if you have trouble arranging the privacy you may need, it may be helpful to use headphones. Try to find a comfortable place where you will not be disturbed.

During the narrative, try to relive the experience; smell, taste, and feel everything as if you are really there. Although this can be scary, in the back of your mind you will know that you are safe. Some people find it helpful to have a trusted family member or friend nearby in another room or available by phone the first time they do the narrative homework alone. If you feel you will not be able to follow through without support, you may make arrangements for someone to be present or easily available to you during the task.

You will use the Subjective Units of Distress (SUDs) during Trauma Narration form, which will be introduced to you during your first in-session narration, to record your "subjective units of distress" (SUDs) immediately before and after the narrative. Also note the highest SUDs level you reached during the narrative. Next, jot down on a copy of Relationship Patterns Worksheet–2 the event described in the narrative and the relationship model you associate with this story. If possible, formulate an alternative way of interacting with others and a relationship model that is more representative of the beliefs you wish to hold about yourself and your relationship with others in the present. If you cannot do this on your own, you and your therapist will complete this work in your next session.

Memory Hierarchy

Number	Memory	SUDS Score

Narrative of First Memory

And suddenly it had come to her . . . that the voice she
was hearing was her own, for the first time in her life.
—ANNA QUINDLEN (1992, p. 393)

In Session 12, the client completes the first trauma narrative. The therapist will help put the client at ease by reviewing the rationale for Narrative Therapy, identifying the client's available coping skills, and reminding the client of the therapist's presence as a support. The client first practices with a neutral memory, in order to become familiar with the structure and pacing of the narration. The same structure and process are then implemented with a selected traumatic memory. The main goal of the session is for the client to experience mastery over the memory, so it is important for the client and therapist to titrate the intensity of the client's emotions carefully during this process, according to the client's strengths.

When the narrative ends, client and therapist conduct grounding exercises if the client needs these. The client then identifies feelings that emerged from the telling, including what parts of the story elicited these feelings and how intense they were. Therapist and client then listen to the recording together. This gives the client some familiarity with the task before the client listens to the recording at home. It also helps the therapist monitor and explore the client's reaction to their own story. We have found that clients experience a range of reactions, many of which appear unavailable when they are engaged in the actual narration. These often include sympathy for themselves and curiosity—as if they are experiencing themselves as people with histories and with interesting stories to tell. Box 22.1 outlines the theme and curriculum for Session 12 of treatment.

CHECK-IN AND REVIEW OF SKILLS PRACTICE

Although this is the first session of Narrative Therapy proper, it begins like previous sessions: with a brief check-in about the client's current emotional state, followed by a review

BOX 22.1

Theme and Curriculum for Session 12
Narrative of First Memory

The client's recollection of the trauma is only a memory, and as such it cannot hurt the client. When the client is able to revisit the memory in a detailed and emotionally alive way, there is an opportunity to help the client experience mastery over the traumatic memory. When the client listens to the recording of the narrative plus the narrative analysis of the memory, they often become aware of feelings that were not available during the telling of the story. These include sympathy for what they have been through, and curiosity about the self as a person with a story to tell.

PLANNING AND PREPARATION

Prepare two completed versions of the Memory Hierarchy (Handout 21.2), one for the client and one for your own use as the therapist. You will need to make a recording of the trauma narrative, both to listen to with the client in session and for the client to bring home. Often this is easiest if done on the client's smartphone, but if the client does not have that capacity, then identify other options for recording the narrative. Bring a copy each of Handouts 22.1 and 22.2, and several copies of the Relationship Patterns Worksheet–2 (Handout 16.4). This session is 60 minutes in duration.

AGENDA

- Check-in and review of skills practice.
- Identify focus of the session.
- Practice narrative of a neutral memory.
- Conduct first narrative of a trauma memory.
- Ground the client in the present.
- Listen to the first narrative recording together.
- Explore beliefs about self and/or others in narrative.
- Summarize the goals of the session.
- Plan skills practice:

(continued)

- Listen to the recording daily; monitor distress with SUDs, using Subjective Units of Distress (SUDs) during Trauma Narration form.
  - Initiate at least one interpersonal situation and practice an alternative relationship model, using a copy of Relationship Patterns Worksheet–2 to record the practice and the results; include emotion regulation skills as relevant to situation.
  - Continue to practice Focused Breathing twice a day.

SESSION HANDOUTS

Two completed copies of Handout 21.1. Memory Hierarchy

Handout 22.1. Subjective Units of Distress (SUDs) during Trauma Narration (several copies)

Handout 22.2. Assessment of Postnarrative Emotional State

Additional copies of Handout 16.4. Relationship Patterns Worksheet–2

---

of the client's skills practice over the week. The planned skills practice from the last session included reviewing Handout 21.1, Overview of Narrative Therapy; depending on what was agreed upon with the client, it may also have included completing distress tolerance exercises, review of their trauma narrative and related themes, practicing Focused Breathing, and practicing other emotion regulation skills as needed. The therapist begins by briefly reviewing whether the client completed all of the planned work, asking for a brief summary of how the practice went, and offering to answer any questions that may have arisen since the preceding session.

IDENTIFY FOCUS OF THE SESSION

The focus of this session is on the narrative of the first memory. Before beginning the first narrative, the therapist reviews in whatever detail is appropriate to the particular client the rationale for Narrative Therapy and the nature of the analysis that follows each narrative. Also, the therapist takes the time to talk with the client about how the client is feeling about starting Narrative Therapy. The therapist reminds the client that they have many more resources now than they did as a child, and that these resources will be available to them as they engage in this challenging work. The client will revisit the past with the strengths and resources of the present. The client will view the experiences of their childhood from the critical and more informed perspective of an adult. The therapist can say something like this:

> "When you experienced your traumas, you were just a child, alone, with limited coping skills, and the experience was overwhelming. Our goal is to create a different experience for you. You will not be alone this time; I will be with you every step of the way.

Part of the rationale for the first module of the treatment was to prepare you for trauma-focused work. As an adult, having gone through this treatment, you have skills and resources you didn't have as a child. You have the resources to confront these memories. Does this make sense to you?"

PRACTICE NARRATIVE OF A NEUTRAL MEMORY

In prolonged exposure (Foa & Rothbaum, 1998), prior to beginning work with traumatic memories, a client first practices with a narrative of a neutral memory. This practice is extremely useful in allowing the client to learn the process and structure of Narrative Therapy before having to confront intense emotions. The therapist explains to the client:

> "Before focusing on your trauma memories, let's practice with a memory from your childhood that is not related to your trauma. Some people choose a memory of a birthday party, or a vacation, or a friend they liked to play with, or their childhood room. Can you think of a memory like that? [The therapist helps the client choose a memory if the client has difficulty. This memory is neutral to positive in valence.] OK, so we will focus on this memory in the same way we will later with a trauma memory. Sit back in your chair in a comfortable position. Close your eyes, or let them rest on an object or location that is comfortable and where you will not get distracted. Tell about this particular incident or person in your life. The story should have a beginning, a middle, and an end. You should describe it in the first person, as if you are there right now—for example, 'When I wake up, I am happy because I remember it is Saturday, which means no school today.' "

As the client talks through the memory, the therapist probes the client for details about what the client sees, hears, smells, and touches. The therapist also asks them what they are feeling and what sensations they experience in the body. A client who forgets to stay in the first person is reminded to do so. When the client has finished, the therapist provides support and continued direction:

> "That was very good. That is exactly what we are going to do again, but this time you will narrate a trauma memory. We are going to start with a memory that is difficult, but one that you think you can manage."

CONDUCT FIRST NARRATIVE OF A TRAUMA MEMORY

Selecting a Memory

The memory selected is the one that elicits the most distress the client feels they can handle at this point. This will ensure that processing for fear reduction is relevant, but that the client will succeed in experiencing distress reduction in the session. Our experience has been that when a client succeeds in managing a high-distress memory, those memories associated with less distress become easy to narrate, and in fact may become uninteresting and irrelevant to the client in their recovery work.

If the client has more than one distressing memory of equal weight, the client picks the one that has the most relevance to problems the client is dealing with in day-to-day life. This also serves the purpose of enriching the postnarrative analysis with particular value. Therapist and client work together in the selection of the memory.

The client goes through the narration of the memory once with no interruptions. The second time the client begins the narration, the therapist reinforces the instructions as needed. For example, the therapist may need to remind the client to stay in the first person if the client has forgotten, to speak more slowly, or to provide more details. The therapist's goal is to help the client make the memory as real as possible, so questions facilitate this process. How this works best depends on the client. For some clients, asking them to provide more detail about sensations (sights, smells) enables them to get deeper into the memory. If a therapist believes that a client is avoiding reexperiencing the feelings associated with the memory, the therapist asks the client how they are feeling. Some general guidelines for the therapist during the session include the following:

1. *Active listening.* Since some clients will have their eyes closed or focused away from you, show that you are listening with vocalizations such as "Uh-huh," "Yes," or "I see."

2. *Be supportive.* If the client demonstrates strong emotions during narrative work, reinforce this by being empathic: "I know this is difficult. It takes courage to do this. I am listening. You are doing well."

3. *Clarification.* If the client moves out of the first person ("I"), rushes through the memory, or doesn't seem to be allowing themselves to relive the experience, clarify the procedure before the client begins the memory the next time.

4. *Details.* Help the client emotionally engage in the memory by asking the client questions about details of the experience, particularly details about sensations (e.g., touch, smell).

5. *Encouragement.* Praise the client for their courage in confronting their traumatic memories: "You can be proud of yourself. You have done something very difficult."

6. *Focus.* If the client becomes distracted (e.g., by noise outside the office), gently remind the client where they were in the memory: "You just said you were falling asleep and your stepfather came into the bedroom." Or sometimes the client will break out of the memory and ask a question. If the client does this, tell the client that you will make a note of it and answer it later. For now, ask the client to return to the memory.

The therapist can begin the process by saying:

"Now we are going to focus on your trauma memory, just like we did a few minutes ago with the memory of your [the therapist describes the neutral memory]. Sit back in the chair, and close your eyes or focus on an image from the memory. We are going to travel back in time to when this memory occurred. Make the memory as real as possible. Talk slowly, in the first person, using 'I,' as if the events were happening to you right now. Describe what you are experiencing, feeling, thinking, tasting, and touching. I may ask you questions along the way to help you make the memory more real. It is sometimes tempting to avoid the memory by speaking quickly and trying to get it over with. If I think you are doing this, I will help you slow down. Remember, I will be here next to you every step of the way. To keep in touch with how you are doing, I will be asking for SUDs ratings every few minutes. I will say, 'Rating,' and then you are to give me your SUDs for how you are feeling in that moment, on the scale from 0 to 100. Does this make sense? When you have finished the memory, I will ask you to start over again. We will cycle through the narrative two or three times. Ready?"

The therapist records the ratings on Handout 22.1, Subjective Units of Distress (SUDs) during Trauma Narration, as the client revisits the trauma memory. The length of the trauma memory will determine how often the therapist asks for a SUDs rating. In the beginning, these memories are often short, so the therapist may ask only once or twice during the memory (every few minutes). After the memories become more elaborate, the therapist usually asks for ratings every 5 minutes, or more often if a client is appearing distressed. The use of SUDs ratings is an excellent way for the client and therapist to stay in touch with the client's emotional movement through the narrative. These ratings become a rapid, rather telegraphic way for clients to communicate their in-the-moment emotions as they narrate the event.

As the client goes through the memory, the therapist notes parts that seem particularly distressing. These parts provide clues to the meaning of the memory for the client, and also point to which parts of the memory the therapist might choose to focus on in later sessions. In addition to SUDs ratings, the therapist records any relevant observations in the "Comments" section on Handout 22.1—for example, any physical reactions, facial expressions, or voice changes noted during the narrative.

When the client has gone through the memory once, the therapist asks the client to go back to the beginning and start again. For instance, the therapist can say this:

"Very good. I know that was hard to do the first time. Now we are going to go through the memory again. This time I am going to ask you more questions, to try to make the memory more real to you."

Number of Repetitions and Duration of Narrative Retelling

The therapist has the client go through the memory at least two or three times. This can take from 10 to 20 minutes, depending on the length of the narrative. It is recommended that the client spend at least 10 minutes engaged in repeated narrations of the memory (or, if the telling of the memory is relatively lengthy, at least one repetition). If the memory takes longer than 20 minutes to describe, client and therapist can work on breaking the memory down into shorter, more emotionally focused, and more manageable narratives.

In later sessions, a narrative may need to be completed only once. This can happen when the SUDs levels are relatively low, or the intensity of the event is no longer as strong as it was when it was first rated. The initial narrative work often diminishes fear reactions to other memories in the hierarchy that have not been described when those memories are related in content or theme. Sometimes rapid fear reduction occurs when the client experiences a significant insight about what has been described. Insight often reduces fear. The client moves from experiencing fear to experiencing excitement, curiosity, or satisfaction.

Ending the Retelling of the Narrative

If the client's distress or anxiety decreases within this session of narrative work, the therapist asks if the client notices a difference (in terms of SUDs ratings) between how they are feeling at the end and how they felt at the beginning of the session:

> "When we started today, you rated your distress at a [SUDs score]; by the end of the session, you were at a [SUDs score]. This is what we talked about earlier: Your distress decreases if you allow yourself to face the memory."

If the client's distress does not decrease, the therapist reminds the client that this happens when someone is struggling with a particularly difficult memory, and praises them for sticking with it:

> "I know this was very difficult today. You showed a lot of courage sticking with the memory, even though it was very difficult. We will be discussing the meaning of the memory, and in doing that, we can identify what makes it so hard. Before that, let's do some distress reduction exercises."

If the therapist and client are interested in obtaining a more detailed picture of the client's emotional reactions at this stage, Handout 22.2, Assessment of Postnarrative Emotional State, can be used. After briefly describing the 1–10 rating scale, the therapist asks the client about the intensity of their feelings in each domain following the initial telling. This form creates a more specific preliminary profile of the client's emotional state, and the therapist and client can also use it in later sessions to guide the narrative work.

GROUND THE CLIENT IN THE PRESENT

The therapist helps the client begin making the transition from narration to analysis by simply stating that the narrative work portion of the session is finished and asking how the client is feeling. These comments or similar sentences signal that the narrative work is over, and that the client is ready for review, discussion, and exploration of the narrative experience. The therapist ensures that the client is clearly in the present, is physically comfortable, and is engaged with the therapist. Although many feelings and thoughts from the narrative work may be resonating with the client, the client also needs to be able to maintain a comfortable distance from the experience.

If the client feels somewhat disoriented, the therapist and client can use several skills to ground the client in the present. These include having the client do Focused Breathing, look around the room and share what they see, drink a hot or cold beverage, rub their hands together, or press their feet into the floor. The client and therapist will at this point have identified the skills the client prefers to use to increase physical comfort and awareness of the immediate environment.

Sometimes the therapist's voice is soothing to the client and can orient them to the present. In addition, the therapist can make several comments that reinforce a sense of safety and of being grounded in the present. The therapist can state that the client is in a safe environment, and that the events described belong to the past.

The therapist also congratulates the client for completing the narrative. The shift from narration to analysis is a passage from immersion in the traumatic past to engagement in the present. This transition is a therapeutic experience in itself: It demonstrates to the client that they have the skills to shift from the past to the present, and that the feelings elicited during the narrative work can be tolerated and diminished. The therapist comments on this by specifically identifying the ways in which the client has been able to manage their feelings and use coping skills—not only during the narration, but also in coming to successful closure on the task.

LISTEN TO THE FIRST NARRATIVE RECORDING TOGETHER

Next, the therapist and client listen to the recording together. Again, it is important to reiterate the purpose of this activity. The therapist can say something like this:

> "At this point, I would like us to listen to the recording together. This is what I will be asking you to do on your own between sessions. Listening to yourself detailing a trauma narrative for the first time can be daunting, so doing it in session first will be helpful in decreasing this initial anxiety and will give us a chance to talk about what it felt like to hear yourself. Often clients have very different reactions to telling the narrative of their trauma versus listening to themselves tell it on the recording."

EXPLORE BELIEFS ABOUT SELF AND/OR OTHERS IN NARRATIVE

After the client has identified and labeled the central feelings emerging from the narration, the client explores what beliefs about self and others are embedded in the narrative. The client can use the feelings they have identified as a springboard for this. At this point in treatment, the therapist and client are aware of many of the client's core relationship models and patterns, based on their work in the STAIR module. However, new, more detailed, or more precise beliefs often emerge from organizing the trauma narrative or from articulating details to which the client has never given thought. The central goal of the analysis is to clarify and repeatedly reinforce the fact that certain beliefs the client holds about the self as a traumatized child are no longer applicable to the client as an adult. Alternative and more adaptive relationship models, along with supporting evidence from current experience, are discussed.

Below is a case illustration of a narrative analysis that occurred after the first telling of the trauma history. We have found that our clients are often full of thoughts, feelings, and observations after the first narrative experience. Clients experience relief, sadness, amazement, and curiosity about what might come next. It is valuable to take an informal approach to the analysis after the first telling and follow a client's lead about important observations. In the example below, the most important observation for Tom was the difference between the therapist's reaction and his ex-boyfriend's reaction. The therapist helped Tom to summarize his insights at the end of the session, using two copies of Relationship Patterns Worksheet–2 (Handout 16.4).

CASE EXAMPLE: TELLING ABOUT THE TRAUMA, THEN AND NOW

In the STAIR module of treatment, Tom's therapist focused during the skills training on helping him develop ways to manage his anxiety and to be more direct in communicating his distress with others. When presented with the rationale and description of the narrative work, Tom reacted strongly: "I feel like what you are saying goes against all of my natural human instincts. It's like you're suggesting I jump off of a cliff." In addition, Tom had never told anyone the whole story of his abuse. The first and only occasion on which he had disclosed what had happened had been about 8 years ago to an ex-boyfriend. Tom described his boyfriend's reaction as "disturbing," because the boyfriend became distressed when he heard about what happened. It started to have a major impact on their relationship, and ultimately his boyfriend broke up with him, stating he "just couldn't handle it." Tom decided never to tell anybody about the abuse again. Tom's therapist spent time discussing his fear of telling about his abuse and reiterated the connection among his symptoms, his problems in relationships, and his trauma experiences. Although Tom was hesitant and frightened to begin narrative work, his distress over his worsening symptoms and their impact on his functioning gave him incentive.

At the beginning of the session in which the narrative work was to begin, Tom continued to express anxiety and skepticism. His therapist repeated the treatment rationale and reviewed the reasons Tom had given for wanting to be in the treatment. At the end of the first narration, Tom saw the experience in a different way and felt much more comfortable with beginning to talk about his abuse. He had experienced some sense of mastery in the process, even during this first time. He compared the process of revisiting his abuse memories to trying to hold onto a handful of sand: "If you hold it tightly, it slips out through your fingers, but if you keep your grip loose, you can actually keep it in your hand."

Tom and his therapist also discussed his strongly held belief that talking about the abuse was dangerous and would have disastrous consequences. Tom linked this belief to his experience with his ex-boyfriend, and he expressed the belief that he would be considered "damaged goods." Tom's therapist focused on the fact that he no longer had to believe that. Instead, he could believe that he could tell about the abuse and expect that at least some people would still be there for him—in fact, would feel closer to him than before. Tom expressed feeling supported and "much lighter" following the disclosure of his abuse to his therapist.

SUMMARIZE THE GOALS OF THE SESSION

This session is profoundly therapeutic in itself for many clients. For some, this will be the first time they talk in detail about their trauma with another person. For others, this will be the first time they have spoken about their trauma and have been truly and compassionately heard. At the end of the session, the therapist briefly summarizes the goals of the session and describes how the goals fit within the larger treatment goals for the specific client. These may include reducing anxiety and PTSD symptoms, and/or reaching a better understanding of how beliefs and feeling related to the trauma influence the client's current life. The therapist checks in with the client to see how they are feeling about completing their first trauma narrative and continuing with other narratives in the next several sessions. The therapist praises the client for the courageous work done in this session and all the work done during the STAIR module, which has strengthened the client's skills and enabled them to begin engaging in the narrative work. The therapist also highlights the importance of listening to the recording of the first trauma narrative between sessions, and briefly reviews the rationale for doing so.

PLAN SKILLS PRACTICE

At the end of the session, the therapist gives the client the recording of the first trauma narrative. The therapist requests that the client listen to it once a day. The therapist also tells the client to record their SUDs ratings and any comments or observations on Handout 22.1 after each listening. As with previous planned skills practice, the therapist spends some time predicting any potential obstacles to the client's completing this work and suggesting ways to make it feasible. In order to maintain the skills the client has developed during the STAIR module, the therapist also assigns the client to initiate at least one interpersonal situation and practice an alternative relationship model, using Relationship Patterns Worksheet-2 (Handout 16.4) to record the practice and the results. The client should also continue to practice Focused Breathing twice a day, as well as other emotion regulation skills relevant to their needs and situations.

The client will need to be able to listen to the recording of the narrative. Clients most commonly use their smartphones for this nowadays, and they may or may not want to listen with headphones. The therapist and client also discusses when it makes the most sense to listen to the recording, taking into consideration the client's schedule and possible times when they are free and can have some privacy. Another consideration is the surrounding environment while listening. A client should not listen to the recording along with other people. However, if the client has identified safe and supportive people, they might enlist these individuals in certain ways (such as calling them before and after listening to the recording, to check in). The client might also make a social plan for after they listen to the recording if this would be helpful.

As always, it is up to the client to decide how much they would like to share with others. For example, some clients feel comfortable sharing details about the treatment process with significant others; other clients want to make contact with other persons without directly involving them in the process; and still others prefer to keep the process a private experience. Whereas some clients prefer to listen to recordings when nobody else is around, others prefer to do it in a place where they feel less isolated (e.g., using headphones at a coffee shop, or doing it at home when others are present in another room). As long as distractions are minimized and a client can devote time to concentrating on the recording, the choice of context is of relatively minor importance and is based on what the client feels would be preferable. After listening to the initial recording, the therapist and client will discuss how the process went and whether the client may want to make any adaptations for listening in the future.

Subjective Units of Distress (SUDs)
during Trauma Narration

This form is to be used when you are listening to the trauma narrative as between-session practice. First, provide a brief description of the memory. Then record the date of practice, along with the subjective units of distress (SUDs; 0–100) ratings for before, highest during, and after listening to the memory.

Brief description of memory: _____

_____

_____

_____

Date	Preexposure SUDs ____ Highest SUDs ____ Postexposure SUDs ____	Comments
Date	Preexposure SUDs ____ Highest SUDs ____ Postexposure SUDs ____	Comments
Date	Preexposure SUDs ____ Highest SUDs ____ Postexposure SUDs ____	Comments
Date	Preexposure SUDs ____ Highest SUDs ____ Postexposure SUDs ____	Comments
Date	Preexposure SUDs ____ Highest SUDs ____ Postexposure SUDs ____	Comments
Date	Preexposure SUDs ____ Highest SUDs ____ Postexposure SUDs ____	Comments
Date	Preexposure SUDs ____ Highest SUDs ____ Postexposure SUDs ____	Comments

Assessment of Postnarrative Emotional State

After completing the narrative of the trauma memory, rate the intensity of each emotion on the scale of 1 to 10 below, with 1 being "the least intense/not at all feeling that emotion" and 10 being "the most intense."

Date: _____ Exposure #: _____ Session #: _____

Rating scale

1	2	3	4	5	6	7	8	9	10
Not at all		Mild		Moderate			Severe		Extreme

Fear/anxiety

1	2	3	4	5	6	7	8	9	10

Numbness

1	2	3	4	5	6	7	8	9	10

Anger

1	2	3	4	5	6	7	8	9	10

Sadness

1	2	3	4	5	6	7	8	9	10

Shame

1	2	3	4	5	6	7	8	9	10

Guilt

1	2	3	4	5	6	7	8	9	10

Strongest feeling: _____

CHAPTER 23

Narratives of Fear

> The patient reproduces instead of remembering. . . . This condition is shifted
> bit by bit within . . . the treatment . . . [W]hile the patient lives it through
> as something real and actual, we have to accomplish the therapeutic task,
> which consist chiefly in translating it back again into terms of the past.
> —SIGMUND FREUD (1914/1963, p. 163)

The sessions following the first narrative (Sessions 13–17) maintain essentially the same structure as Session 12. This includes a review of the feelings elicited by the narrative, an identification of the relationship patterns embedded in the story, a critical analysis comparing the patterns of the traumatic past with the client's current situation, and applications of new models to current life difficulties. These procedures will become routine, and the sessions will move fluidly from one activity to the next. Clients will progress from one memory to the next, repeating this cycle of activities.

Some clients will have difficulty making progress, however, because they tend to react to fear with avoidance or dissociative responses to fear-laden memories. This chapter describes strategies for managing such reactions, to be used as needed. This chapter also describes the benefit of close and sensitive attention to, and possible revision of, relationship patterns. In narration, as the particulars of trauma histories are told, a better understanding of critical interpersonal experiences emerges and can lead to more precise, "emotionally real" versions of established relationship patterns. The strategies for management of fear-laden reactions, sustained emotional involvement in the narration, and the evolution of relationship patterns all share the recognition that these experiences belong to the past. Although memories have extraordinary power to influence current behavior, they nevertheless have, by definition, one weakness: They belong to the past. The client, in contrast, has one major strength, which is that they live in the present.

The client's capacity to live in and feel the power of the present will provide an important resource in putting distance between the client's self and their memories, and developing a perspective on the limited influence these events need to have. Accordingly, a basic principle of the work is for the therapist to maintain the client's engagement in and appreciation for the present. The therapist and client work together to maximize the resource of the here and now. This can be done through words, through sensory exercises, and through repeatedly contrasting the past with present living conditions and opportunities. Negative beliefs about self and others belonging to the traumatic past can be countered with alternative models and experientially based demonstrations that disconfirm these beliefs and support new formulations about the self. As this effort proceeds, the client will begin developing a sense of a historical self—a self with a past that is distinct from the present. Box 23.1 outlines the theme and curriculum for working with narratives of fear in Sessions 13–17 of treatment.

CHECK-IN AND REVIEW OF SKILLS PRACTICE

During Narrative Therapy, the therapist begins each session by checking in with the client about their reaction to listening to the recording made in the preceding session. This will help identify the next step in the narrative work. After the review is complete, the therapist can remind the client that the ability to think about and discuss painful memories is a skill, and can congratulate the client on their efforts. This ability will allow them to become free of their past, and will give them the energy and ability to focus on the present and plan for the future.

If the client did not listen to the recording or only listened once or twice between sessions, the therapist works with the client to identify what interfered with completing the task. For example, did something unexpected happen that interfered with the assignment, such as an unplanned family visit or illness? Or was the client avoiding listening out of fear or anxiety? If the latter was the case, the therapist will want to work with the client to identify and address the specific fears or anxieties that interfered with listening to the recording. The therapist may need to revisit the rationale for listening to the recording as well. If the client's concerns center around feeling distressed or overwhelmed during or after listening to the recording, the therapist problem-solves with the client in regard to these concerns, and then reviews the skills the client finds most effective when they find themselves distressed (e.g., Focused Breathing).

Often a client will identify parts of the narrative that were particularly difficult. A brief discussion will determine whether the memory should be further explored. The therapist can review the pattern of SUDs ratings with the client and determine whether they should go on to a new memory, repeat the memory, or focus on a particular aspect of the memory. Before this is decided, the therapist elicits from the client any insights the client might have had as a result of listening to the recording—about their feelings, views of self, or relationship patterns they have identified. This will also help inform the therapist whether the client feels "done" with the memory. In addition, the therapist explores whether the client had any interpersonal difficulties during the week, especially ones relating to the narrative work, and briefly problem-solve in regard to these issues. More detailed discussion of using skills can be interwoven during the session as appropriate.

Theme and Curriculum for Sessions 13–17
Narratives of Fear

Clients quickly learn the structure and process of Narrative Therapy. The five sessions that follow Session 12 involve conducting repeated narratives of the most distressing aspects of a particular traumatic event, or moving to other events that would have been too distressing with which to begin the narrative work. The resolution of fear reactions results in large part from the realization that the trauma belongs to the past, and as such cannot hurt the client. The client begins to experience control over their memories and is actively working to organize them. The client also begins to assess the memories' influence over the client's current attitudes and behaviors. Consequently, the narrative work is a form of self-reflection and the beginning of the development of a historical sense of self. The repeated narration of an organized past, and identification of its relationship to the present, establish and reinforce an experience of continuity in the self.

PLANNING AND PREPARATION

Bring therapist's copy of completed Memory Hierarchy (Handout 21.2), and ensure that the client has a way to record the narrative processing. Bring other handouts as listed below. This session is 60 minutes in duration.

AGENDA

- Check-in and review of skills practice.
- Identify focus of the session.
- Complete narrative of fear memory.
- Work with avoidance behaviors.
- Manage dissociative reactions.
- Conduct narrative analysis.
- Summarize the goals of the session.

(continued)

* Plan skills practice:
  - Listen to recording daily; monitor distress with Subjective Units of Distress (SUDs) during Trauma Narration form.
  - Initiate at least one interpersonal situation and practice alternative relationship model(s), using Relationship Patterns Worksheet–2 to record the practice and results; include emotion regulation skills as relevant to situation.
  - Continue to practice Focused Breathing twice a day, and other emotion regulation skills as relevant.

SESSION HANDOUTS

Completed copy of Handout 21.2. Memory Hierarchy

Additional copies of Handout 22.1. Subjective Units of Distress (SUDs) during Trauma Narration

At least one additional copy of Handout 22.2. Assessment of Postnarrative Emotional State

Additional copies of Handout 16.4. Relationship Patterns Worksheet–2

IDENTIFY FOCUS OF THE SESSION

The focus of Session 13 and subsequent sessions is the processing of fear memories. An important component of these sessions is memory selection. The therapist takes the time to talk with the client about how the client is feeling about processing their traumatic memories. The therapist will often find it helpful to remind the client that they have many more resources now, having completed the STAIR module, and that these resources will be available to them as they engage in this challenging work. The client may find it useful to review the skills they found most helpful in the STAIR module, to help them cope with feelings that arise when processing their traumatic memories.

COMPLETE NARRATIVE OF FEAR MEMORY

This and the next four sessions will begin with memory selection and then move to narrative processing.

Select a Memory

The decision to move on to a new memory is determined by the amount of fear the client still experiences when revisiting the memory, as well as the client's satisfaction with their understanding of it. The therapist and client review the SUDs ratings the client reported on each day the client listened to the recording. Ratings of 30 or below indicate low fear responses, suggesting that the therapist and client can select a new memory. If there are particular areas of difficulties, indicated by the client's report and high SUDs ratings for only certain sections of the narrative, the next portion of narrative work can be a repetition and analysis of these "high-distress" sections. If the client did not listen to the recording between sessions or did not record their SUDS ratings, the therapist will likely want to continue focusing on the memory from the preceding session.

The selection procedure is the same for each new memory: The client and therapist select the memory that has the highest SUDs rating the client believes they can manage. The choice is also influenced by the relevance of particular memories to the client's day-to-day life. A memory with an initially low rating may become relevant to the further elaboration of a theme in a memory, or may become more significant due to life circumstances. For example, if a client identifies a theme of chronic fear of suffocation from narratives of adolescent sexual abuse memories, the client may eventually recognize the same theme in a less intense memory of an early childhood molestation. Alternatively, a memory of physical abuse by the client's mother may be reactivated upon a visit from or some news about the mother. The memory thus becomes more salient to the client and should be addressed. SUDs ratings for this memory can be revised accordingly.

Complete Narrative

The procedures for conducting the narrative are identical to those described for the first narrative in Session 12 (see Chapter 22). These include orienting the client to the task, recording the narrative, following the client with SUDs ratings, occasionally inquiring about details, and determining the number of repetitions. When the client is done, the recording is shut off, and grounding exercises are conducted as needed. This is followed by analysis (which is also recorded) of feelings in the narrative.

Assess Feelings in the Narrative

The therapist facilitates activities that label and contain the traumatic feelings and associated material. These include literally labeling the recording of the narrative with a title selected by the client. The title can provide clarity of feeling and some distance from the event via humor (albeit black humor)—for example, "Trapped in the Closet: Part III."

In addition, the therapist inquires about the client's specific feeling states, such as fear/anxiety, numbness, anger, sadness, shame, and guilt. Handout 22.2, Assessment of Postnarrative Emotional State, is again used as an in-session worksheet for this activity. After briefly reviewing the 1–10 rating scale in this handout, the therapist inquires about the intensity of the client's feelings in each domain after the narrative work. This creates a specific profile of the client's feeling states, which informs both client and therapist about the key feelings that have emerged as a result of this narrative work.

The therapist will be able to compare this profile to others that have been elicited from the same memory. It is likely that there will be reductions in the severity of fear and anxiety states in this first narrative. The therapist identifies these changes to the client as examples of the client's growing mastery of the trauma memory. An essential part of narrative work includes explicit recognition of mastery over overwhelming reactions to the trauma memory. This highlights the client's progress in an essential aspect of trauma recovery.

In the following sections, we address common challenges that arise in Narrative Therapy with our clients, including avoidance behaviors and dissociation.

WORK WITH AVOIDANCE BEHAVIORS

Avoidance behaviors are behaviors that distract the client from approaching a distressing aspect of the trauma. They are often evident in the client's speech or gestures. A client may hesitate before moving to the next word or sentence in their narrative, or may turn away or look down at certain segments of the narrative. Over time, the therapist will become familiar with these "clues." The therapist may initially simply observe these behaviors if the overall level of emotional engagement in the narrative is strong. However, if the client seems to have habituated to many fear-related elements of the story and seems to be going through the story in a rote fashion, the therapist gently inquires at the moment the behavior is observed: "I noticed that you hesitated. Was there something you thought or felt?" This can be enough to orient the client to pursue a detail they would have otherwise discarded. The therapist can also prompt the client by asking them what particular feeling or image they are having, which can lead to better engagement in meaningful aspects of the trauma.

CASE EXAMPLE 1: IDENTIFYING A HIGH-DISTRESS MOMENT IN THE NARRATIVE

Avoidance behaviors can be "flags" for identifying aspects of a narrative that are particularly distressing and have not been addressed in sufficient detail or possibly at all. A therapist can facilitate identification of high-distress, high-conflict memories by becoming familiar with a client's particular patterns of avoidance and bringing them to the client's attention. Some of these patterns can be subtle.

For example, a client, Jillian, was observed turning her body away when she described how her older brother slid into her bed before he raped her. Initially the therapist didn't comment, but this behavior continued in the repeated narrations. The therapist then called Jillian's attention to this behavior, and she was able to move further into the details of the story. It became clear that Jillian had been avoiding a key aspect of her trauma. Jillian described the moment when she turned around in her bed, looked into her brother's face, and saw "someone whom I did not know." This had been a very frightening moment. As she described it, her world completely crumbled. Her brother became a stranger to her. She felt she had "lost" her brother, who was the only member of the family still living in their abandoned household and on whom she depended in every way. She was able to describe this moment in detail in one of her final narrations of this event:

"I am feeling mortified, dirty, scared, angry, revolted. My heart is absolutely pounding. Still, I am afraid of running away. I am paralyzed with fear. It is like moving through molasses. If I try to get up and leave, it will be acknowledging that this is really happening. And I can't do that. It will send me over the edge."

Jillian noted that from then on, she knew she was "pretty much alone in the world," although at the time she would not have identified the source of this belief as the assault by her brother. In reflecting on her experience at the time, she added an important postscript:

"A few days later, I told him that I was moving out. At the time, I did not think it was because of what had happened. I was very shut down. If someone had told me it had happened, I would not have believed them, even though I knew it had."

Completing the narrative with access to a greater range of feelings led Jillian to recognize the devastating impact the assault had on her relationship with her brother, where she lived and why, and how she conducted herself in her adolescent years. This was difficult. But telling about this aspect of the trauma led to greater clarity about one of Jillian's principal relationship patterns, which was "If you rely on someone, then that person will just exploit and abandon you." This relationship pattern had previously been a free-floating belief that had been, to her, a self-evident truth about the world. Pinning the origins of this belief on this particular moment with her brother allowed her to consider limiting this belief to the context of the abuse. Once this relationship pattern was anchored in a particular episode in her life, she was able both to make sense of this belief and to consider that it might not be generally applicable to all relationships.

MANAGE DISSOCIATIVE REACTIONS

As the narrative work moves toward the client's more challenging memories, the client will be facing their worst fears and worst experiences. Some clients respond to high-stress material by dissociating. Below, we provide guidelines for managing, and ideally preventing, these kinds of reactions.

Dissociation and Trauma Narration

The best intervention for dissociation is prevention. A guiding principle of our narrative work is that the emotional intensity of the experience must be titrated so that the client always remains in the here and now and retains control of the process, particularly in the modulation of their fear. The purpose of the narrative is for the client to confront the trauma and to experience mastery of the memory. A successful narrative exercise is an empirical demonstration of the client's mastery over their trauma and emotional experiences. A key aspect of the client's initial trauma (and indeed of the very definition of trauma) is loss of mastery and control. During the trauma, the client did not have the ability to control the event or its outcome. Narration of the traumatic memory is therapeutic because it demonstrates to the client that although the client was helpless to stop the trauma as it happened, they can now regain control of the event via its influence on their memory and emotional reactivity. This success can lead to remarkably rapid resolution of PTSD symptoms.

Dissociation, in contrast, indicates that the traumatic material overwhelms the client. This is countertherapeutic, as it reinforces the client's experience of the self as having little control over the memories—an experience similar to the loss of control during the trauma itself. Indeed, this type of experience can be retraumatizing or can become a new trauma in its own right. The battle between the client and their PTSD symptoms is the battle between the power of the memory and the power of the client to confront and manage the memory.

Strategies for Managing Dissociation

When working with a client who has a tendency to dissociate, the therapist talks with the client about it, reassures the client that the therapist is aware of it, and identifies specific strategies for dealing with it.

We have found it helpful if the therapist and client agree on a signal for indicating that the client is feeling vulnerable to dissociation. This can be as simple as having the client raise their hand. The client and therapist can use such a gesture as a signal to reduce the emotional intensity of the narrative or to back away from certain material.

In addition, clients may exhibit specific automatic behaviors indicating that they have reached their maximum coping capacity and may be at risk for breaking off emotional or cognitive engagement with the present. These include small gestures such as rubbing their fingers together, "pilling" the fabric of their clothing, rapid blinking, or other kinds of eye or hand movements.

Perhaps the most powerful intervention in reducing dissociative experiencing is to remind the client regularly that the traumatic event is in the past. This can be done in a straightforward statement at the end of the narrative, such as "All of this happened in the past." This reality will be elaborated in relation to the client's particular core fears, and reinforced through role play in sessions and experiential exercises outside of sessions.

Additional Grounding Techniques to Orient Client to Present

Some survivors of trauma have strong fears of physical injury or death, particularly if their trauma was life-threatening or chronic (i.e., sustained and regular injury was inflicted). Other common are fears are of the perpetrators' coming after them, intruding upon them, and violating their bodies. Perhaps most particular to chronic interpersonal trauma—such as abuse by caregivers or relationship violence, which often happens over years—are clients' fears that they will never "get away" from their perpetrators because the perpetrators "live inside" them. This is evidenced not only in nightmares and images, but in their own day-to-day emotional reactions and behaviors that remind them of their perpetrators.

These fears are often effectively resolved through the repeated narration of the trauma and habituation to the fear associated with particular aspects of the traumas. After the narration, repeated reminders of differences between the conditions of a client's childhood and the present create a "life history" in which to contextualize the trauma as an event of the past. A client can be told, "You are no longer in your father's house. You have a home of your own," or "Your mother can't hurt you any more. She is old and feeble," or "Your ex-partner can't get you any more. He is in jail."

Exercises in mastery that invite contrast to the traumatic memory can provide evidence supporting these statements. If the client experienced abuse in childhood, this may include visiting the old neighborhood or house that the client lived in when the abuse occurred. Often the power of this environment is much diminished when it is actually viewed from the perspective of the adult survivor. If the client experienced abuse in childhood, fears of being physically overwhelmed by the perpetrator can be addressed in a similar way, by looking at pictures of the perpetrator as that person is now or was in the past. The perpetrator's size and strength are usually much less impressive from the adult survivor's perspective. Similar exercises can also be used if the client experienced chronic interpersonal trauma in adulthood. However, the therapist will want to ensure the client's safety before proceeding with exercises such as visiting a former neighborhood. In addition, the therapist helps the client recognize their own physical strength and resources. The client may also be encouraged to engage in activities that reinforce development and awareness of physical strength. This might include engagement in sports, yoga, martial arts, or any activity that creates awareness of physical integrity and agency. Such an activity can be as simple as walking or stretching, or using Focused Breathing.

CONDUCT NARRATIVE ANALYSIS

Relationship patterns identified during STAIR may be based solely on problematic behaviors and beliefs identified in day-to-day difficulties. Often very good progress can be made in the development of alternative relationship patterns and their implementation in role plays and between-session exercises. However, sometimes alternative relationship patterns and role plays do not elicit any significant change in a client's behaviors and are resisted by the client.

Under these circumstances, it is worthwhile to consider that the relationship pattern formulation is not quite accurate or conflicts with other fear-based relationship patterns. Little progress may occur during this time, but it is worthwhile for the therapist to keep tracking the expression of behaviors claimed to be associated with this relationship pattern. Reformulation of the relationship pattern can occur during Narrative Therapy, where, in the context of narrative work, previously unidentified feelings and memories will inform the "grain of truth" that was in the first relationship pattern. The relationship pattern identified as embedded in the narrative may be a more accurate and precise formulation of the beliefs and feelings driving the client's problematic behaviors. A more substantial and relevant alternative relationship pattern can then be formulated, and shifts in behavior can be more easily accomplished. An example of this process is provided below.

CASE EXAMPLE 2: REFORMULATING RELATIONSHIP PATTERNS

Identify Fear-Related Relationship Models in Narrative

During the STAIR module of treatment, Rose and her therapist had identified some maladaptive relationship patterns that kept her from asking for things she wanted. The initial identified relationship pattern was "If I love you, then I put your needs first." The behaviors associated with this relationship pattern of putting others' needs before hers had created conflict in Rose's marital relationship. Her husband, a likeable and easygoing person, did not particularly share her beliefs. Thus he did not engage in giving things he needed to his wife; nor was he particularly observant of her efforts to "sacrifice her needs" as expressions of her love for him. As a consequence of her husband's lack of response to her efforts, Rose felt angry, disregarded, and unimportant.

Rose and her therapist critically examined this relationship pattern, and an alternative was developed that explored an opposite principle: "If I love you, then I share my feelings and needs with you." The therapist and client engaged in assertiveness role plays in which Rose asked her husband for things and sometimes simply told her husband she was going to do things in accord with her own wishes. Both in life and in role plays, the husband was agreeable to these changes and to the more equal sharing of responsibilities and resources. Still, these activities were only modestly successful and yielded little change in the relationship.

Develop Alternative Relationship Models during Narrative Therapy

During Narrative Therapy, Rose described many different episodes of having been physically abused by her mother. The mother had in fact terrorized all of her children. Rose recalled her mother coming home in a drunken state in the middle of the night and rousing all of the children to look for her cigarettes or to clean out the bathroom. Rose also described some frightening scenes in her childhood home, which involved random demands by her mother that were enforced with physical violence. These demands included giving up food on their plates to their father. The narration of each of these stories was followed by an analysis of the relationship patterns embedded in the narrative.

The relationship pattern that had first been articulated during STAIR was eventually, in the context of Rose's abuse history, developed and refined into a much more meaningful belief: "If I make demands, then I am just like my cruel and crazy mother."

The therapist and client then discussed ways in which Rose was unlike her mother. Rose, having reached the age of 47 years, had never been physically abusive to her husband, nieces, and nephews. She was consistently kind and considerate of others. She was articulate and had a sense of humor, unlike her mother, who had been surly and had spoken rarely (and generally incoherently). Her mother had been addicted to alcohol; Rose was not. Her mother tended to like dark rooms, while Rose thrived in sunlight and open spaces. Distinguishing herself from her mother, and distinguishing appropriately assertive request behaviors from abusive demand behaviors, freed Rose to approach request behaviors in a more healthy and positive way.

Conduct Role Play

During both the STAIR and Narrative Therapy modules of treatment, a therapist and client continue to engage in assertiveness role-play practice at the end of sessions. In Rose's case, one role play with particular relevance to the narrative described above concerned Rose's reported difficulty in distributing food on the table and uncertainty about how much to give herself compared to her husband. Rose and the therapist practiced scenarios (with appropriate language, tone of voice, and behavior) that allowed Rose to engage in a variety of exchanges with her husband. In one, she gave all of the remaining food to her husband; in another, she shared the remaining food. Finally, in a third, Rose was to express her desire for the remaining items to her husband, make an explicit request to her agreeable husband ("I really would like those two baked potatoes"), and engage in the behavior of placing the food on her plate. The client was in fact unable to complete the third scenario in the initial attempts. First she disavowed her desire ("You know what? I am really not that hungry. Why don't you have some more?"). In the second effort, when she began reaching for the platter, she asked her husband, "Do you want me to cook you up something else?" even when he stated he was already finished with his meal.

It was not until Rose and her therapist had elaborated the initial relationship pattern to include its relevance to her perceptions of her mother's behavior that she was able to participate in this role play effectively. The final alternative relationship patterns generated from this effort were "If I make demands, then I can still be a good person," and a more emphatic variation, "I must identify my needs to be a good person." In a complementary fashion, Rose's perceptions about her husband's view of her were also changing. Her earlier assumption that her husband would view her as selfish, mean, and abusive was altered to this expectation of what he would think: "He will still love me (maybe even respect me more) if I ask for what I want." (See Box 23.2.)

Apply New Relationship Model to Current Life

Over time, Rose was able to view her some of her current beliefs as related to her childhood abuse experiences, and consequently as not particularly valuable or adaptive for living in the present. Through a review of some of her family history, and with the help of the therapist, it became apparent that her mother might have had a significant psychiatric illness; the mother had been hospitalized at least twice, according to the reports of her siblings. This information helped Rose create a way of understanding her mother's behavior and of seeing herself as quite different from her mother. The narrative work gave her a more organized, coherent, and understandable version of her childhood. It also helped her understand why she was "where she was at" in the present. Awareness of the particular ways that the past influenced her present—for example, her difficulty in expressing her needs—gave her the ability to critically analyze the necessity and value of this behavior. She also importantly recognized that she now had the skills and resources to change her current behavior and plan her future, guided by different expectations of herself and others.

BOX 23.2

Rose's Completed Relationship Patterns Worksheet–2

Interpersonal situation	What did I feel and think about myself?		What were my expectations about the other person?		My resulting behavior
What happened?	**My feelings**	**My thoughts**	**Their feelings**	**Their thoughts**	**What did I do?**
There were only two potatoes left on the platter.	Angry. Disregarded. Unimportant.	If I love you, I put your needs first.	Selfish. Mean. Abusive.	If I do not attend to his needs, I am a selfish, mean, bad person.	Gave husband both potatoes.

Relationship model: "If _I make demands_____, then _I am just like my cruel and crazy mother_____"

Interpersonal goals for situation	Alternative beliefs and feelings about myself: What else could I . . .		Alternative beliefs and feelings about the other person: What else could I expect the other person . . .		Alternative actions
What are my goals in this situation?	**. . . feel about myself?**	**. . . think about myself?**	**. . . to feel?**	**. . . to think?**	**What else could I do?**
Maintain loving relationship while asking for my needs to be met.	Curious. Confident.	I can ask for my needs to be met and still be a good person. I am not my mother.	Happy. Grateful.	My husband is a grown man. He will tell me if he wants more to eat. He will still love me (maybe even respect me more) if I ask for what I want.	**What else might they do?** Share the potatoes. Ask for potato and help myself.

Alternative relationship model: "If _I make demands_____,

then _I can still be a good person_____"

SUMMARIZE THE GOALS OF THE SESSION

At the end of the session, the therapist briefly summarizes the goals of the session and discusses how the goals fit within the larger treatment goals for the specific client. These may include reducing anxiety and PTSD symptoms, and/or reaching a better understanding of how beliefs and feeling related to the trauma influence the client's current life. The therapist checks in with the client to see how they are feeling about completing their narrative(s) and continuing with other narratives in the next several sessions. The therapist praises the client for the courageous work done in this session and all the work done during the STAIR module, which has provided the client with the skills to enable them to engage in the narrative work. The therapist highlights the importance of listening to the recording of the trauma narrative between sessions, and briefly reviews the rationale for doing so.

PLAN SKILLS PRACTICE

The skills practice will be similar to that assigned after Session 12. At the end of the session, the client will have their recording of the narrative(s). The therapist requests that the client listen to it once a day. The client therapist reminds the client to record their SUDs ratings and any comments or observations on Handout 22.1, Subjective Units of Distress (SUDs) during Trauma Narration, after each listening. As with previous planned skills practice, the therapist spends time predicting any potential obstacles to the client's completing this work and suggesting ways to make it feasible.

The therapist will also assign specific between-session work. In Rose's case, appropriate between-session work included implementation of the new relationship pattern "I can ask for my needs to be met and still be a good person" with her husband in situations other than negotiating at the dinner table. The client, for example, had significant health problems that she had not even disclosed to her husband, let alone asked for his help in managing. The particular conversations and requests inviting him into her life would need to be titrated in a way that would not overwhelm him and disappoint her. Rose jotted down her successes on additional copies of Relationship Patterns Worksheet–2. She also continued to practice Focused Breathing, particularly to deal with her anxiety in confronting her health problems and making an appointment to see a doctor. Finally, as part of her continued emotion regulation skills practice, she scheduled a pleasurable activity: going for a walk around a local lake with a friend.

Narratives of Shame

> If the client is ashamed of her past, she cannot create
> an integrated life history.
> —JUDITH HERMAN (2007)

Shame is an inevitable and salient consequence of interpersonal trauma, particularly childhood abuse and neglect, but it can be difficult to explore deeply in therapy. As one survivor wryly observed, "We have shame about feeling shamed." Clients often feel profound shame about their victimization because they think that they deserved or provoked it in some way. The ensuing feelings of shame often serve as self-confirmation of their own wrongdoing, creating a vicious cycle. The present chapter provides information to share with the client about how shame influences the survivor, as well as reasons for telling about shameful experiences. It also includes suggestions about the therapist's reactions to disclosure of shaming events, the importance of the therapist's positive regard for the client, and guidelines for sensitively conducting narrative retelling and analyses with shame themes. Box 24.1 outlines the theme and curriculum for this session.

Guidelines for Therapists' Response to Disclosure of Shaming Events

The aspects of the trauma about which the client is most ashamed tend to emerge only in the later part of the therapy, during the narrative work. Disclosure of shaming experiences creates a variety of risks, and so a client may delay or avoid doing so. A client may fear that disclosing an experience in which they were diminished will lead the listener to view them in a diminished way. They may worry that the listener will be disgusted and repelled by the event, and so will be disgusted and repelled by them. They may worry that they will be stigmatized not only for the event, but also for not having stopped the event; for not having had the capacity to do so; or for having maintained, provoked, or encouraged the traumatic events in some way. A client's disclosure of these events risks the revision of the therapist's view of them as "less"—of less value, interest, or importance to the therapist. The client may

Theme and Curriculum for Sessions 13–17
Narratives of Shame

Often the most difficult aspects of a trauma story involve themes of shame. Effective work with shame involves several aspects, the most important of which is repairing the client's diminished sense of worth. Ways in which this can be accomplished are critically analyzing the sources for the client's shame, building alternative relationship models in which they feel competent and valued, and developing opportunities for building self-confidence and for having positive experiences with others who value the client. The therapist also accomplishes this through direct expressions of positive regard for the client.

PLANNING AND PREPARATION

Bring therapist's copy of completed Memory Hierarchy (Handout 21.2); at least one copy of Assessment of Postnarrative Emotional State (Handout 22.2); and several copies each of Subjective Units of Distress (SUDs) during Trauma Narration (Handout 22.1) and Relationship Patterns Worksheet–2 (Handout 16.4). This session is 60 minutes in duration.

AGENDA

- Check-in and review of skills practice.
- Identify focus of the session.
- Discuss value of telling. Complete narrative about shame.
- Conduct narrative analysis.
- Provide support: Express positive regard.
- Summarize the goals of the session.
- Plan skills practice:
  - Listen to recording daily; monitor distress with Subjective Units of Distress (SUDs) during Trauma Narration form.
  - Initiate at least one interpersonal situation and practice alternative relationship model(s), using Relationship Patterns Worksheet–2 to record the practice and results; include emotion regulation skills as relevant to situation.
  - Practice Focused Breathing twice a day, and other emotion regulation skills as relevant.

(continued)

> **SESSION HANDOUTS**
>
> Completed copy of Handout 21.2. Memory Hierarchy
>
> Additional copies of Handout 22.1. Subjective Units of Distress (SUDs) during Trauma Narration
>
> At least one additional copy of Handout 22.2. Assessment of Postnarrative Emotional State
>
> Additional copies of Handout 16.4. Relationship Patterns Worksheet–2

assume that the human connection (so difficult to forge in the first place) will be broken, and that they will be worse off than before.

A supportive, compassionate, and practical response to the client's shaming experience is integral to helping the client resolve negative attitudes about the self. In the experience of shame, a person fears the negative opinion and evaluation of another. The client expects that disclosing events in which they were demeaned will make the therapist see them in a negative light. The repeated responses by a therapist of continued support and positive regard will help disconfirm this expectation, facilitating the client's capacity to think in other ways about their experiences and themselves. This attitude will be reinforced as the therapist proposes alternative relationship models that help the client identify their own value, and as the therapist helps them identify opportunities for building competence and having positive experiences with others who value them.

CHECK-IN AND REVIEW OF SKILLS PRACTICE

The therapist begins any of these sessions with the same structure as in previous Narrative Therapy sessions: by checking in with the client about ways they practiced emotional or relationship skills over the week, and then by focusing on what they experienced while listening to the narrative recording from the preceding session. The therapist reviews patterns of SUDs ratings and discusses any reactions, observations, or challenges the client may have had. After the review is complete, the therapist can once again remind the client that the ability to think about and discuss painful memories is a skill, and can congratulate the client on their efforts.

IDENTIFY FOCUS OF THE SESSION

Any type of victimization leads to feelings of shame, because such events are often interpreted as signs of weakness, defeat, worthlessness, or inferiority (see Chapter 7). Childhood abuse and neglect impose added burdens on the victim because of the social stigma associated with violation, especially sexual violation. The therapist can identify shame themes when stories involve the client's self-description as feeling "small," "humiliated," "weak," "inferior," "worthless," "defective," or "nonexistent." After a narrative, a client may judge the earlier self in the story as a pathetic or despicable person.

Though the client has already learned by this point in the treatment that avoiding emotions only makes them stronger and feel more out of control, they will often resist exploring feelings of shame. In fact, however, a powerful antidote to feelings of shame can be the satisfactory disclosure of these painful experiences.

The therapist opens up the discussion by clearly articulating the several benefits of telling about shameful experiences. It is important for the therapist to be aware that their own reactions and comments will be relevant to the client's ability to benefit from this process. The therapist can note any of the benefits below that apply to a particular client.

DISCUSS VALUE OF TELLING

Reducing Feelings of Alienation

Shame burdens a person with a feeling of being different from others. The client may believe that "if you knew I was victimized in this particular way, you would not connect with me." Telling about the trauma, and receiving a response of understanding and recognition, can dissipate the feeling of having an "outsider status." The client's belief that the experiences they have undergone are "beyond the range of normal" can be revised when the therapist conveys that what happened was terrible, but that they are not alone in their experiences. Even when the client believes the particulars of the experience to be unique, the client can come to realize that their feelings are experienced and understood by many.

Reducing Strength of Bond to Perpetrator

The client's traumatization has been one of the defining experiences of their life. Often, because of the secrecy in which the trauma (particularly sexual and sometimes physical abuse) takes place, the reality of the trauma is shared only with the perpetrator. To the extent that the client's self-definition is reflected in this shared reality, the client remains psychologically bonded to the perpetrator for a feeling of authenticity. The survivor may feel that the only person who knows everything or perhaps the worst about them is the perpetrator, and thus that the perpetrator is the only person who knows the "real me." By telling about the trauma, the client is able to dissolve that link and become independent of the perpetrator for their sense of authentic personal history. The client becomes free to experience their "real" self in full with others.

Enhancing Self-Compassion

A survivor's shame often arises from belief that the trauma or their inability to escape from it indicates that they were inherently weak, deserving of the victimization, or even inviting of it. These beliefs are often the result of the client's childhood view of the self as "frozen in time" and the feeling that they are responsible for the things that happened around them.

Reevaluation of this conclusion, perhaps prompted by observation of children in day-to-day life, can lead the client to understand the essential vulnerability of children. In addition, listening to the recordings of their trauma can provide the client with sufficient distance from their own experience to give them sympathy for what they have lived through. Listening to the recording can also provide a different perspective about the locus of responsibilities and shame. The narrative is a story of what happened to the client, and it includes not only the client but also the perpetrator. Shifting focus or widening the perspective of the story can help the client understand the active role of the perpetrator, the perpetrator's own motivations, and the powerful forces that the client was up against.

Gaining Appreciation and Awareness

The experience of self-compassion is particularly beneficial if the client is able to appreciate their capacity to have survived as they did in very difficult circumstances. A more positive, more open, and less defensive attitude about the self will allow the survivor to understand their own motivations and vulnerabilities with greater clarity (e.g., relationship models based on efforts to avoid shame, or perceptions of shaming behaviors). It will provide insight about the meaning of their feelings, actions, and reactions, and help the client map out strategies for effective change.

Improving Interpersonal Relationships

Survivors' negative and critical views of themselves also affect their evaluation of others. Survivors who internalize the ideas that vulnerability is weakness and that weakness is bad not only view themselves negatively, but often judge others in the same fashion. These attitudes diminish opportunities for positive social experiences and the development of sustained interpersonal relationships. The growth of self-compassion allows clients to live much more easily with themselves, and perhaps even to feel some pride and enthusiasm. This more positive and more generous process of self-evaluation may lead to more generous appraisal of others. Positive changes in self-regard go hand in hand with positive changes in regard for others. Clients thus benefit in their relationships with others, as well as in relationship to themselves.

Experiencing Agency and Facilitating Growth

Narration is an action, and as such can be an effective antidote to shame. Shame, which often arises from a sense of being ineffectual, is countered by the experience of agency in the creation of the story. A common, immediate, and understandable reaction to shame is silence. But in silence, many aspects of a person's experience and identity are left misunderstood or are not understood at all. The client's personal history is reduced to a simplistic and incomplete version of what they have experienced. In contrast, disclosure of the trauma story can liberate the client from the burden of secrecy that often paralyzes the capacity for self-expression and growth. If the client can tell about the trauma, even the shameful parts, they can tell about anything. The client's feelings and imagination are liberated and can be harnessed as resources for understanding their needs and for planning their present and future.

COMPLETE NARRATIVE ABOUT SHAME

In the way that narratives of fear must be titrated so that the client experiences mastery over fear rather than a reinstatement of it, so too narratives of shame need to be titrated so that the client experiences dignity rather than humiliation in the telling. Attention to feelings of shame can derive from the client's description of these feelings during the narrative or the review of it (see Chapter 20). The therapist can suggest further exploration of events related to these feelings, or can support the client's interest in doing so.

In shame-based narrative work, the greater portions of effort, time, and energy are spent on the analysis of the narrative after it has been completed and an appraisal of its meaning. Repeated telling of the story is useful to elicit details of the experience that produced the critical moments of shame. However, the transformation of shame lies in an exploration of the client's understanding of what happened and why, and a purposeful designation of its value to the client now. A client's shame may arise from having engaged in reprehensible acts during the course of the traumatic event(s), such as active participation in one's own abuse or the abuse of others. The therapeutic task is to help the client realistically evaluate the context in which these events occurred, which often involve dire circumstances and limited choices. Shame also arises from the perceived lack of action or inability to act in ways that would have averted or ended the trauma. Here too, the therapeutic goal is to help the client toward a realistic and compassionate evaluation of their circumstances.

The transformation of shame requires continual reference to the essential worth of individuals as they confront the ways in which they have been humiliated and diminished. This cannot be done in a naive or simplistic way that directs clients to attend to their "positive qualities." Rather, this process involves recognition of the psychological harm and accumulated losses that are results of the trauma, and an attendant and emerging sense of compassion for the person in the narrative and for the person who tells the story. In this way, clients can more readily explore the past in a respectful way and can simultaneously work toward seeing value in themselves now.

Perhaps the strongest feelings of shame emanate from circumstances in which a client reports obtaining physical pleasure from sexual abuse, or actively participating in such abuse by initiating abuse events or engaging in the established sexual activities that constituted the abuse scenario. When a client repeats that they felt compelled to submit to either sexual or physical abuse, the client's feelings of self-blame are often fairly easy for the therapist to counter. A child is outmaneuvered emotionally, cognitively, and physically by an abuser. However, in situations where the client reports initiating or provoking events, the therapist may have more difficulty in articulating this reality. From our perspective, however, a child's active engagement in abuse scenarios typically represents the extreme end of the abuser's domination over the child's life and the child's effort to exert a sense of personal control—and, in some cases, to secure their own survival when other avenues are closed off. The following case provides an example of such a situation and describes effective therapeutic interventions.

CASE EXAMPLE 1:
CLIENT AS ACTIVELY INVOLVED IN HER OWN ABUSE

Shanique had completed three narratives of physical and sexual abuse committed by her older brother when she was between the ages of 4 and 8. She believed that before she was born, her brother had been physically and sexually abused by her father. Her father took off shortly after she was born, and all she knew of him was that he had spent a lot of time in jail for drug-related offenses. She now began telling of another period of abuse in her early teen years. At this time, her brother was in his mid-20s.

> "When I was about 9, my brother enlisted in the armed forces. So the sexual abuse by my brother ended for a while. But things were still pretty bad for me at home. My mother was having long periods of depression where she stayed in bed for days, just staring at the ceiling. I'd have to take care of myself—borrow money from one of my aunts, and do the food shopping, cleaning, and cooking. When she was up and about, she just went out for days at a time, looking for drugs.
>
> "About the time I was 12, my brother came back. The armed forces hadn't done much for his temper or attitude. He was just a lot bigger now. My mother did not seem to notice one way or the other that he was back. I was terrified. I thought I had escaped from his torture, but no. I thought about how he had sodomized and beat me until I was a bloody mess. I knew there was no one I could go to. Then (*starts crying*)—I feel terrible to tell about this—I just gave up fighting him. It's worse. I started getting involved with him, anticipating his moods. He'd get this glassy-eyed look, and I knew it was time for me to give him a blow job. Sometimes I'd even bring it on more, doing the things he liked or telling him how I liked it.
>
> "It makes me sick. It makes me hate myself. After about 5 months of this, I realized he was settling into the house for good. Seeing how things were going, I convinced my best girlfriend to let me move in with her family. When I turned 18, I joined the armed forces. I got out of there ASAP. I still hate myself, though. What I did was sick, and it makes me sick to my stomach to think about."

Admission of her active involvement in her own abuse was a shameful component of Shanique's story, and it took several narratives before this aspect of the experience emerged. The therapist knew Shanique fairly well at this point and was able to articulate several reasons for this behavior. She presented them to Shanique, with compassion for her situation and support for how well she had done under those circumstances.

When her brother returned from his military service, Shanique was thrown back into a situation she thought she had escaped. At that point, she literally feared for her life and knew, without a doubt, that she could not count on anyone (including her mother) to help her survive her brother's presence. After a few years of relative peace and independence, and just as she was entering her early teens, she was desperate for a sense of control over her body and her environment. Her active efforts in prompting and participating in the abuse was a way to experience control over being abused, so that she did not feel so dominated and terrified. It was a "counterphobic" response, similar to the one many individuals engage in when confronted with a fear (such as heights or flying). Shanique hated being at the mercy of her fear and her brother. Her behavior gave her a sense of mastery. Unfortunately, in "matching" her brother, she also became, like him, a perpetrator of abuse—her own abuse. This left her with feelings of self-loathing and an inescapable core belief in herself as evil and bad.

By emphasizing the purpose of Shanique's behavior, the therapist was able to provide a way for Shanique to be more sympathetic to herself. Shanique was not being masochistic; she was engaged in reaching a goal that most people wish for and attain relatively easily—self-control and mastery of her body. Shanique had few if any other options to reach this goal. The alternative for her risked complete physical dominance and subjugation.

In addition, Shanique's past experience with her brother had informed her that he was capable of severe violence. Now he was bigger and angrier. Shanique believed, probably accurately, that he could kill her. She protected herself by anticipating his needs, essentially acting like an external mood modulator. If he was not angry, he was less likely to hurt her. She took the situation into her own hands as best she could. Taking care of his needs kept her alive.

The therapist acknowledged the horrors that Shanique had gone through. She noted especially that Shanique had been a survivor in the most basic meaning of the word: She had probably saved her own life. Shanique had also effectively used the resources she had at hand. As soon as she was able, she found other accommodations for herself with a friend's family, again showing her resilience in this situation. In reviewing her story with the therapist, Shanique understood that she had done the best she could, which was very good. She had held on to her life, to emerge at another time and place where things were very different. She now had the gift of life and a choice about how to live her life in freedom and with future opportunity.

CONDUCT NARRATIVE ANALYSIS

Clients who have experienced interpersonal trauma, particularly childhood abuse and neglect, can have long-held negative beliefs about themselves and deeply entrenched maladaptive behavioral patterns. Change is difficult and can be frightening. Although there is a desire for new and better ways of living, there is also resistance to leaving behind the comfort of the familiar. This work can be very challenging for both the client and the therapist. Narrative analysis in cases of shame involves several aspects. First, therapist and client identify shame-related relationship models that emerge through the client's telling, and determine how they developed in the context of the client's specific environment and traumatic experiences.

Next, the therapist assists the client in developing alternative relationship models that can be explored and applied in the present. To be successful, the development of alternatives to shame-driven relationship models (and their role plays) requires the regular identification, development, and support of psychological, practical, and emotional resources that reinforce the client's sense of value. Active efforts to demonstrate the client's value and current competencies include explicit identification of latent positive characteristics in the client and the enhancement of these characteristics in the STAIR activities.

The testing and application of alternative relationship models may utilize—and may in fact require—circumstances in which the client has confidence in an identified ability and the opportunity to share this skill with interested others. Role plays help clients practice presenting themselves in ways previously unimagined. Below, we present the case of Jerome, which illustrates these components of narrative analysis and demonstrates how to put it all together.

CASE EXAMPLE 2: POWERLESS OR A PERPETRATOR?

Throughout his entire life, Jerome carried a huge sense of guilt and shame related to the childhood abuse he endured at the hands of his father. Not only did his father physically abuse him, but he was forced to witness the abuse of his mother and little brother as well. He believed that he should have been able to protect his mother and brother, but that he failed to do so. Viewing himself and others as either victims or perpetrators with no roles in between, Jerome had experienced a series of failed romantic relationships, difficulty keeping a steady job, and constant disappointment in most aspects of his life. Below, we describe each intervention that helped Jerome to move toward the goal of reevaluating his history, resolving some of the shame he felt about himself, reorganizing his view of himself and others, and exploring new behaviors and attitudes.

Jerome believed that he was essentially a bad person, and that this was why he had been abused and failed to save those he loved from also experiencing trauma. He believed that he was a failure as a man, and that he was entirely responsible for the violence his family had endured. Several steps were taken to explore the source, viability, and adaptive nature of these beliefs. These steps included (1) listening to the recordings of his narratives, from the perspective of an adult listening to the story of a child and revising views of himself as "bad"; (2) engaging in critical analyses of relationship patterns by reevaluating the sources of blame for the traumatic events; and (3) proposing alternative interpersonal patterns and behaviors that would support connection to others and the development of healthy models of relating.

Identify Shame-Related Relationship Models in Narrative

Jerome's view of his abuse was that he must have deserved it (i.e., been a bad child), or that he was bad because he had "let the abuse happen" to him and his family. After the childhood abuse narratives were completed, the therapist explored the reasons for these beliefs.

Jerome's belief that he was a bad child stemmed from being told that he was bad by his father. This label organized and explained his experience; it created consistency between what was happening to him (how he was treated) and who he thought he was. Jerome's belief that he was bad for "letting himself" be physically abused as a child was being maintained by a distorted sense of his own culpability in the situation.

The therapist and Jerome reviewed the logic of these beliefs from the perspective of an adult rather than a child. For years, Jerome had believed that he was bad for "letting the abuse happen" because he had held on to the childhood perception that he was in control of the events of his early life. The therapist explained that children have relatively underdeveloped cognitive and emotional resources to control events; rather, they depend on adults who are charged with the responsibility to care for and protect them. However, what was most striking to Jerome was engaging in a between-session assignment to watch neighborhood children approximately the same age as he was (between 5 and 8 years) when he was abused. Watching them play and interact with adults provided very concrete and realistic information about the significant levels of dependency and trust children exhibit toward adults. Hearing his own voice on the recordings, Jerome began to have immense compassion for that little boy who was being abused by his father. Rather than deeming him somehow responsible for the violence inflicted upon him when he was a young, dependent child, he began to see that in fact he had done absolutely nothing to "cause" or "deserve" his father's abuse.

Develop Alternative Relationship Models

Jerome had already been working in the earlier portion of treatment to reassess underlying relationship expectations, notably the pattern "If I assert myself, then others will hurt me." His therapist helped him generate an alternative approach: "If I assert myself, then others may *not* hurt me." Over time, and with more successful assertiveness practice (including stating which restaurant he wanted to go to, asking for directions, and even telling a friend no), he was able to extend this belief to "If I assert myself, then others can still respect me."

This underlying relationship pattern took on a whole different meaning and significance in the context of Narrative Therapy. In the course of describing one particular memory in which his father abruptly switched from physically abusing him to abusing his brother instead, Jerome confided, for the first time ever, that part of him was relieved his father gave him a break and focused on his brother instead of him. This initial relief only lasted a split second, and then Jerome felt intense shame about his reaction. Now not only did he view himself as bad because he allowed this to happen to his brother; he also viewed himself as a perpetrator because part of him was glad.

As Jerome completed the memory, he recalled that he had actually run in between his father and his brother and attempted to stop his father's violent behavior. Instead, his father yelled at him, and then grabbed his mother and began to hit her too. Again, Jerome felt like a perpetrator, because from his child's perspective he had caused his mother to be hurt as well. Rather than using this as further ammunition against himself, the therapist helped him see that he actually was trying to *save* his brother. He was not a perpetrator at all; in fact, he was quite the opposite. Again, for the first time in his life, Jerome began to develop a sense of compassion for that little boy who had tried in vain to protect his brother and his mother.

When Jerome first told this narrative to his therapist, he spoke so quietly the therapist could barely hear him, with his head hung low and his entire body slumped over in his chair. The therapist validated his reaction and did not judge him or castigate him, as he had anticipated. He was heartened by the therapist's response to his deepest, darkest secret. She explained that it was perfectly natural that he would feel an initial sense of relief that he had a brief reprieve from the hurt his father inflicted. Then when Jerome explained that it felt even worse seeing and hearing his poor brother be hurt, the therapist could understand how he would feel that way, too. She had him retell his narrative, but this time while sitting up straight and using a louder, more direct tone of voice. When they processed the memory afterward, she asked him to do his best to maintain eye contact with her. He saw her acceptance and understanding, rather than the hatred and disgust he had expected. With each repeated telling of this story, Jerome felt the burden of shame grow less and less.

As part of the narrative analysis, Jerome identified another related trauma-generated relationship pattern: "If I assert my needs, then others will be hurt." He had linked his attempts to protect himself and his family with not only his own punishment, but punishment of those he cared about. The alternative pattern—"If I assert my needs, then others can still respect me"—took on extended meaning as he reassured himself that in the present, standing up for oneself did not equal terrible things happening.

Determine Resources

With a new perspective on his abuse history, Jerome turned to building capacities in the present. Armed with the realization that he had not caused his abuse, and that he was not a failure because he could not protect his mother and brother, he continued to experiment with new, revised relationship patterns that were more applicable to the here and now. He continued to make requests and express his opinions and feelings. He reminded himself repeatedly, "That was then; this is now," when he worried about the consequences of being assertive.

His budding sense of compassion for himself and what he had been through allowed him to finally consider that people actually meant it when they said they liked him or liked his work. Jerome was a very skilled carpenter, but he had never pursued this as a career interest, because he did not believe the positive feedback he received. He always gave away his work for free, assuming that he did not deserve to get paid for his efforts. Furthermore, he had never before entertained the possibility that he could be self-employed doing something he truly loved. He was now interested in exploring the possibility of starting his own carpentry business and began advertising his services.

Jerome also wanted to challenge himself in what he called "the final frontier"—romantic relationships. He had never sought out anyone; all of his relationships had developed from women who had approached him. For years he had been interested in Tonia, a friend of his cousin. He had recently asked her out on a date, and much to his delight, she said yes.

He was now trying to enact alternative relationship patterns with her, such as "If I express my opinions, people will be interested." He was starting to believe that friendships and romantic relationships could be resources for coping with life's difficulties and for experiencing life's pleasures.

Conduct Role Play

Jerome had the opportunity to test these new relationship beliefs when he accepted a potential job: building a bookcase for an acquaintance. The acquaintance, however, offered to pay him less than what it would cost for him to purchase the materials. He was not sure how to handle this, and he brought in a completed Relationship Patterns Worksheet–2 to discuss with his therapist (see Box 24.2).

When the therapist proposed that he negotiate for more money, his first reaction was "I am being selfish. They are probably just doing me a favor, anyway." The therapist pointed out that this way of thinking was based upon a trauma-based relationship pattern: "If I am assertive, then others will hurt me." Together, they developed new ways of approaching this situation, focused on the acknowledgment that it was OK for Jerome to ask for a fee that was commensurate with his effort and time. This capitalized on the new relationship pattern: "If I assertive, then others might respect me."

Jerome and the therapist engaged in a role play so that he could practice negotiating a reasonable fee. Initially he was very apologetic and explained how the cost of lumber had risen exponentially in recent weeks; he also spoke in a quiet and subdued tone while looking down at the floor. The therapist praised some aspects of the role play, but also pointed out that Jerome need not apologize for the price of lumber—that he had the right to ask for a fair fee in a way that was direct and clear. The therapist then modeled how he might ask for the fee in a respectful yet unapologetic manner. Jerome reminded himself that being assertive would not automatically lead to something terrible happening, and he then tried the role play again. This time he adopted a bit of the therapist's style in a way that felt comfortable to him, and he requested a reasonable fee in a more confident fashion. Now that he had practiced this in session, he was ready to try it out in the real world.

PROVIDE SUPPORT: EXPRESS POSITIVE REGARD

The therapist's capacity to convey their continued perception of the client's positive value can counter the client's incipient feelings of shame provoked by struggles in meeting the challenges in the treatment work. These struggles may include difficulties in completing the narratives, assimilating new relationship models, and/or practicing self-enhancing exercises. The therapist makes observations about what the client has felt, said, or done that support the positive valuation of the client. This valuation is reinforced by working steadfastly with the client on the tasks of the therapy with hope and vigor.

A therapist's positive regard for a client is generally viewed as a "nonspecific" positive aspect of the therapy. Some of our own research, however, suggests that the therapist's

BOX 24.2

Jerome's Completed Relationship Patterns Worksheet–2

Interpersonal situation	What did I feel and think about myself?		What were my expectations about the other person?		My resulting behavior
What happened?	**My feelings**	**My thoughts**	**Their feelings**	**Their thoughts**	**What did I do?**
A customer wants me to make a custom bookcase for him for less than the price of supplies.	Scared. Embarrassed.	I should count myself lucky that anyone would want me to make something.	Anger. Disdain.	He is just trying to do me a favor. Who do I think I am?	Froze and said I would think about it.

Relationship model: "If I am assertive _____, then will hurt me."

Interpersonal goals for situation	Alternative beliefs and feelings about myself: What else could I . . .		Alternative beliefs and feelings about the other person: What else could I expect the other person . . .		Alternative actions
What are my goals in this situation?	**. . . feel about myself?**	**. . . think about myself?**	**. . . to feel?**	**. . . to think?**	**What else could I do? What else might they do?**
Get a fair price. Respect myself and the customer too.	A little nervous, but also confident.	I do very good work.	Appreciative.	He may really want me to make him a bookcase.	Assertively and respectfully negotiate a fair fee with him.

Alternative relationship model: "If I am assertive

then others might respect me _____."

402

positive regard for the client does not exist in a vacuum, but is part of a collaborative working relationship, which is expressed through active engagement in competency-enhancing activities (Cloitre et al., 2004). The experience of someone (in this case, a therapist) expending effort on behalf of a client and showing interest in their problems may contribute to persuading the client of their own value.

Challenge: When Clients Don't Tell

Clients in short-term treatment may not have the opportunity, readiness, or inclination to reveal humiliating details of what has happened to them. There is a risk that if clients withhold something important about themselves, they will discount the therapist's good opinion of them and the value of the work they have completed. A client may think, "If the therapist really knew who I was, they would not think well of me," or "If the therapist knew what happened then, they would realize I am 'damaged goods.' " This outcome may be avoided by saying something to the client that acknowledges and "normalizes" the possibility that they may not be able to disclose particularly painful or humiliating aspects of their trauma. Here is an example:

> "I understand that there may be some things that are very difficult for you to say, and that you may in fact not be able to tell about them right now. Many people have this experience. This will not in any way reduce the value of your efforts here or the progress you have made. You can identify important trauma-based relationship models without necessarily stating or even knowing all of the reasons you hold these beliefs. Similarly, the new relationship models you have developed are valuable and consistent with the person you are now and are becoming. You have gone through terrible things. You deserve to live a good life now, and as best as you are able."

Role of Therapeutic Relationship in Transforming Shame

The therapist's behavior plays a particularly important role in the client's recovery from shame. As described in some detail in the case of Jerome, the therapist actively works with the client in implementing the interventions of the treatment to identify and revise shame-based relationship models and behaviors. In addition, the therapist's *attitude* of compassion about what has been shaming for the client is itself a therapeutic intervention. It contradicts the expectation that when the client discloses events of gross humiliation, the therapist will be appalled, think less of them, or create distance or a break in the relationship. Shameful events engender not only a fear of rejection, but, in the big picture, fear of permanent dislocation outside the mainstream of ordinary life. The positive interaction between the therapist and client upon disclosure of demeaning stories models for the client the possibility of acceptance by another. When the therapist describes the client's circumstances with respect and compassion, the client understands their own experience in a new way, through the therapist's eyes. The client's experience of shame is transformed into one of self-respect.

SUMMARIZE THE GOALS OF THE SESSION

At the end of the session, the therapist briefly summarizes the goals of the session and discusses how the goals fit within the larger treatment goals for the specific client. These include exploring feelings of shame that are the consequence of the client's interpersonal trauma, and beginning to rework negative beliefs that the client was somehow deserving of or to blame for their victimization, which have perpetuated isolation. The therapist checks in with the client to see how they are feeling about completing their narrative(s), especially in regard to telling about the aspects of which they have been most ashamed. The therapist expresses admiration for the courageous work done as well as appreciation for the risks that the client has taken by sharing in this session. The therapist highlights the importance of listening to the recording of the trauma narrative between sessions, and again briefly reviews the rationale for doing so.

PLAN SKILLS PRACTICE

The client is instructed to listen to the recording of the latest narrative daily during the week, and to identify relationship models of shame they hear in the narrative. The therapist and client have already identified some of these models and role-played some alternative formulations of them. Now the client and therapist can also determine a real-life circumstance in which the client can practice alternative relationship models, using a copy of Relationship Patterns Worksheet–2 (Handout 16.4) to record the results. Practice of Focused Breathing twice a day, as well as of other emotion regulation skills as relevant, continues. The therapist and client can determine collaboratively the skills that make the most sense for the client to practice at this point in the treatment.

Narratives of Loss

> Grieving for . . . lost opportunities, for lost childhood, for lost
> innocence, for losses of long ago and far away is quite difficult. . . .
> for traumatic losses that do not involve immediate death, grieving
> is often an uncharted and socially unsupported wilderness.
> —SANDRA L. BLOOM AND MICHAEL REICHERT (1998, p. 193)

The experience of loss, like that of shame, has not always been directly addressed in traditional trauma treatments. In part, this is because feelings of loss often emerge relatively late in the working through of trauma, particularly childhood abuse and neglect. In order to truly understand and mourn losses suffered in the context of interpersonal trauma, one must first feel deserving of the care, protection, and resources that were not available at the time of the event(s). The belief among some clients that their traumatic experiences were deserved or are in some way "normative" interferes with the development of self-compassion and a healthy sense of entitlement, both of which are relevant to the grieving process.

In addition, the grief for "what never was and never can be" is often very acute and can amplify other negative trauma-related feelings, such as shame. Typically, survivors have warded off feelings of sadness about their histories through avoidance and numbing, or through focusing solely on their anger. As one client put it, "If I let myself really feel how sad my life has been, I would never stop crying. I would turn to mush, and you would have to peel me off the floor."

However, until a client can conceptualize what their past might or should have been, and can allow for sorrow associated with this recognition, it is likely that they will remain stuck in this past. In contrast, helping the client to tolerate and process feelings of sadness and grief associated with interpersonal trauma and its costs can, over time, serve to further decrease symptoms of numbing and avoidance. It can also increase the possibility of developing a more positive and meaningful personal identity and better connections with others. Box 25.1 outlines the theme and curriculum for working with narratives of loss in Sessions 13–17 of treatment.

BOX 25.1

Theme and Curriculum for Sessions 13–17
Narratives of Loss

Themes of loss tend to emerge during narrative work. This emergence provides a valuable opportunity to help the client initiate the grief process. Successful engagement in this effort can result in decreased avoidance and numbing symptoms, increased self-compassion, and increased intimacy and openness in relationships. The therapist listens for ways sadness and loss are expressed in narratives (e.g., loss of protective parent figure, loss of childhood, loss of time), and describes potential long-term benefits of tolerating and processing painful trauma-related loss experiences. The therapist provides support and containment while encouraging the client to elaborate on feelings and to mourn losses. The therapist also helps the client to identify the impact of loss experiences on current relationships through relationship models, and to generate and practice alternative models that will increase positive connections with others in the present.

PLANNING AND PREPARATION

Bring therapist's copy of completed Memory Hierarchy (Handout 21.2); at least one copy of Assessment of Postnarrative Emotional State (Handout 22.2); and several copies each of Subjective Units of Distress (SUDs) during Trauma Narration (Handout 22.1) and Relationship Patterns Worksheet–2 (Handout 16.4). This session is 60 minutes in duration.

AGENDA

- Check-in and review of skills practice.
- Identify focus of the session.
- Explore reasons to discuss loss and to grieve.
- Complete narrative about loss.
- Conduct narrative analysis.
- Provide support: Share the burden of pain.
- Summarize the goals of the session.

(continued)

- Plan skills practice:
  - Listen to recording daily; monitor stress with Subjective Units of Distress (SUDs) during Trauma Narration form.
  - Initiate at least one interpersonal situation and practice alternative relationship model(s), using Relationship Patterns Worksheet–2 to record the practice and results; include emotion regulation skills as relevant to situation.
  - Practice Focused Breathing twice a day, and other emotion regulation skills as relevant.

SESSION HANDOUTS

Completed copy of Handout 21.2. Memory Hierarchy

Additional copies of Handout 22.1. Subjective Units of Distress (SUDs) during Trauma Narration

At least one additional copy of Handout 22.2. Assessment of Postnarrative Emotional State

Additional copies of Handout 16.4. Relationship Patterns Worksheet–2

CHECK-IN AND REVIEW OF SKILLS PRACTICE

The therapist begins with checking in about ways the client practiced emotion or relationship skills over the week, and then by focusing on what the client experienced in terms of listening to narrative recordings from last session, including a review of SUDs ratings as well as any reactions, observations, or challenges the client encountered. After the review is complete, the therapist can again remind the client that the ability to think about and discuss painful memories is a skill, and can congratulate them on their efforts.

IDENTIFY FOCUS OF THE SESSION

The therapist needs to listen for how themes and layers of loss (e.g., loss of protective parental figure, loss of childhood, loss of time) are expressed in narratives, and to observe these with the client. The therapist elicits the client's own observations of these themes as they listen to recordings of narratives both in and outside of sessions. Often clients have been too busy recruiting their emotional and cognitive resources to manage fear reactions, which typically carry with them a sense of urgency and crisis, and have not attended to their experiences of loss.

As they often are with feelings of fear, clients may be somewhat avoidant of, or reluctant to deal with, feelings of sadness. If themes of loss are present in a narrative, the therapist may broach the theme by making comments such as "It sounds like such a sad and terrible thing to have happened." Sometimes a client's feelings of anger indicate an awareness or belief that the trauma has "cheated" them of what they should have had. If so, the therapist asks the client to articulate what specifically makes them angry about what has happened. Typically underneath anger are feelings of sadness and hurt.

Sometimes clients who were maltreated as children say they feel angry or sad when they think or tell about their abuse or neglect, but cannot specify what makes them feel that way. One exercise that can be helpful in this regard is to ask such a client between sessions to observe a child who is about the same age as they were at the time of the abuse or neglect. The client watches how a "normal," nonmaltreating caregiver interacts with the child, and then wonders, "What does that child have or do that I did not?" This exercise often evokes powerful loss-related feelings.

EXPLORE REASONS TO DISCUSS LOSS AND TO GRIEVE

Though the client has already learned by this point in the treatment that avoiding emotions only makes the emotions feel stronger and more out of control, many questions and anxieties are still often raised: "Why do I have to feel sad about it?", "How is that going to help me?", "What good is feeling sorry for myself?", and the like. The therapist must acknowledge the pain and distress involved in this process, empathize with the client's fears about delving into feelings of sadness, and understand their skepticism about how this will be helpful. In response to the implicit or explicit question "Why should I grieve?", the therapist articulates clearly to the client potential important long-term benefits of doing this work, described below.

Liberate Emotional and Physical Energies

Giving voice to feelings of underlying sadness and grief can provide tremendous relief and decrease the level of mental energy the client has been consistently expending to avoid feelings and reminders of the past. This makes more energy available for the client to develop their life in the present. Since it is not possible to numb only negative feelings, allowing sadness to come to the surface also increases the possibility of experiencing more positive emotions, such as happiness. In this way, the grief process ultimately facilitates the availability of a fuller spectrum of feelings, where previously there was access to only a constricted range.

Disrupt Links between Loss/Grief and PTSD Symptoms

As appropriate, the therapist helps the client recognize ways that unprocessed loss feelings may be keeping them stuck and perpetuating PTSD symptoms. When difficult feelings from the past are expressed in the present, their power to disrupt the future may be decreased.

Cultivate Self-Compassion

Often even if a survivor is no longer in a traumatic relationship, they are still perpetuating these experiences through self-blame, intolerance of their emotions, and invalidation of their life experiences. One of the main goals of grieving is to gain more compassion toward oneself and to cultivate respect for what one has endured.

Increase Capacity for Meaningful Interpersonal Relationships

As self-compassion develops, a client also has the possibility of forming more meaningful interpersonal connections. Being dismissive of one's own emotional experiences can make it difficult to be understanding and remain open to those of others. Being locked in a self-protective mode breeds isolation and alienation. In contrast, becoming more empathic toward the self often translates into becoming more empathic toward others. The increase in openness and authenticity that often accompanies the grief process is likely to elicit more responsiveness and engagement on the part of others.

Find Value in the Present

Developing a deeper understanding of what has been missing can allow a client to put more value on the things they do have in the present and could have in the future. The distress associated with loss can provide a powerful impetus for making life changes, so that at least some of what has been lost can be balanced by what can be had in the present. The alternative—avoidance of grief—keeps the client emotionally paralyzed and prevents growth.

COMPLETE NARRATIVE ABOUT LOSS

Although a client may accept the value of grieving and be aware of their sadness, they still may not have a clear understanding of what exactly they have lost and feel sad about. By revisiting the trauma, the client can experience greater clarity about what makes them sad. Telling about the losses will help clarify events that were significant to the client and the impact that these experiences have had on both their beliefs about the self and their current behaviors. Procedures for conducting loss narratives are the same as those described in Chapter 22.

Narratives of loss, like all trauma narratives, also provide the client with the opportunity to have someone bear witness to the loss and share in remembrance of the child who once was before the trauma, or who never was and could have been. This may lead to ways of creating some aspects of the imagined but lost self, or identified experiential losses, through planned activities in the present.

CONDUCT NARRATIVE ANALYSIS

Grieving for the losses engendered by interpersonal trauma requires that they first be recognized. This recognition is often hampered by a client's critical and self-blaming attributions about their history. The therapist can make efforts to promote respect and understanding of the experiences the client has endured. Often listening to recordings provides useful distance, which can be effective in helping the client develop self-compassion (e.g., "I felt sorry for that little girl"). If the client is still having difficulty accessing feelings of sadness, sharing the impact that hearing the narrative has had on the therapist can be an effective catalyst (e.g., "When I was listening, I was aware of how desperate and abandoned that little girl sounded, and it made me feel very sad that nobody was taking care of her"). In this context, the client will be able to identify relationship models they developed that reflect themes of loss and that perpetuate associated painful feelings in their present relationships.

The therapist helps the client understand how their feelings of loss typically get reactivated and reenacted, and identify current relationships in which this is most likely to happen. The development of alternative relationship models will emphasize changes that decrease the sense of loss and increase social connection. This may include the client's either distancing/detaching from, or making changes in, particular relationships that tend to trigger loss feelings. Covert modeling and role playing can be used in sessions to experiment with different ways of interacting, so as to identify how the client could increase feelings of connection and decrease feelings of detachment in interpersonal interactions. A description of this process is provided in the case example below.

Coming to terms with trauma-related losses can be more tolerable if clients can gain a sense that some good can come in the present from having had to endure such painful experiences in the past. Clients may benefit from considering how their loss experiences give them a unique ability to value and appreciate certain things others may waste or take for granted. Clients can also gain from realizing what they have lost by identifying areas in their lives where they want to make changes. For example, clients who feel they have lost time because of the trauma can work on turning that feeling around by better valuing and making use of the time they still do have.

Role plays associated with grief usually reflect fears of intimacy and of abandonment. Role plays about building relationships are successful when a client is guided by strategies that allow them to go slowly and in an informed way ("Who is this person?", "What do I do?") in seeking out the companionship and friendship of others. The case of Juanita demonstrates this process.

CASE EXAMPLE: LAYERS OF LOSS

The case of Juanita, a 67-year-old single woman with a history of sexual abuse and long-standing PTSD symptoms, serves to illustrate some common ways loss themes emerge in narratives and how they can be worked with in the treatment.

Juanita's mother was a single parent who worked long hours to support the family. Juanita's uncle lived nearby and often helped out by doing repairs around the house and caring for the kids. When she was 10, her uncle began molesting her. After the first few times, Juanita told her mother that she no longer wanted to be left alone with him. Juanita's mother found her change in attitude toward her uncle surprising, but did not make much of it and also felt that there was no alternative to relying on the uncle for help. Over the next few months, her uncle began forcing himself on her more frequently, and Juanita realized that she would have to explain what was going on if there was to be any change: "I didn't want to tell her about the things he was doing to me, because I knew she would be upset, but I wanted it to stop." According to Juanita, her mother initially dismissed it by saying, "Your uncle loves you and would never hurt you or me." Juanita persisted and got more specific about the abuse. In shock and disbelief, her mother asked Juanita for more details and began shaking upon hearing them. Juanita remembers her mother desperately grabbing her and sobbing as she said things like "How could he do this to me?" and "How could I not have known?"

Juanita felt incredibly guilty and frightened by her mother's reaction. In order to stop her own mounting anxiety and dread, she told her mother that she had made it all up. Juanita's mother accepted this explanation, asked no further questions, and never brought it up again. Juanita's uncle continued to spend time around the house and continued to molest her until she was 16, at which time he moved to another state. Juanita did not try to tell her mother or anyone else about the abuse again, figuring it would be in everyone's best interest if she pretended it never happened.

Identify Loss-Related Relationship Models in Narrative

Loss of parental protector

Juanita remembered idealizing her uncle prior to the abuse and viewing him as a surrogate father—someone she loved and could turn to if she needed help. Her subsequent abuse experiences with him led her to believe that trusting others in relationships was dangerous and likely to end in betrayal of that trust. The way she managed her feelings of bewilderment and anger at this betrayal by someone she had been raised to believe loved her and had her best interests at heart was to "turn off" all thoughts and feelings about it. The unprocessed anger and grief that emerged during the narrative process, though at times overwhelming, did not surprise Juanita: "I always knew it was there, but was afraid to face it." With the support of her therapist, and equipped with improved emotion regulation skills, Juanita was able to verbalize and move through some of these feelings. Over time, they lost some of their power over her.

What caught Juanita off guard were her intense and complicated feelings toward her mother, which also emerged through the narratives. Prior to this phase of the treatment, Juanita had remained protective of her mother, feeling that she had done her best with limited resources. Juanita said she had forgiven her mother for "not knowing" that the abuse was going on, and felt that it was in large part her own fault for making the decision to take back her original report of the molestation.

During Juanita's telling of the abuse during the narrative portion of treatment, the deep loss she felt with regard to her mother became apparent to both the therapist and herself. It was Juanita's sense that after she disclosed the abuse, there was a change in her relationship with her mother. For example, she felt that her mother spent less time alone with her and avoided asking her what was going on when Juanita seemed upset. The therapist was able to identify how these experiences formed the basis for another of Juanita's relationship models—the expectation that if she were to tell others about pain she was experiencing, they would be likely to become overwhelmed and withdraw from her. Juanita became very panicky as feelings about being abandoned by her mother came to the forefront in the treatment. The therapist worked with Juanita to integrate and accept her previously unexpressed feelings of anger and grief about her mother's absence and her failure to protect Juanita, allowing them to coexist with the knowledge that her mother was fragile and depressed. It was important for Juanita to realize the extent of her losses: She had in effect been abandoned not by one of her central caregivers, but by both. This knowledge and understanding allowed her to feel more tolerant of her continued difficulties in putting her childhood abuse behind her.

Loss of childhood

In one of her narratives, Juanita vividly recalled being able to hear kids from the neighborhood laughing and playing outside while her uncle was having sex with her. This memory tapped into the reservoir of grief she felt about not having had a "normal," carefree childhood. Because she had been victimized and forced into having sex prematurely by a trusted adult, she was not afforded the period of dormant sexuality and innocence most children have during their early preadolescent years. Juanita went on to share how knowing more than she should about sex made her feel very different and isolated from other kids her age, which was another source of great sadness to her: "While other kids were playing tag with friends, I was inside having sex." Juanita described her transformation from a happy and trusting little girl to a scared, shy, and strange one. Prior to the narrative analysis, this dramatic shift in her demeanor had been incomprehensible and had been viewed by Juanita as further evidence of her "defectiveness"—which drove her anxiety about being exposed, and which continued in the present to minimize the degree to which she was willing to let other people get to know her. Being able to link these changes to her trauma experiences provided her with a way to challenge her belief that she had been at fault for taking back her original story. Instead, Juanita was able to see how she did in fact continue to try to communicate to others that something was very wrong. This understanding of events and their sequence also provided Juanita with a sense of order and meaning about what had previously felt confusing and mysterious to her.

Loss of time

Symptoms of avoidance and the loss-related relationship models Juanita had developed perpetuated her social discomfort, mistrust, and disappointment in others, and continued to affect Juanita in numerous ways in adulthood. Though she was likeable and often sought out, Juanita had very few close relationships. The friends she did have, she kept at arm's length; she rarely socialized and did not invite anyone over to her house. She had been intimately involved with one man when she was in her late 20s, but according to Juanita, this relationship had been a constant source of pain. She described a cycle in which he often made plans and promises that he did not keep, which left Juanita feeling "needy" and "deserted." Juanita had trouble understanding why, instead of ending the relationship, she continued to hold out hope for so long that she would get what she wanted from him. After he eventually ended the relationship, Juanita made the decision that she would not give another person the power to hurt her so deeply. As a result, she did not pursue any potential romantic situations when they arose, because she felt much more comfortable being on her own. However, she was now acutely aware of the consequences of shutting herself off in this way, and she began to feel despair at never having had children and created a family of her own.

Instead, Juanita had thrown herself into her work, which she described as her "relationship." She volunteered to take on extra duties and work extra hours, and she explained that her work was her greatest source of fulfillment. Now that she was on the cusp of retirement, however, she was feeling very anxious about how she would spend her time. Most importantly, she was now realizing how lonely she was, and she could not help wondering how her life might have been different if she had not experienced trauma.

Through narrative analysis, Juanita's growing awareness of the connection between her abuse experiences and current interpersonal difficulties compounded her anger and grief. She wondered how she would ever be able to make up for the time and life experiences she had lost. She also felt depressed that her early abuse experiences were continuing to have such an impact on her life. Juanita's therapist worked with her on accepting that what had been lost could not be reclaimed, but also on identifying ways in which these losses could be used to make meaningful changes in the present. Though it was quite distressing for Juanita to face just how much her trauma experiences were continuing to "rob" her in the present, this awareness ultimately provided tremendous motivation for her to finally begin making some important life changes, including taking more risks in relationships.

Juanita also began to recognize that though her trauma-related losses would always be there, they could become more manageable and ebb and flow at different times, rather than remain at such an intense and disorganizing level. Also critical was her belief in her therapist's rationale that the grief related to the past would lessen as she became more engaged in the present.

Develop Alternative Relationship Models

Accessing her loss and grief feelings in Narrative Therapy provided Juanita with more clarity about the emotional context in which her models of relationships were developed. Based on her experiences, Juanita had learned to expect that people she trusted would use or abandon her, and that expressing her needs would ultimately lead to loss of relationships. In order to cope with these contingencies, Juanita had learned to be extremely guarded and to maintain a façade of independence and self-sufficiency. Though this strategy had once served an adaptive function, it was no longer useful, as evidenced by her ongoing PTSD symptoms, depression, and isolation.

Juanita's therapist worked with her to identify the benefits and costs of this method of self-protection that had become so ingrained. Through continued use of both Relationship Patterns Worksheets, she could observe concretely how at present these models, rather than sparing her emotional pain, actually perpetuated her feelings of disappointment/abandonment and confirmed her belief that others could never fill the void created by earlier losses. Though she did not give others much opportunity and sent strong signals for others to keep their distance, she still often felt abandoned by others and believed that they should figure out what she was really needing or wanting. The therapist was also able to work with Juanita on noticing how her assumptions about others were based on the past and not necessarily applicable to some of her current relationships. She began to consider the idea that rather than driving others away or setting herself up for hurt, being more open and less guarded could actually result in others' feeling more connected and interested in her.

Conduct Role Play

An opportunity soon became available for Juanita to experiment with an alternative way of interacting. One consequence of Juanita's taking more social risks was that she began getting more invitations. When a long-time acquaintance, Ben, asked her out on a date, Juanita was taken off guard. She told him she would get back to him, but then avoided contacting him and stopped going to places they both frequented. She reported feeling guilty and "like a coward."

Using a copy of Relationship Patterns Worksheet–2 (see Box 25.2), Juanita and her therapist were able to break down and examine her beliefs and expectations of the situation that were driving her avoidance behavior. Juanita said that she was interested in Ben, but felt she could not afford to risk being hurt: "He thinks he wants to get to know me better, but what if he does and then decides he doesn't like me?" In addition to prematurely preparing for a negative outcome, Juanita was also assuming that if things did not work out, she would be unable to handle it. Juanita's automatic beliefs about Ben were that he probably did not know many other single women and was really just desperate.

When asked about her interpersonal goals, Juanita identified her desire to break her cycle of avoidance and stop basing her behavior on negative expectations from the past. Juanita agreed that if nothing else, the situation with Ben could be a good practice opportunity. When asked about her alternative beliefs, she said she could believe it possible to take the risk to go out on a date and potentially get to know someone. She could also try to trust that if it did not work out, she would be able to cope. Juanita and her therapist discussed how this potential "loss" would be different from past losses, given that she was now an adult with coping skills who did not need to rely on others to take care of her. In terms of Ben's intentions, Juanita felt she could believe that he was not out to use her, but that maybe he was interested in actually getting to know her. Juanita and her therapist did some role playing of a scenario in which Juanita called Ben, expressed an interest in a date, and offered an apology for not getting back to him sooner. Also, the therapist and Juanita agreed that it would be important for her to determine the parameters that were comfortable for her, and to take it slowly by keeping the date brief and casual.

This example shows the importance of encouraging a client toward new behaviors in seemingly safe situations, while keeping in mind that other people's responses are not in the client's control. In this case, Juanita's alternative belief that she could handle it even if things did not work out kept the emphasis on her own role in the interaction. Luckily, Juanita's willingness to take this work outside of the session resulted in her getting positive feedback from Ben. Thus, as Juanita was in the process of mourning past losses, she was also simultaneously building more opportunities for intimacy in the present. These therapeutic

BOX 25.2

Juanita's Completed Relationship Patterns Worksheet-2

Interpersonal situation	What did I feel and think about myself?		What were my expectations about the other person?		My resulting behavior
What happened?	**My feelings**	**My thoughts**	**Their feelings**	**Their thoughts**	**What did I do?**
I was asked out on a date by Ben, someone I have known for a very long time.	I am really scared.	Why would he want to be with me? I want to say no. I couldn't take it if I connected with him and then he rejected me.	He probably feels sorry for me (pity).	He doesn't really have any other options right now, so he might as well go out with me.	Avoided giving him an answer, stopped going to places he might be. Felt like a coward.

Relationship model: "If _I open up to him_____, then _he will reject me_____."

Interpersonal goals for situation	Alternative beliefs and feelings about myself: What else could I . . .		Alternative beliefs and feelings about the other person: What else could I expect the other person . . .		Alternative actions
What are my goals in this situation?	**. . . feel about myself?**	**. . . think about myself?**	**. . . to feel?**	**. . . to think?**	**What else could I do? What else might they do?**
To take more social risks and try to develop relationships with people. To make an active decision rather than just avoid. Not to base decision on fear or negative expectations.	I am capable of taking the risk to get to know someone. If it does not work out, I will be able to handle it.	I am a different person than I was in the past. I now have coping skills and resources.	He may be interested in actually getting to know me.	He may not be out to use me.	Agree to go on date, but keep it casual and brief.

Alternative relationship model: "If _I take a risk to get to know him_, then _he will be interested in getting to know me_____."

activities reinforced each other and provided the needed momentum for continued progress in treatment.

PROVIDE SUPPORT: SHARE THE BURDEN OF PAIN

The therapist's role is to offer a consistent source of containment, support, and empathy while the client elaborates on loss experiences and begins mourning. This involves reminding the client that they do not have to bear their pain alone, and identifying ways they can keep this in mind between sessions (e.g., letting other trusted people in their life know what is going on; reading something written in the clinician's handwriting; or keeping a symbolic token from the therapist with them, such as a paperweight or stone). This also involves reminding the client of coping strategies they have learned earlier in the treatment (e.g., distress tolerance) to deal with intense feelings that may arise.

SUMMARIZE THE GOALS OF THE SESSION

As in previous sessions, the therapist briefly summarizes the session goals at the end, and how they fit within the larger treatment goals for the specific client. These include helping the client to identify and process feelings of sadness associated with their interpersonal trauma history, and to understand how their losses may continue to impact current relationships. The therapist checks in with the client to see how they are feeling about completing their narrative(s). The therapist also acknowledges the courageous work done by the client in this session around facing grief, which will ultimately allow them to be more present and connected to others. The therapist reiterates the importance of listening to the trauma narrative recording between sessions, and if needed, again briefly reviews the rationale for it.

PLAN SKILLS PRACTICE

As in other Narrative Therapy sessions, the client is directed to listen to the recording of the latest narrative daily during the week and to monitor stress with the Subjective Units of Distress (SUDs) during Trauma Narration form (Handout 22.1). This time the client will focus on recognizing relationship models of loss as they come up in the narrative. The therapist and client have already identified and begun work on revising these models through the role plays; they can now determine how the client can build on this work in interpersonal interactions outside of treatment, using copies of Relationship Patterns Worksheet–2 (Handout 16.4) to record the results. Practice of Focused Breathing twice a day continues, as well as practice of emotion regulation skills, with specific exercises being based on the individual client's needs and circumstances.

The Final Session

Freedom is what you do with what's been done to you.
—Jean-Paul Sartre (quoted by Steinem, 1992, p. 63)

The goals of the final session are to summarize and reflect on the client's progress, identify relapse risks and associated recovery strategies, and plan for the client's next steps in their journey. Above all, the therapist gives recognition to the survivor for their accomplishments in the treatment, and conveys a sincere appreciation for the courage and strength that this work has involved. The therapist spends time reflecting beforehand and adapts the session contents and time spent on each domain to the needs of the particular client. Some clients will be well prepared for this final session; others will feel very anxious and may even experience reactivated fears of abandonment. Some clients will prefer to spend time reflecting on the process of therapy and will be prepared to articulate their feelings; others will want to focus on the future in general and on what comes next after weekly therapy ends in particular. The therapist's ability to respond openly to whatever the client needs to discuss in this final session models a compassionate and flexible attitude that can be healing for the client, no matter what they bring to the process of ending the treatment. Box 26.1 outlines the core content of this session (with corresponding flexibility to adapt to the client's needs).

CHECK-IN AND REVIEW OF SKILLS PRACTICE

Even though this session marks the final session of STAIR Narrative Therapy, it begins as others do: with a brief check-in about the client's current emotional state, followed by a review of the client's between-session practice. The agreed-upon practice from the previous session included emotion regulation and interpersonal skills relevant to the client's goals and needs, as well as the client's ongoing review of their trauma narrative and related themes. The therapist begins by briefly reviewing whether the client completed all of the planned

BOX 26.1

Theme and Curriculum for Session 18
The Final Session

The goals of the final session are to summarize the client's progress, identify any relapse risks and highlight relevant coping skills for risk management and recovery, and plan next steps for the client's ongoing recovery. Most importantly, the therapist gives recognition to the client for their specific accomplishments and shows sincere appreciation of the courage and strength that this work has involved.

PLANNING AND PREPARATION

Create a summary of the client's progress. Create list of resources for next steps and relapse recovery. Bring a copy each of Handout 26.1 and 19.3, along with copies of additional handouts as needed (see list below). This session is 60 minutes in duration.

AGENDA

- Check-in and review of skills practice.
- Identify focus of the session.
- Reflect on client's change and progress.
- Prepare and plan for client's independent skills maintenance.
- Identify plans for next steps.
- Review relapse risk and associated management/recovery strategies.
- Indicate respect for pace of change and role of ongoing self-compassion.
- Provide resources for transition and future needs.
- Present completion certificate.
- Say good-bye.

SESSION HANDOUTS

Handout 26.1. Summary of Accomplishments

Handout 19.3. STAIR Skills for Continued Practice

Individualized resource list (to be compiled by therapist)

Additional copies of Handout 11.3. Feelings Monitoring Form and/or Handout 16.4. Relationship Patterns Worksheet–2, if desired by or helpful for client work, asking for a brief summary of how the practice went, and offering to answer any questions that may have arisen since the last session. Reviewing changes in SUDs scores from the trauma narrative practice can be done briefly, as a broader discussion of overall progress in treatment (of which SUDs and other markers of change are reflections) will take place later in this session.

IDENTIFY FOCUS OF THE SESSION

Because this session is the final session of Narrative Therapy and of the STAIR Narrative Therapy program as a whole, the session serves to integrate themes from all previous sessions, with a particular focus on the narrative work that has just been completed. The importance of compassion is reintroduced to mark this important transition; this topic plays a part similar to the role it played in the final session of the STAIR module. The main goal is to reflect on and appreciate the client's accomplishments and to prepare them for continued independent work after ending treatment.

REFLECT ON CLIENT'S CHANGE AND PROGRESS

Among the most important tasks of the final session are to identify the progress the client has made and to give positive recognition of this progress to the client. The client, of course, will have their own ideas about which aspects of the work they are most proud of and most satisfied with, and the therapist elicits these appraisals. As needed, the therapist can prompt the client to consider changes in their symptoms, emotion regulation skills, interpersonal functioning, general life functioning, and experience of self since the beginning of treatment, as well as to compare the client's overall past and present states.

Typically, the client has done more work and has changed more than they are able to see and experience. The therapist, as an observer, has had the benefit of a different vantage point and thus may be able to identify further accomplishments, or to elaborate on and give depth to the changes the client has identified. To accommodate this common pattern, it is especially helpful for the therapist to prepare beforehand in reviewing the client's progress over the course of treatment, including reviewing therapy notes, the client's problems and goals, and the results of any formal symptom assessments over time.

Creating a summary of accomplishments can be especially helpful, because (as mentioned in Chapter 19 in connection with the end of the STAIR module) clients with a history of trauma tend to diminish their gains (at least partially) and to focus on their shortcomings and limitations. As at the end of STAIR, the therapist organizes such a summary of accomplishments to highlight where the client first started and how far they have come. If time allows and the client has completed assessments regularly in treatment, graphing the scores across the course of treatment can provide a nice visual summary to use in session with the client. For clients who have completed both key components of this intervention (the STAIR and Narrative Therapy modules), this conversation can also consider how the individual responded to each of these modules. The therapist can use the review of data to refresh the client's memories of important events and changes, and add observations about changes that the client may have forgotten or overlooked.

For any client who has completed Narrative Therapy, Handout 26.1, Summary of Accomplishments, can help guide the conversation and even give the client something to bring home and use as a reminder in future times of distress and moments of reflection. Below are recommendations of how to have this type of conversation and how to guide it to the specific treatment targets of the STAIR and Narrative Therapy modules. The nature of the conversation and amount of time spent on each domain with any given client will depend on the specific client's personal goals and course of treatment.

Note Decreases in Severity of PTSD/CPTSD Symptoms

By the end of this treatment, pronounced changes are likely to have occurred in the frequency and severity of PTSD/CPTSD symptoms. If completing a measure of these symptoms has not already been a routine practice during sessions, it is useful in the week preceding or at the beginning of the final session to have the client fill out a symptom questionnaire identical to the one completed during the initial assessment. The client may have forgotten the significant distress they were experiencing when they entered treatment; if so, they are likely to discount the amount of symptom reduction there has been. A comparison of the total PTSD/CPTSD scores before and after treatment is an effective way to summarize and demonstrate this change.

Reflect on Improved Emotion Regulation Skills

The therapist elicits, and participates with the client in, an enumeration of the improvements the client has experienced in emotion regulation and emotional experiencing. Changes in emotional experiencing to discuss include the following:

- General acceptance of emotions as normal and as containers of information.
- Ability to face fear and anxiety.
- Ability to manage angry feelings with specific skills.
- Ability to tolerate sadness and reduce the amount of time spent in a depressed state.
- Reductions in dissociative experiencing (less spacing out, derealization, and depersonalization).

Note Changes in Interpersonal Skills

Changes in interpersonal functioning are often best reviewed by referring to experiential exercises or other specific skills practices that were successfully completed. It is unrealistic to believe that interpersonal functioning can be entirely transformed within just a few months; such behaviors are strongly ingrained habits. However, the therapy has provided three important interventions that will help the client maintain and continue the change process. These interventions align with the "triple A's" of awareness, alternatives, and actions that have been explored across different interpersonal themes and types of relationships.

1. *Awareness* of interpersonal patterns is the first step in changing behavior. Interpersonal patterns of behavior have been clearly identified. They are no longer automatic behaviors, out of the client's awareness. The client has learned that with awareness comes the opportunity to intervene and choose alternative ways of thinking and alternative behaviors. Sometimes the insights may occur "post hoc" after particularly triggering interpersonal encounters, but with continued practice, the client will gain more and more control in the moment.

2. *Alternatives* to interpersonal patterns from the past have been formulated. The client has begun developing alternative templates for ways of thinking about relationships in the form of more adaptive interpersonal models ("If . . . , then . . ."). These new templates can guide the client in analyzing difficult situations, identifying interpersonal goals, and organizing alternative behaviors to reach these goals well beyond the end of treatment.

3. *Actions* have demonstrated the client's capacity for change. The client has developed and successfully practiced alternative behaviors. These new behaviors provide building blocks for new situations as they emerge. They have also demonstrated the client's capacity for genuine change, which might have seemed impossible before treatment. Knowledge of this capacity gives the client confidence in experimenting with new behaviors and seeking out new people. The world opens up in exciting ways when a person realizes they possess a sense of agency and choice, independent of the fears and perceived constraints that have previously held them back in life.

Reflect on Client's New Experience of Self

Moving from more concrete treatment targets, the conversation can expand to the more abstract but no less important target of improving the client's sense of self. The therapist elicits from and explores with the client their subjective experiences during each component of the treatment. How did the client feel about themselves during the STAIR module? What about during the Narrative Therapy module? Were there times when they felt the treatment was just right for them and resonated with their goals? Were there times when they disliked the treatment, or felt alienated from the tasks, methods, or goals? How did they experience each of the components as a change or growth experience? Each of these questions elicit reflections on the client's experience, likes, dislikes, personal values, and independent perspective—all of which reinforce a stronger, more integrated sense of self. The therapist's nonjudgmental, open stance during this conversation allows the client to be simply who they are. That alone may be a new experience different from how their caregivers or significant others have treated them in the past.

The STAIR module's interventions have provided the client with tools for behaving, thinking, and feeling in more positive and competent ways. As such, this module has laid the groundwork for the possibility of continued positive change. In contrast, the Narrative Therapy module has required going back to the past and telling about events in the distant past with emotional depth and intensity. The process has returned the client to a traumatic early life history and led to the recognition of the far-reaching influence these formative experiences have had on the trajectory of their life. Together, the two components of treatment have helped the client integrate the past with the present and with a sense of the future, giving the client a sense of a coherent self that was not possible before.

Honestly grappling with the pain, shame, and loss generated by these experiences deepens a person's inner emotional life. Recognizing and experiencing a gamut of feelings, and surviving them, lead to renewed emotional strength. Increased capacity for openness in emotional experiencing also provides the opportunity for authentic connection with others. These connections are supported by the very necessary skills of self-management and social competence that have been in practice throughout the treatment. In this way, the STAIR and Narrative Therapy components of treatment are necessary, complementary partners for a truly comprehensive recovery process. The client who reaches this final session has completed both parts of the treatment, so they are well prepared to continue to use these skills to express who they are and who they hope to become as they move forward in their life.

Congratulate the Client on Progress

After reviewing all relevant data and reflecting on the course of treatment, the therapist congratulates the client on their hard work and accomplishments, including any positive experiences outside of sessions. The therapist can include any additional observations of change that they have wanted to share but might not have had the opportunity to share before now. Either in the previous conversation or at this point in the session, the therapist can highlight specific, memorable moments of success from the client's treatment, even if they have already provided positive feedback on the example in previous sessions (which may have occurred several weeks prior to this final session).

PREPARE AND PLAN FOR CLIENT'S INDEPENDENT SKILLS MAINTENANCE

Some clients may have entered this treatment expecting therapy to be something done to them, passively accepted, then completed, and finally left to the past. STAIR Narrative Therapy, however, has introduced these clients to a more active and collaborative role in therapy and in making major life changes. This sense of motivation, engagement, and responsibility is crucial to maintain for success in sustaining and expanding the gains made in therapy. A therapist and client will both benefit from openly discussing how the client can continue to make progress without the therapist's presence or the sessions that provided structure for the initial skill acquisition. The client may share some concerns about how to do all this independently, and the therapist works to normalize some of this anxiety, while also reinforcing the client's sense of ownership for what they have accomplished. The therapist can remind the client of specific examples of the client's use of skills during difficult moments, and/or of successes that occurred because of the client's actions outside the therapy room.

Which skills are practiced independently after treatment will differ from person to person. The client is ultimately the primary creator of the plan, with guidance from the therapist as needed. In many cases, continuing to work on emotion regulation and communication skills will be a core component of the plan. As in Session 10 of STAIR, Handout 19.3, STAIR Skills for Continued Practice, provides good guidance to selecting skills across the three channels of emotion, as well as the interpersonal skill domains. Some clients may also prefer to use the structure of the Feelings Monitoring Form (Handout 11.3) or Relationship Patterns Worksheet–2 (Handout 16.4) to reflect on their experience. For these clients, the therapist can provide extra copies of the requested worksheets. Any additional psychoeducational handouts or copies of worksheets given by the therapist to the client also support the idea that the work is not over. In other words, this transition marks primarily the move to independent practice and skills maintenance, and not the abandonment of lessons learned with the therapist's help.

IDENTIFY PLANS FOR NEXT STEPS

There will inevitably be many tasks and areas of growth remaining for the survivor of trauma as they move out of this treatment. The client and therapist identify the client's goals during this transition and for the near future. These goals can include emotional and interpersonal goals, such as "being kinder to myself when I make mistakes" or "being more assertive with my friends about plans for what I like to do." They may also include specific ways to apply insights made during the trauma narrative work. For each kind of goal, it is useful to clarify which skills or resources the client has that will allow them to reach these goals and maintain progress as it is made. The therapist and client can take some time to jot down these goals and potential strategies for reaching them (see the second page of Handout 19.3). During periods of depression or demoralization, the client may forget the goals they have set for themselves and may not recall that they do have the basic capacity and knowledge to tackle new challenges. Handout 19.3 can serve as a reminder and morale booster during such periods.

In addition, the client may have concerns about dealing with the exacerbation and management of symptoms—particularly PTSD or depression symptoms; feelings of anger, anxiety and sadness; and dissociative phenomena. Here again, the therapist and client review which skills they have learned work best to help the client navigate these difficulties.

REVIEW RELAPSE RISK AND ASSOCIATED MANAGEMENT/ RECOVERY STRATEGIES

It is inevitable that the client will experience additional stressful life events in the future. It is therefore useful to identify any such events that seem likely, particularly those situations the client is fearful of managing. Examples include confronting the perpetrator of interpersonal trauma, disclosing the experience of this trauma to friends or family members, becoming a parent, or making a relationship commitment. Again, written guidelines for effective management of these stressors are useful to create now, so that they will be available when the client needs them but may be less able to formulate them effectively. The spaces on the second page of Handout 19.3 for outlining goals and skills to meet the goals can also be used to outline specific plans related to these ongoing or potential future stressors.

Other practical preparations for managing setbacks can be made ahead of time. These preparations may include keeping medication prescriptions up to date or checking regularly with a physician, and identifying which friends are best at helping with which type of crisis and reaching out for help accordingly.

The therapist articulates general principles for coping with setbacks. First, the client can accept and remember that relapses into old behaviors and symptom exacerbations are inevitable and manageable; they are not signs of failure. A second general guideline is for the client to avoid putting energy into self-criticism, languishing in humiliation, or viewing any relapse into old patterns as meaning that all progress is lost. The therapist encourages the client to adopt a healthy, compassionate response to any relapse, and immediately to begin (or prepare to begin) a plan to recover from any effects of the relapse. The client can remind themselves that they have accomplished many things in therapy, and that these successes demonstrate their capacity to manage difficult and emotionally demanding situations. If they were successful in making healthy changes in the past, then they can succeed at this again!

INDICATE RESPECT FOR PACE OF CHANGE AND ROLE OF ONGOING SELF-COMPASSION

A client may feel unsure of their readiness to continue their recovery without the structure of weekly therapy or without the therapist's presence. The therapist can convey that this anxiety is natural and understandable. After all, the client's experience of success—sometimes the first such experience they have had with their symptoms—has occurred in the context of treatment with a therapist. Often the therapist can effectively respond to a client's anxiety about making the transition out of therapy by repeating the many successes that the client has achieved. The therapist has supported the client's achievements, but the client has done the real work of putting to practice in the "real world" the skills they have learned in the therapy room.

A particularly skeptical client may respond to the therapist's sharing a summary of interview feedback with clients who participated in STAIR or STAIR Narrative Therapy programs as part of one of the published research studies (e.g., Cloitre et al., 2010). These data indicate that after treatment ends, clients continue to improve even further—generalizing the gains they have made as they encounter new opportunities to master their skills and put these into practice. Introducing the data should not distract from the client's emotional experience, so the therapist works primarily to ensure that the client feels sufficiently satisfied to go forth in the world and try their new skills independently. They can be their own scientist and let their experience speak for itself, adapt to what arises for them, and reach out for support if needed.

For some clients, especially those with multiple traumas, the work accomplished during the therapy may seem like a "drop in the bucket." Such a client and their therapist can concretely evaluate outstanding problem areas. If the opportunity exists in the clinical setting to extend treatment and the client is willing to do so, this option may be considered. One approach within this option may be to titrate the frequency of sessions over time to encourage greater levels of independence. For example, the therapist may see the client again in 2 weeks, then again in 3 weeks, then again after a month, and so on until the client feels comfortable about the transition. This approach has the added benefit of paralleling the development of a more secure attachment: Such an attachment allows independence and exploration of the world, without the need to be near the attachment figure at all times. Throughout this treatment, the client has likely internalized the therapist as a secure base; with this gradual transition, the client can learn to rely more and more on the internalized therapist even when contact with the therapist lessens in frequency. This process is a key one for the ending of more intense therapies like STAIR Narrative Therapy. Alternatively, the therapist may be able to make recommendations for continuing treatment in a program or modality that best suits the client at this point in their recovery.

Handout 19.1, Compassion: Recovery Is a Journey, is a helpful handout to review in this session. Completing the Self-Compassion Meditation again in session may also be beneficial to the client, but the therapist uses their clinical judgment and discusses collaboratively whether this practice would be helpful for the particular client. Encouraging the client to continue their practice and exploration of compassion is an important aspect of starting the client on the independent journey toward continued growth and recovery.

PROVIDE RESOURCES FOR TRANSITION AND FUTURE NEEDS

The therapist provides a list of local services or programs that the client may find to be useful resources in the transition or in the near future. This list can include information about programs related to the client's identified goals or continued recovery needs, such as Twelve-Step groups, legal services, employment skills training programs, or other community services. It can also include basic resources, such as telephone numbers for the client's local emergency room, domestic violence bureau, or crisis hotline.

For many clients, a reminder of the skills learned can be especially helpful. For clients with smartphones, STAIR Emotion Coach is a free app available on iOS and Android that lets people practice skills "on demand" in the moment and on the go (see Chapter 27 for a fuller description). This resource may be most beneficial for clients who are already familiar with STAIR skills and thus do not need a therapist to review the skills and how to use them.

PRESENT COMPLETION CERTIFICATE

Many clients appreciate receiving an official completion certificate as a concrete symbol of their hard work and accomplishments. This certificate may also act as a reminder in the future for when they need to refocus on their personal goals, skills, and well-being. In the last moments of the session, the therapist can provide such a certificate and congratulate the client one last time. As we have noted at the end of Option 2 in Chapter 19, some clients like the idea of "graduating" from treatment, but others may prefer to view this transition as the beginning of a new stage of treatment—one in which they act as their own therapists and make further use in their lives of the many skills they have learned in their initial work. Either way, this moment is a meaningful one, so the therapist shows respect for the emotional importance it likely holds for the client.

SAY GOOD-BYE

Throughout this session, the therapist has had opportunities to summarize their appreciation of the client's hard work. If anything has been left unsaid, the therapist can communicate these messages in the final moments of the session when saying good-bye. They generally extend a message of hope and good wishes for the client's next steps.

The issue of future contact with the therapist is likely to be brought forward by the client at some point. If it is not, the therapist can address this issue here or earlier in the session (as relevant), since most clients do wonder about contact after therapy has ended (even if they do not verbalize this question). There is no "right" decision in this situation. It depends on many factors, including the nature of the treatment setting, the client's needs and preferences, and the therapist's own guidelines in their work and their own personal and professional boundaries. The discussion is guided, however, by the therapist's awareness that the client has shared some of the most intimate details of their life. The therapist has borne witness to this history and is also now a guardian of it. Therefore, whatever the particulars of the ensuing discussion, it is important for the therapist to express respect for the client's history, appreciation for having learned about their life, and gratitude for having had the opportunity to learn from them.

After saying their final words, the client and therapist may shake hands, hug, wave good-bye, or smile as they part ways. Once again, the decision about how to proceed depends on both the therapist's and the client's personal boundaries, cultural expectations, ethics, and needs. No matter what makes sense for the two parties involved, the moment offers a sense of warmth, conclusion, and pride in what has been accomplished. Congratulations are in order for both!

Summary of Accomplishments

Let's review all the things you've learned and accomplished during this treatment!

- We discussed how trauma affects emotion and how it affected you.

> *Before STAIR, how did you experience your emotions?*

- We then explored skills that could change how you coped with your emotions. Later today, we'll select the skills from the three channels of emotion (body, thought, behavior) that you want to continue practicing. For now, consider:

> *What are ways you're experiencing your emotions differently from before starting treatment?*

- We also explored how trauma affects relationships, and we identified different ways to approach and manage relationships—with flexibility, assertiveness, power, intimacy, and compassion.

> *What are ways you're approaching relationships differently in what you believe, feel, and do?*

(continued)

Summary of Accomplishments *(page 2 of 2)*

- In the last series of sessions, we explored your traumatic memories and ways to create new meanings from them, while also exploring themes of fear, shame, and loss.

What are ways you're viewing your traumatic memories/experiences, and yourself, differently? How are these changes influencing what you believe, feel, and do?

- As you prepare to move on to the next chapter of your life and recovery, let's reflect on the progress you've made.

What are the most important lessons you've learned?	
What lessons felt most helpful?	
How have your thoughts, emotions, and behaviors changed?	
How have you changed your relationship with your traumatic memories and experiences?	
How will you continue to build on the progress you've made so far?	

CHAPTER 27

New Developments for STAIR Narrative Therapy

> Adaptability enforces creativity,
> and creativity is adaptability.
> —PEARL ZHU (2016)

Since the first edition of this book was published, we have adapted STAIR Narrative Therapy for use with different client populations, clinical settings, and delivery modalities. These adaptations have often been the results of requests by clinicians or community leaders who have identified the potential benefits of the STAIR interventions for their specific client populations, services, or communities. STAIR, in particular, has been popular because its focus on skills training differs from those of various other trauma-focused treatments. We view this interest from other professionals as reflecting a broader recognition of the importance of emotion regulation and relational capacities in daily life and in trauma recovery. In this new chapter, we briefly review current adaptations of STAIR and describe how they fit within the larger framework of mental health care service delivery. We also share published research related to each adaptation when such research is available. Box 27.1 provides an overview and summary of these adaptations.

CLINICAL TREATMENT ADAPTATIONS

The specific clinical adaptations of STAIR Narrative Therapy have evolved from a broadened understanding of different delivery models and different client populations that can benefit from specific areas of focus. The adaptations discussed here are examples of programs that have matured past the initial development and brainstorming phases, with many having supporting data.

Adaptations and Extensions of STAIR

Specific Adaptation	Length	Format	Target Population	Intervention Focus
Group STAIR	12 sessions	Group	Adults with PTSD and/or depression	Emotion regulation and interpersonal skills
STAIR-A	Variable (three 90-minute modules vs. 16 sessions)	Group or individual	Adolescents with PTSD and/or depression	Emotion regulation and interpersonal skills, with or without written trauma narrative homework
STAIR-PC	5 sessions	Individual	Adults with PTSD or depression	Emotion regulation and social support skills individualized to personal goals
STAIR-R	5 sessions	Individual	Refugees with PTSD or depression	Emotion regulation and social support skills individualized to personal goals
Parenting STAIR	5+ sessions (usually 5–8)	Individual, family (parents only), or group	Parents who have children at home and have completed STAIR	Parenting skills in teaching emotion regulation and good communication to children
STAIR Emotion Coach	Variable (user choice)	Self-guided	Clients who are currently in STAIR and/or have completed the intervention	A mobile app (Apple iOS and Android) that offers guided tools, symptom and goal tracking, and brief psychoeducation
webSTAIR with coaching	10 online interactive lessons + 5–10 coaching sessions	Self-guided + coach support	Adults with subthreshold to mild PTSD or depression symptoms	An online web-based therapy program with guided psychoeducation and skills exercises
Telehealth delivery	Variable (depending on version of STAIR Narrative Therapy)	Individual or group	Clients with mental health treatment access issues (distance, mobility, etc.)	Variable (depending on version of STAIR Narrative Therapy)

Group STAIR

Perhaps the most often requested adaptation for STAIR has been a group version. Group STAIR (Cloitre et al., 2019) is a 12-session version of the skills training module and follows the session work as outlined in Chapters 10–19 of this book, with two important exceptions. First, the group program introduces and organizes the emotion regulation skills within the "three channels of emotion" framework one channel at a time, instead of combining the thought and behavior channels; it thus divides individual STAIR's Session 4 into the third and fourth group sessions. This change helps with the conceptual organization of the program and allows more time and attention for the individuals in the group to generate examples of situations and engage in skills practice. Second, an additional introductory session for the interpersonal work expands the concept of changing relationship patterns before diving into the specific relational themes of assertiveness, power, and intimacy/closeness. This session introduces the idea of healthy boundaries, which individual STAIR explores in Session 9 (see Chapter 18).

There are several benefits to delivering STAIR in a group format. First, it can increase access to care by allowing a greater number of clients to engage in treatment and reduce the wait time for limited numbers of individual therapy time slots. In addition, group delivery requires only one or two trained therapists to serve 3–10 clients. These two benefits can save a great deal of clinical and system time and costs. Beyond the pragmatic aspects of group delivery, this format also allows important group processes to emerge that provide fertile ground for experiential learning of interpersonal communication skills and boundary setting. Learning occurs not only through the process of group therapy; it also occurs in more explicit ways. For example, group members can participate in role-playing scenarios; can learn from other members' experiences, perspectives, and practices; and can brainstorm together how to approach different socioemotional situations with their new skills. If the therapist(s) can establish group safety and cohesion (a necessary and occasionally complex task), the group experience can enliven the work of STAIR in impressive ways. Some clinics have broken down the STAIR work into two groups, one for the emotion regulation skills training (six sessions) and the other for the interpersonal skills training (six sessions). The limited number of sessions seems to support commitment to and completion of the groups. Clients also like having the option of either repeating the emotion regulation skills group as needed or "graduating" to the interpersonal skills group.

As expected, Group STAIR does not include a Narrative Therapy component, due to the highly individualized nature of this kind of intervention and the risk of distress resulting from exposure to other group members' trauma accounts. We recommend individual therapy for the narrative work, which can occur concurrently with or after the group work, depending on each client's interests and abilities.

Three published studies have reported good outcomes associated with Group STAIR. The first study was a comparative trial of Group STAIR with a treatment-as-usual (TAU; supportive therapy) comparison group in an adult inpatient unit for individuals with treatment-resistant schizophrenia and schizoaffective disorders (Trappler & Newville, 2007). The participants in the study had diagnoses of both a psychotic disorder and PTSD.

Results indicated that compared to those in the supportive group, participants who received Group STAIR showed greater improvements in symptoms of PTSD and psychosis alongside increases in various outcomes related to emotion regulation, including fewer angry outbursts and less behavioral overactivation.

MacIntosh, Cloitre, Kortis, Peck, and Weiss (2018) completed an open trial evaluating both the implementation satisfaction and symptom outcome of Group STAIR in a community-based outpatient setting treating adult survivors of childhood sexual trauma. Of note, this trial included relatively limited training in STAIR delivery for study therapists—one workshop followed by weekly supervision of a local leader who had access to the trainer. The aim of the study was to evaluate the ease of integration of a structured, manualized treatment in a community setting. Pre–post treatment analyses indicated significant reductions in PTSD symptoms, emotion dysregulation, and interpersonal difficulties. Standardized interviews with study therapists indicated that they viewed the treatment as easy to deliver and relevant to their clients' needs; both of these views resolved their concerns about using a manualized treatment approach. Clients in the group expressed high satisfaction with the approach and a strong sense of validation in seeing how trauma had played a "huge role" in their day-to-day life functioning (MacIntosh et al., 2018, p. 599).

Similar findings emerged from a recent open-trial study in a Department of Veterans Affairs (VA) outpatient PTSD clinic serving veterans with various types of trauma, including military sexual trauma (Jackson, Weiss, & Cloitre, 2019). This study provided group treatment in a mixed-gender format, and to our knowledge was the first study to do so within the VA system. Results indicated significant decreases for veterans in PTSD symptoms. However, while both male and female veterans showed declines in general distress symptoms, these findings were significant only for the men in the group. This result may reflect the impact of being in a mixed-gender group, especially given the high incidence of military sexual trauma among women veterans. Despite the significant barriers women veterans face in the male-dominant VA health care setting, these results were encouraging about the option of offering mixed-gender STAIR groups.

STAIR for Adolescents

Because STAIR is a developmentally informed treatment, adapting it for the treatment of trauma-exposed adolescents has been a natural extension of the program. In a case–control study, STAIR for Adolescents (STAIR-A) was delivered to girls in a public high school serving a low-socioeconomic-status catchment area. The STAIR-A treatment group was compared to a control group that received assessments only and was matched by age, trauma exposure, and baseline symptoms (Gudiño, Leonard, & Cloitre, 2016). Results indicated that girls in STAIR-A experienced greater improvements in depression and management of social stress than did those in the assessment-only group. There was little change in PTSD scores across both groups. Baseline PTSD scores were relatively low, however, which may have resulted in "floor effects."

A second study evaluated the implementation of a weekly three-session STAIR-A program in an inpatient setting. To our knowledge, STAIR-A is the only trauma-informed treatment to be delivered and tested in an adolescent inpatient setting (Gudiño et al., 2014). Results indicated that at discharge the adolescents experienced a reduction in PTSD and depression symptoms, as well as greater self-efficacy in coping with life stressors.

STAIR for Primary Care

Over the years, models of mental health care have shifted away from ones focused on specialty care clinics separated from general medical care settings. These specialty clinics still have a place in larger models of care delivery, but the emphasis on primary care integration has expanded greatly. In response to this updated model, we have created a five-session version of STAIR for Primary Care (STAIR-PC), which focuses on emotion regulation skills development individualized to client's specific needs (Cloitre, Ortigo, & Gupta, 2018c). A randomized controlled trial (RCT) evaluated STAIR-PC as compared to TAU among veterans with a positive screen for PTSD or depression in a VA primary care clinic (Cloitre, Gimeno, Ortigo, Weiss, & Jain, 2018a). The treatment was delivered in person and by a mix of providers, including psychology technicians (including trained peers), mental health trainees, and professionals (social workers and psychologists).

On the first visit, guided by a worksheet, therapists and veterans collaborated in identifying the symptoms or problems that would be the focus of the treatment (e.g., depression, posttraumatic stress, anxiety, insomnia, panic attacks, social isolation) and then matching skills to address these problems via STAIR's three channels of emotion. Sessions 2, 3, and 4 explored the body, thought, and behavior channels of emotion, with relevant skills chosen collaboratively by the therapist and the client. Session 4 also included optional behavioral skills related to interpersonal communication to expand the focus to relationships, if this was appropriate to the client's goals. The final session summarized skills learned and introduced the role of compassion as the client prepared for either independent practice or moving to a more intense treatment. A clinical psychologist (Dr. Kile M. Ortigo) provided weekly group supervision to study therapists, focused on succinct case conceptualization to aid the brief, efficient model of care and skills acquisition. Results indicated that compared to TAU, STAIR-PC provided greater reductions in PTSD symptoms, depression symptoms, emotion dysregulation, and social engagement problems; all gains were maintained at a 3-month follow-up. These study results suggest that a brief version of STAIR in coordination with good case conceptualization and an individualized treatment plan can have a positive impact on patients in settings where mental health issues are frequently seen, yet often insufficiently addressed.

STAIR for Refugees

Refugees experience substantial and chronic psychosocial stressors, many related to separation from family members and uncertain legal status, alongside high rates of trauma exposure. STAIR has accordingly been adapted for refugees and asylum seekers. In STAIR for Refugees (STAIR-R), the treatment focuses predominantly on emotion regulation skills to manage daily stressors, and on the development of social and communication skills to facilitate the resolution of challenging daily life difficulties and the expansion of social support networks. Typical problems refugees experience include (but are not limited to) uncertainty about asylum status, interactions with the local government, long-distance communication with family members remaining in their countries of origin, and challenges in finding employment and developing new occupational skills. The treatment has been adapted to and is respectful of specific cultural idioms and concepts, via a client narrative describing the ways in which clients can use STAIR in meaningful ways that are relevant and meaningful in their individual situations.

STAIR-R is currently being tested in a government-funded RCT in Australia, where STAIR-R plus Narrative Exposure Therapy (NET; Schauer, Neuner, & Elbert, 2011) is being compared to general problem-solving therapy with NET (Nickerson et al., 2016; Nickerson, Cloitre, & O'Donnell, 2018–2022).

Parenting STAIR

Parenting STAIR is designed specifically for survivors of trauma who have completed STAIR in some other format, but are still struggling with difficulties in their parent–child relationships (Cloitre & Makin-Byrd, 2018). Because parenting presents a unique set of challenges beyond caring for oneself, survivors who are also parents may feel overwhelmed by the responsibilities and emotional experiences inherent in nurturing and raising a child. Parenting can be especially problematic for survivors whose social competencies feel limited because of early life trauma or abuse. Bowlby (1969, 1984) identified attachment and caregiving as two separate but related behavioral systems, and the interventions in Parenting STAIR attend to concerns related to both the attachment and caregiving or skills training aspects of parenting. Parenting STAIR thus focuses on improving both the clients' parent–child relationships and their parenting skills in teaching children good emotion regulation via instruction, role modeling, and bonding activities with the children. The intervention is geared toward STAIR completers, because it builds upon on an earlier-established foundation of key concepts and tools learned through the core STAIR intervention. In addition, because the parenting role may be occupied by biological parents, adoptive parents, stepparents, or grandparents, the intervention deems any person in a parenting role as potentially appropriate. The program was developed with the support of the VA Women's Mental Health, Military Sexual Trauma Support, and Family Services teams, but it is applicable to parents in the general community as well.

TECHNOLOGICAL ADAPTATIONS

Alongside adaptations of the STAIR intervention to different formats, populations, and settings, efforts to utilize technology in the service of further broadening care delivery options for the intervention have shown great promise. Below, we describe a few recent examples of these efforts.

Telehealth Delivery

Delivery of treatment via telehealth is gaining new acceptance and use (Backhaus et al., 2012). An open trial of STAIR delivered to women veterans in their own homes via telehealth found the treatment both highly satisfactory and effective in reducing PTSD, depression, social engagement problems, and functional impairment (Weiss, Azevedo, Webb, Gimeno, & Cloitre, 2018). The study provided strong support for the adaptability of this treatment to a telehealth delivery model, which would benefit many individuals with various barriers to getting into in-person care.

STAIR Emotion Coach

Technology offers opportunities beyond traditional psychotherapeutic approaches, and from a public health standpoint, the creation of applications ("apps") for smartphones and tablets is one of the most promising new domains of exploration for mental health care. Apps give "users" (the field-appropriate term for anyone who downloads and uses apps) on-demand access to psychoeducation, interactive exercises, skills, and symptom tracking—and at least in the case of STAIR Emotion Coach, it can be free of charge and completely confidential. The original app, STAIR Coach, was developed for Apple devices (iOS) at the National Center for PTSD, where two of us (Dr. Marylene Cloitre and Dr. Kile Ortigo) work (Vigil Dombeck et al., 2017). This center focuses on technology innovations to serve veterans with PTSD, but because it is a federally funded research think tank, all products are free to the public regardless of veteran or military status.

STAIR Emotion Coach contains several features that allow individuals to track their PTSD symptoms, rate their emotional experiences (using a simplified Feelings Monitoring Form), and read brief psychoeducational materials in line with the STAIR philosophy of emotions and relationships. In addition, guided practice of skills such as Focused Breathing and "I Messages" provides hands-on experience with key STAIR interventions. The app is generally most useful for clients undergoing STAIR Narrative Therapy in any of its formats, but it is also available for interested people who want to learn more about the impact of trauma on emotional and interpersonal functioning. A new revision is currently underway and will be launched alongside an Android version to allow access to both Apple and Android users. This version will feature a guided learning plan for people to access parts of the app in small chunks, which aid learning and the systematic building of knowledge and skills. More information can be found at *https://mobile.va.gov/app/stair-coach*.

Web-Based STAIR

Resulting from another collaboration with the National Center for PTSD and the Office of Rural Health, a web-based version of STAIR has been developed and is currently being evaluated in a national program targeting primarily rural women veterans with a history of military sexual trauma. The full online program, called webSTAIR, consists of 10 core treatment lessons that largely coincide with the STAIR module as described in this book (see *www.webstair.org*, developed by Ortigo, Cloitre, Jackson, Weiss, & Schmidt, 2019). Each lesson is interactive and offers a mix of psychoeducation, guided skills practice, and tracking of the user's symptoms across time. A dashboard orients the user to unlocked skills for continued practice, worksheets and other resources, graphs for tracking progress, and an area for the user to enter messages. The program also incorporates elements of "gami-fication" (i.e., the use of behavioral reward models often seen in video games) to increase independent engagement, more consistent use, and ongoing skills practice. These elements are reflected visually in the awarding of digital achievements for meeting certain conditions (e.g., learning about all three channels of emotion) and in the "charging" of skills as the user practices each one multiple times over a period of time.

In the national webSTAIR evaluation project, trained mental health professionals serve as "coaches" in helping veterans stay engaged and apply the skills to their lives. The evaluation plan for the program includes quantitative interviews, online self-report measures, web usage data, and qualitative interviews with both coaches and veterans. Initial findings have been very promising in demonstrating the program's feasibility and effectiveness (Ortigo & Cloitre, 2018). A free version is planned for launching within a year of this book's publication, and it will feature the core course content for free without tracking user data to protect privacy.

FUTURE DIRECTIONS

The future is bright for the creative, theory-driven, and evidence-informed expansions of STAIR Narrative Therapy. Instead of a static or rigid model for treating childhood and relational trauma, STAIR Narrative Therapy's evolution reflects an ever-growing and improving approach to care for survivors of such trauma. Over the years since the first edition of this book appeared, we ourselves have evolved as trauma specialists, researchers, and therapists, and our expanding team of collaborators and approaches reflects this evolution. What will unfold in the next decade-plus of innovation is unknown, but the prospects are intriguing indeed!

References

Agosti, V., & Stewart, J. W. (1998). Social functioning and residual symptomatology among outpatients who responded to treatment and recovered from major depression. *Journal of Affective Disorders, 47,* 207–210.

Alaggia, R. (2002). Balancing acts: Reconceptualizing support in maternal response to intrafamilial child sexual abuse. *Clinical Social Work Journal, 30,* 41–56.

Allen, J. G. (1995). *Coping with trauma: A guide to self-understanding.* Washington, DC: American Psychiatric Press.

American Psychiatric Association. (2000). *Diagnostic and statistical manual of mental disorders* (4th ed., text rev.). Washington, DC: Author.

American Psychiatric Association. (2013). *Diagnostic and statistical manual of mental disorders* (5th ed.). Arlington, VA: Author.

Ammaniti, M., & Ferrari, P. (2013). Vitality affects in Daniel Stern's thinking—A psychological and neurobiological perspective. *Infant Mental Health Journal, 34*(5), 367–375.

Amstadter, A. B., Elwood, L. S., Begle, A. M., Gudmundsdottir, B., Smith, D. W., Resnick, H. S., et al. (2011). Predictors of physical assault victimization: Findings from the National Survey of Adolescents. *Addictive Behaviors, 36,* 814–820.

Andalibi, N., Haimson, O. L., De Choudhury, M., & Forte, A. (2016, May). Understanding social media disclosures of sexual abuse through the lenses of support seeking and anonymity. In *Proceedings of the 2016 CHI Conference on Human Factors in Computing Systems* (pp. 3906–3918). New York: Association for Computing Machinery.

Anderson, R. E., Edwards, L. J., Silver, K. E., & Johnson, D. M. (2018). Intergenerational transmission of child abuse: Predictors of child abuse potential among racially diverse women residing in domestic violence shelters. *Child Abuse and Neglect, 85,* 80–90.

Andrews, B., Brewin, C. R., Rose, S., & Kirk, M. (2000). Predicting post-traumatic stress disorder symptoms in victims of violent crime: The role of shame, anger and childhood abuse. *Journal of Abnormal Psychology, 109,* 69–73.

Backhaus, A., Agha, Z., Maglione, M. L., Repp, A., Ross, B., Zuest, D., et al. (2012). Videoconferencing psychotherapy: A systematic review. *Psychological Services, 9,* 111–131.

Baird, K., & Kracen, A. C. (2006). Vicarious traumatization and secondary traumatic stress: A research synthesis. *Counselling Psychology Quarterly, 19,* 181–188.

Baker, E. K. (2003). *Caring for ourselves: A therapist's guide to personal and professional well-being.* Washington, DC: American Psychological Association.

Bakermans-Kranenburg, M. J., & van IJzendoorn, M. H. (2009). The first 10,000 Adult Attachment Interviews: Distributions of adult attachment representations in clinical and non-clinical groups. *Attachment and Human Development, 11,* 223–263.

Barkham, M., Hardy, G. E., & Startup, M. (1996). The IIP-32: A short version of the Inventory of Interpersonal Problems. *British Journal of Clinical Psychology, 35,* 21–35.

Barlé, N., Wortman, C. B., & Latack, J. A. (2017). Traumatic bereavement: Basic research and clinical implications. *Journal of Psychotherapy Integration, 27*(2), 127–139.

Baumann, B. L., & Kolko, D. J. (2002). A comparison of

abusive and nonabusive mothers of abused children. *Child Maltreatment, 7*(4), 369–376.

Beckham, J. C., Roodman, A. A., Barefoot, J. C., Haney, T. L., Helms, M. J., Fairbank, J. A., et al. (1996). Interpersonal and self-reported hostility among combat veterans with and without posttraumatic stress disorder. *Journal of Traumatic Stress, 9*, 335–342.

Benjet, C., Bromet, E., Karam, E. G., Kessler, R. C., McLaughlin, K. A., Ruscio, A. M., et al. (2016). The epidemiology of traumatic event exposure worldwide: Results from the World Mental Health Survey Consortium. *Psycholological Medicine, 46*, 327–343.

Bennett, D. S., Sullivan, M. W., & Lewis, M. (2005). Young children's adjustment as a function of maltreatment, shame, and anger. *Child Maltreatment, 10*, 311–323.

Bisson, J. I., Brewin, C. R., Cloitre, M., & Maercker, A. (2020). PTSD and complex PTSD: Diagnosis, assessment and screening. In D. Forbes, D. C. Monson, L. Berliner, & J. I. Bisson (Eds.), *Effective treatments for PTSD: Practice guidelines from the International Society for Traumatic Stress Studies* (3rd ed.). New York: Guilford Press.

Bjureberg, J., Ljótsson, B., Tull, M. T., Hedman, E., Sahlin, H., Lundh, L. G., et al. (2016). Development and validation of a brief version of the Difficulties in Emotion Regulation Scale: The DERS-16. *Journal of Psychopathology and Behavioral Assessment, 38*, 284–296.

Blieberg, K. L. (2000). *The disclosure of childhood sexual abuse and post-traumatic stress disorder and related symptoms of cognitive and affective impairment*. Garden City, NY: Adelphi University.

Bloom, S. L., & Reichert, M. (1998). *Bearing witness: Violence and collective responsibility*. Binghamton, NY: Haworth Press.

Bonanno, G., Çolak, D., Keltner, D., Shiota, M. N., Papa, A., Noll, J. G., et al. (2007). Context matters: The benefits and costs of expressing positive emotion among survivors of childhood sexual abuse. *Emotion, 7*, 824–837.

Boudewyns, P. A., & Hyer, L. A. (1990). Physiological response to combat veterans and preliminary treatment outcome in Vietnam veteran posttraumatic stress disorder patients treated with direct therapeutic exposure. *Behavior Therapy, 21*, 63–87.

Bourne, E. J. (1999). *The anxiety and phobia workbook*. Oakland, CA: New Harbinger.

Bouton, M. E., & Swartzentruber, D. (1991). Sources of relapse after extinction in Pavlovian and instrumental learning. *Clinical Psychology Review, 11*, 123–140.

Bowers, M. E., & Yehuda, R. (2016). Intergenerational transmission of stress in humans. *Neuropsychopharmacology, 41*, 232–244.

Bowlby, J. (1969). *Attachment and loss: Vol. 1. Attachment*. New York: Basic Books.

Bowlby, J. (1984). Violence in the family as a disorder of the attachment and caregiving systems. *American Journal of Psychoanalysis, 44*, 9–27.

Bowlby, J. (1988). *A secure base: Clinical applications of attachment theory*. London and New York: Routledge.

Brewin, C. R. (2003). *Posttraumatic stress disorder: Malady or myth?* New Haven, CT: Yale University Press.

Brewin, C. R., Cloitre, M., Hyland, P., Shevlin, M., Maercker, A., Bryant, R. A., et al. (2017). A review of current evidence regarding the ICD-11 proposals for diagnosing PTSD and complex PTSD. *Clinical Psychology Review, 58*, 1–15.

Briere, J. (1992). *Child abuse trauma: Theory and treatment of the lasting effects*. Newbury Park, CA: SAGE.

Briere, J., & Rickards, S. (2007). Self-awareness, affect regulation, and relatedness: Differential sequels of childhood versus adult victimization experiences. *Journal of Nervous and Mental Disease, 195*, 497–503.

Briere, J., & Runtz, M. (1990). Differential adult symptomology associated with three types of child abuse histories. *Child Abuse and Neglect, 14*, 357–364.

Brodsky, B., Cloitre, M., & Dulit, R. (1995). The relationship of dissociation to self-mutilation and childhood abuse in borderline personality disorder. *American Journal of Psychiatry, 12*, 1788–1792.

Brown, B. (2010). *The gifts of imperfection: Let go of who you think you're supposed to be and embrace who you are*. Center City, MN: Hazelden.

Burroughs, A. R. (2003). *Dry: A memoir*. New York: St. Martin's Press.

Carey-Trefzer, C. J. (1949). The results of a clinical study of war-damaged children who attended the Child Guidance Clinic, the Hospital for Sick Children, Great Ormond Street, London. *Journal of Mental Science, 95*, 535–559.

Carliner, H., Gary, D., McLaughlin, K. A., & Keyes, K. M. (2017). Trauma exposure and externalizing disorders in adolescents: Results from the National Comorbidity Survey Adolescent Supplement. *Journal of the American Academy of Child Adolescent Psychiatry, 56*, 755–764.

Carlson, V., Cicchetti, D., Barnett, D., & Braunwald, K. (1989). Disorganized/disoriented attachment relationships in maltreated infants. *Developmental Psychology, 25*, 525–531.

Carson, R. C. (1969). *Interaction concepts of personality*. Chicago: Aldine.

Chaplin, T. C., Rice, M. E., & Harris, G. T. (1995). Salient victim suffering and the sexual responses of child molesters. *Journal of Consulting and Clinical Psychology, 63*, 249–255.

Chauhan, P., Schuck, A. M., & Widom, C. S. (2017). Child maltreatment, problem behaviors, and neighborhood attainment. *American Journal of Community Psychology, 60,* 555–567.

Chauhan, P., & Widom, C. S. (2012). Childhood maltreatment and illicit drug use in middle adulthood: The role of neighborhood characteristics. *Developmental Psychopathology, 24,* 723–738.

Chemtob, C. M., Novaco, R. W., Hamada, R. N., & Gross, D. (1997). Cognitive-behavioral treatment of severe anger in posttraumatic stress disorder. *Journal of Consulting and Cllinical Psychology, 65,* 184–189.

Cicchetti, D., & Toth, S. L. (2015). Child maltreatment. In M. E. Lamb (Vol. Ed.) & R. M. Lerner (Series Ed.), *Handbook of child psychology and developmental science: Vol. 3. Socioemotional processes* (7th ed., pp. 513–563). Hoboken, NJ: Wiley.

Cicchetti, D., & White, J. (1990). Emotion and developmental psychopathology. In L. N. L. Stein & T. Trabasso (Eds.), *Psychological approaches to emotion* (pp. 359–382). Hillsdale, NJ: Erlbaum.

Cloitre, M. (1998). Sexual revictimization: Risk factors and prevention. In V. M. Follette, J. I. Ruzek, & F. R. Abueg (Eds.), *Cognitive-behavioral therapies for trauma* (pp. 278–304). New York: Guilford Press.

Cloitre, M. (2015). The "one size fits all" approach to trauma treatment: should we be satisfied? *European Journal of Psychotraumatology, 6.*

Cloitre, M., Cohen, L. R., & Scarvalone, P. (2002a). Understanding revictimization among childhood sexual abuse survivors: An interpersonal schema approach. *Journal of Cognitive Psychotherapy: An International Quarterly, 16,* 91–111.

Cloitre, M., Garvert, D. W., Brewin, C. R., Bryant, R. A., & Maercker, A. (2013, May). Evidence for proposed ICD-11 PTSD and complex PTSD: A latent profile analysis. *European Journal of Psychotraumatology, 4.*

Cloitre, M., Gimeno, J., Ortigo, K. M., Weiss, B., & Jain, S. (2018a, November). STAIR as a stand-alone treatment: Results from a randomized controlled trial. In C. Rosen (Chair), *What if we don't talk about trauma?: Evidence-based alternatives to trauma-focused psychotherapy.* Symposium conducted at the annual conference of the International Society of Traumatic Stress Studies, Washington, DC.

Cloitre, M., Khan, C., Mackintosh, M. A., Garvert, D. W., Henn-Haase, C. M., Falvey, E. C., et al. (2019). Emotion regulation mediates the relationship between ACES and physical and mental health. *Psychological Trauma, 11,* 82–89.

Cloitre, M., & Koenen, K. C. (2001). The impact of borderline personality disorder on process group outcome among women with posttraumatic stress disorder related to childhood abuse. *International Journal of Group Psychotherapy, 51,* 379–397.

Cloitre, M., Koenen, K. C., Cohen, L. R., & Han, H. (2002b). Skills training in affective and interpersonal regulation followed by exposure: A phase-based treatment for PTSD related to childhood abuse. *Journal of Consulting and Clinical Psychology, 70,* 1067–1074.

Cloitre, M., Levitt, J., Davis, L., & Miranda, R. (2003, November). Bringing a manualized treatment for PTSD to the community. In R. Bryant (Chair), *Improving treatment of posttraumatic stress disorder.* Symposium conducted at the 19th annual meeting of the International Society for Traumatic Stress Studies, Chicago, IL.

Cloitre, M., & Makin-Byrd, K. (2018). *Parenting Skills Training in Affective and Interpersonal Regulation for Primary Care (Parenting STAIR) essentials.* Unpublished manual, Department of Veterans Affairs.

Cloitre, M., Miranda, R., Stovall-McClough, C., & Han, H. (2005). Beyond PTSD: Emotion regulation and interpersonal problems as predictors of functional impairment in survivors of childhood abuse. *Behavior Therapy, 36,* 119–124.

Cloitre, M., Ortigo, K. M., & Gupta, C. (2018c). *Skills Training in Affective and Interpersonal Regulation for Primary Care (STAIR-PC) essentials* (Version 1.6). Unpublished manual, Department of Veterans Affairs.

Cloitre, M., Scarvalone, P., & Difede, J. A. (1997). Posttraumatic stress disorder, self and interpersonal dysfunction among sexually retraumatized women. *Journal of Traumatic Stress, 10,* 437–452.

Cloitre, M., Shevlin, M., Brewin, C. R., Bisson, J. I., Roberts, N. P., Maercker, A., et al. (2018d). The International Trauma Questionnaire: Development of a self-report measure of ICD-11 PTSD and complex PTSD. *Acta Psychiatrica Scandinavica, 138,* 536–546.

Cloitre, M., Stolbach, B. C., Herman, J. L., van der Kolk, B., Pynoos, R., Wang, J., & Petkova, E. (2009). A developmental approach to complex PTSD: Childhood and adult cumulative trauma as predictors of symptom complexity. *Journal of Traumatic Stress, 22,* 399–408.

Cloitre, M., Stovall-McClough, K. C., Miranda, R., & Chemtob, C. M. (2004). Therapeutic alliance, negative mood regulation, and treatment outcome in child abuse-related posttraumatic stress disorder. *Journal of Consulting and Clinical Psychology, 72,* 411–416.

Cloitre, M., Stovall-McClough, K. C., Nooner, K., Zorbas, P., Cherry, S., Jackson C. L., et al. (2010). Treatment for PTSD related to childhood abuse: A randomized controlled trial. *American Journal of Psychiatry, 167,* 915–924.

Cloitre, M., Stovall-McClough, K. C., Zorbas, P., & Charuvastra, A. (2008). Childhood maltreatment, adult attachment status, and psychosocial adjustment: Attachment organization, emotion regulation, and expectations of support in a clinical sample of women with childhood abuse histories. *Journal of Traumatic Stress: Official Publication of The International Society for Traumatic Stress Studies, 21*(3), 282–289.

Cloitre, M., Tardiff, K., Marzuk, P. M., Leon, A. C., & Portera, L. (1996). Childhood abuse and subsequent sexual assault among female inpatients. *Journal of Traumatic Stress, 9,* 473–482.

Coid, J., Petruckevitch, A., Feder, G., Chung, W. S., Richardson, J., & Moorey, S. (2001). Relation between childhood sexual and physical abuse and risk of revictimisation in women: A cross-sectional survey. *The Lancet, 358*(9280), 450–454.

Conte, J., Wolfe, R. R., & Smith, T. (1989). What sexual offenders tell us about prevention strategies. *Child Abuse and Neglect, 13,* 293–301.

Cooper, N., & Clum, G. (1989). Imaginal flooding as a supplementary treatment for PTSD in combat veterans: A controlled study. *Behavior Therapy, 10,* 381–391.

Coryell, W., Scheftner, W., Keller, M., Endicott, J., Maser, J., & Klerman, G. (1993). The enduring psychological consequences of mania and depression. *American Journal of Psychiatry, 150,* 720–726.

Davis, M., Eshelman, E. R., & McKay, M. (1995). *The relaxation and stress reduction workbook.* Oakland, CA: New Harbinger.

DePrince, A. P., Brown, L. S., Cheit, R. E., Freyd, J. J., Gold, S. N., Pezdek, K., et al. (2012). Motivated forgetting and misremembering: Perspectives from betrayal trauma theory. *Nebraska Symposium on Motivation, 58,* 193–242.

Desai, S., Arias, I., Thompson, M. P., & Basile, K. C. (2002). Childhood victimization and subsequent adult revictimization assessed in a nationally representative sample of women and men. *Violence and Victims, 17,* 639–653.

Doyle, C., & Cicchetti, D. (2017). From the cradle to the grave: The effect of adverse caregiving environments on attachment and relationships throughout the lifespan. *Clinical Psychology: Science and Practice, 24*(2), 203–221.

Ehlers, A., & Clark, D. M. (2000). A cognitive model of posttraumatic stress disorder. *Behaviour Research and Therapy, 38,* 319–345.

Ehlers, A., & Wild, J. (2015). Cognitive therapy for PTSD: Updating memories and meanings of trauma. In U. Schnyder & M. Cloitre (Eds.), *Evidence-based treatments for trauma-related psychological disorders* (pp. 161–187). Cham, Switzerland: Springer International.

Erickson, M. F., Egeland, B., & Pianta, R. (1989). The effects of maltreatment on the development of young children. In D. Cicchetti & V. Carlson (Eds.), *Child maltreatment: Theory and research on the causes and consequences of child abuse and neglect* (pp. 674–684). New York: Cambridge University Press.

Fanning, P., & O'Neill, J. T. (1996). *The addiction workbook.* Oakland, CA: New Harbinger.

Feiring, C., Taska, L., & Chen, K. (2002). Trying to understand why horrible things happen: Attribution, shame, and symptom development following sexual abuse. *Child Maltreatment, 7,* 25–39.

Figley, C. R., & Ludick, M. (2017). Secondary traumatization and compassion fatigue. In S. Gold (Ed.), *Handbook of trauma psychology* (Vol. 1, pp. 573–593). Washington, DC: American Psychological Association.

Finkelhor, D. (1980). Sex among siblings: A survey on prevalence, variety and effects. *Archives of Sexual Behavior, 9,* 171–194.

Finkelhor, D. (1994). Current information on the scope and nature of child sexual abuse. *The Future of Children, 4,* 31–53.

Finkelhor, D., Turner, H. A., Shattuck, A., & Hamby, S. L. (2013). Violence, crime, and abuse exposure in a national sample of children and youth: An update. *JAMA Pediatrics, 167*(7), 614–621.

Foa, E. B., Dancu, C. V., Hembree, E. A., Jaycox, L. H., & Meadows, E. A. (1999). A comparison of exposure therapy, stress inoculation training, and their combination for reducing posttraumatic stress disorder in female assault victims. *Journal of Consulting and Clinical Psychology, 67,* 194–200.

Foa, E. B., Riggs, D. S., Massie, E. D., & Yarczower, M. (1995). The impact of fear activation and anger on the efficacy of exposure treatment for posttraumatic stress disorder. *Behavior Therapy, 26,* 487–499.

Foa, E. B., & Rothbaum, B. O. (1998). *Treating the trauma of rape: Cognitive-behavioral therapy for PTSD.* New York: Guilford Press.

Ford, J. D., Fisher, P., & Larson, L. (1997). Object relations as a predictor of treatment outcome with chronic posttraumatic stress disorder. *Journal of Consulting and Clinical Psychology, 65,* 547–559.

Ford, J. D., & Kidd, P. (1998). Early childhood trauma and disorders of extreme stress as predictors of treatment outcome with chronic posttraumatic stress disorder. *Journal of Traumatic Stress, 11,* 743–761.

Fosha, D. (2000). *The transforming power of affect: A model for accelerated change.* New York: Basic Books.

Freud, S. (1955). Beyond the pleasure principle. In J. Strachey (Ed. & Trans.), *The standard edition of the complete psychological works of Sigmund Freud* (Vol. 18, pp. 3–64). London: Hogarth Press. (Original work published 1920)

Freud, S. (1963). Further recommendations in the technique of psychoanalysis: Recollection, repetition and working through. In P. Reiff (Ed.), *Therapy and technique.* New York: Macmillan. (Original work published 1914)

Frewen, P. A., Dozois, D. J. A., Neufeld, R. W. J., & Lanius, R. A. (2008). Meta-analysis of alexithymia in posttraumatic stress disorder. *Journal of Traumatic Stress, 21*(2), 243–246.

Freyd, J. J. (1996). *Betrayal trauma: The logic of forgetting childhood abuse.* Cambridge, MA: Harvard University Press.

Funari, D., Piekarski, A., & Sherwood, R. (1991). Treatment outcomes of Vietnam veterans with posttraumatic stress disorder. *Psychological Reports, 68,* 571–578.

Gapen, M., Cross, D., Ortigo, K. M., Graham, A., Johnson, E., Evces, M., et al. (2011). Perceived neighborhood disorder, community cohesion, and PTSD symptoms among low-income African Americans in an urban health setting. *American Journal of Orthopsychiatry, 81,* 31–37.

Gergely, G. (2004). The role of contingency detection in early affect-regulative interactions and in the development of different types of infant attachment. *Social Development, 13,* 468–478.

Gergely, G., & Watson, J. (1996). The social biofeedback theory of parental affect-mirroring: The development of emotional self-awareness and self-control in infancy. *International Journal of Psycho-Analysis, 77,* 1181–1212.

Giaconia, R. M., Reinherz, H. Z., Silverman, A. B., Pakiz, B., Frost, A. K., & Cohen, E. (1995). Traumas and posttraumatic stress disorder in a community population of older adolescents. *Journal of the American Academy of Child and Adolescent Psychiatry, 34,* 1369–1380.

Gidycz, C. A., Hanson, K., & Layman, M. J. (1995). A prospective analysis of the relationships among sexual assault experiences. *Psychology of Women Quarterly, 19,* 5–29.

Gilbert, P. (2010). *Compassion focused therapy.* Hove, UK: Routledge.

Gilmore, M. (1994). *Shot in the heart.* New York: Doubleday.

Gold, S. N. (2000). *Not trauma alone: Therapy for child abuse survivors in family and social context.* Philadelphia: Brunner/Routledge.

Golden, O. (2000). The federal response to child abuse and neglect. *American Journal of Psychiatry, 55,* 1050–1053.

Goleman, D. (1995). *Emotional intelligence.* New York: Bantam Books.

Gudiño, O. G., Leonard, S., & Cloitre, M. (2016). STAIR-A for girls: A pilot study of a skills-based group for traumatized youth in an urban school setting. *Journal of Child and Adolescent Trauma, 9,* 67–79.

Gudiño, O. G., Leonard, S., Stiles, A. A., Havens, J. F., & Cloitre, M. (2017). STAIR Narrative Therapy for adolescents. In M. Landolt, M. Cloitre, & U. Schnyder (Eds.), *Evidence-based treatments for trauma-related disorders in children and adolescents* (pp. 251–272). Cham, Switzerland: Springer International.

Gudiño, O. G., Weis, J. R., Havens, J. F., Biggs, E. A., Diamond, U. N., Marr, M., et al. (2014). Group trauma-informed treatment for adolescent psychiatric inpatients: A preliminary uncontrolled trial. *Journal of Traumatic Stress, 27,* 1–5.

Gurewitsch, B. (Ed.). (1998). *Mothers, sisters, resisters: Oral histories of women who survived the Holocaust.* Tuscaloosa: University of Alabama Press.

Harvey, M. R., Liang, B., Harney, P., & Koenen, K. C. (2003). A multidimensional approach to the measurement of trauma recovery and resiliency. *Journal of Aggression, Maltreatment and Trauma, 6,* 87–109.

Haskett, M. E., Smith Scott, S., & Ward, C. S. (2004). Subgroups of physically abusive parents based on cluster analysis of parenting behavior and affect. *American Journal of Orthopsychiatry, 74,* 436–447.

Heriot, J. (1996). Maternal protectiveness following the disclosure of intrafamilial child sexual abuse. *Journal of Interpersonal Violence, 11,* 181–194.

Herman, J. L. (1992). *Trauma and recovery: The aftermath of violence from domestic to political terror.* New York: Basic Books.

Herman, J. L. (2007, March 10). *Shattered shame states and their repair.* The John Bowlby Memorial Lecture, presented in the Department of Psychiatry, Harvard Medical School, Boston.

Hien, D., & Honeyman, T. (2000). A closer look at the drug abuse–maternal aggression link. *Journal of Interpersonal Violence, 15,* 503–522.

Hill, C. R., & Safran, J. D. (1994). Assessing interpersonal schemas: Anticipated responses of significant others. *Journal of Social and Clinical Psychology, 13,* 366–379.

Hobfoll, S. E., Mancini, A. D., Hall, B. J., Canetti, D., & Bonanno, G. A. (2011). The limits of resilience: Distress following chronic political violence among Palestinians. *Social Science and Medicine, 72,* 1400–1408.

Hollifield, M., Gory, A., Siedjak, J., Nguyen, L., Holmgreen, L., & Hobfoll, S. (2016). The benefit of conserving and gaining resources after trauma: A systematic review. *Journal of Clinical Medicine, 5*(11), 104.

Holmes, J. (2001). *The search for the secure base: Attachment theory and psychotherapy.* Philadelphia: Brunner/Routledge.

Horan, J. M., & Widom, C. S. (2015). Cumulative childhood risk and adult functioning in abused and neglected children grown up. *Developmental Psychopathology, 27*(3), 927–941.

Horowitz, K., Weine, S., & Jekel, J. (1995). Posttraumatic stress disorder symptoms in urban adolescent girls: Compounded community trauma. *Journal of the American Academy of Child and Adolescent Psychiatry, 34,* 1353–1361.

Horvath, A. O., & Symonds, D. B. (1991). Relation between working alliance and outcome in psychotherapy: A meta-analysis. *Journal of Counseling Psychology, 36,* 223–233.

How America defines child abuse: National poll reveals most who witness child abuse do nothing about it. (1999, June 3). *PRNewswire.* Retrieved October 14, 2019, from *nospank.net/n-e62.htm.*

International Society for Traumatic Stress Studies

(ISTSS). (2019a). New ISTSS prevention and treatment guidelines. Retrieved February 9, 2019, from *www.istss.org/treating-trauma/new-istss-guidelines.aspx*.

International Society for Traumatic Stress Studies (ISTSS). (2019b). ISTSS guidelines position paper on complex PTSD in adults. Retrieved February 17, 2019, from *www.istss.org/getattachment/treating-trauma/new-istss-prevention-and-treatment-guidelines/istss_cptsd-position-paper-(adults)_fnl.pdf.aspx*.

Jackson, C., Weiss, B. J., & Cloitre, M. (2018). STAIR group treatment for veterans with PTSD: Efficacy and impact of gender on outcome. *Military Medicine, 184*, e143–e147.

Jacobs, W. J., & Nadel, L. (1985). Stress induced recovery of fears and phobias. *Psychological Review, 92*, 512–531.

Jaffe, A. E., DiLillo, D., Gratz, K. L., & Messman-Moore, T. L. (2019). Risk for revictimization following interpersonal and noninterpersonal trauma: Clarifying the role of posttraumatic stress symptoms and trauma-related cognitions. *Journal of Traumatic Stress, 32*(1), 42–55.

Jaffee, S. R. (2017). Child maltreatment and risk for psychopathology in childhood and adulthood. *Annual Review of Clinical Psychology, 13*, 525–551.

Janoff-Bulman, R. (1992). *Shattered assumptions: Towards a new psychology of trauma.* New York: Free Press.

Jung, C. G. (1989). *Memories, dreams, reflections* (A. Jaffe, Ed. & C. Winston, Trans.). New York: Vintage Books. (Original work published 1963)

Kagan, J. (1980). Perspectives on continuity. In O. G. Brin, Jr. & J. Kagan (Eds.), *Constancy and change in human development* (pp. 26–74). Cambridge, MA: Harvard University Press.

Kaplan, S. J., Sunday, S. R., Labruna, V., Pelcovitz, D., & Salzinger, S. (2009). Psychiatric disorders of parents of physically abused adolescents. *Journal of Family Violence, 24*, 273–281.

Karatzias, T., Murphy, P., Cloitre, M., Bisson, J. I., Roberts, N. P., Shevlin, M., et al. (2019). Psychological interventions for ICD-11 Complex PTSD symptoms: Systematic review and meta-analysis. *Psychological Medicine, 49*(11), 1761–1775.

Karen, R. (1998). *Becoming attached: First relationships and how they shape our capacity to love.* New York: Oxford University Press.

Keane, T. M., Fairbank, J., Caddell, J., & Zimmering, R. (1989). Implosive (flooding) therapy reduces symptoms of PTSD in Vietnam combat veterans. *Behavior Therapy, 20*, 246–260.

Keenan, K. (2000). Emotion dysregulation as a risk factor for child psychopathology. *Clinical Psychology: Science and Practice, 7*, 418–434.

Kessler, R. C., Aguilar-Gaxiola, S., Alonso, J., Benjet, C., Bromet, E. J., Cardoso, G., et al. (2017). Trauma and PTSD in the WHO World Mental Health Surveys. *European Journal of Psychotraumatology, 8*(Suppl. 5), 1353383.

Kiesler, D. J. (1983). The 1982 interpersonal circle: A taxonomy for complementarity in human transactions. *Psychological Review, 90*, 185–214.

Kilpatrick, D. G., Ruggiero, K. J., Acierno, R., Saunders, B. E., Resnick, H. S., & Best, C. L. (2003). Violence and risk of PTSD, major depression, substance abuse/dependence, and comorbidity: Results from the National Survey of Adolescents. *Journal of Consulting and Clinical Psychology, 71*(4), 692–700.

Kim, K., Mennen, F. E., & Trickett, P. K. (2017). Patterns and correlates of co-occurrence among multiple types of child maltreatment. *Child and Family Social Work, 22*(1), 492–502.

Kolko, D. J., Brown, E. J., & Berliner, L. (2002). Children's perceptions of their abusive experience: Measurement and preliminary findings. *Child Maltreatment, 7*, 41–53.

Konrath, S. H., Chopik, W. J., Hsing, C. K., & O'Brien, E. (2014). Changes in adult attachment styles in American college students over time: A meta-analysis. *Personality and Social Psychology Review, 18*, 326–348.

Krahe, B., Sheinberger-Olwig, R., Waizenhofer, E., & Koplin, S. (1999). Childhood sexual abuse revictimization in adolescence. *Child Abuse and Neglect, 4*, 383–394.

Krupnick, J. L., Sotsky, S. M., Simmons, S., Moyer, J., Elkin, I., & Watkins, J. (1996). The role of the therapeutic alliance in psychotherapy and pharmacotherapy outcome: Findings in the NIMH Collaborative Research Programme. *Journal of Consulting and Clinical Psychology, 64*, 532–539.

Kubany, E. S., Ownes, J. A., McCaig, M. A., Hill, E. E., Iannce-Spencer, C., & Tremayne, K. J. (2004). Cognitive trauma therapy for battered women with PTSD (CTT-BW). *Journal of Consulting and Clinical Psychology, 72*, 3–18.

Langton, L., Berzofsky, M., Krebs, C., & Smiley-McDonald, H. (2012, August). *Victimizations not reported to the police 2006–2010.* Washington, DC: U.S. Department of Justice, Bureau of Justice Statistics. Retrieved from *bjs.gov/content/pub.pdf/vnrp0610.pdf*.

Larsen, S. E., Stirman, S. W., Smith, B. N., & Resick, P. A. (2016). Symptom exacerbations in trauma-focused treatments: Associations with treatment outcome and non-completion. *Behaviour Research and Therapy, 77*, 68–77.

Layne, C. M., Kaplow, J. B., Oosterhoff, B., Hill, R. M., & Pynoos, R. S. (2018). The interplay between posttraumatic stress and grief reactions in traumatically bereaved adolescents: When trauma, bereavement, and adolescence converge. *Adolescent Psychiatry, 7*, 266–285.

Leary, T. (1957). *Interpersonal diagnosis of personality.* New York: Ronald Press.

LeDoux, J. E. (1998). *The emotional brain.* London: Weidenfeld & Nicolson.

Leskela, J., Dieperink, M., & Thuras, P. (2002). Shame and posttraumatic stress disorder. *Journal of Traumatic Stress, 15*(3), 223–226.

Levitt, J. T., & Cloitre, M. (2005). A clinician's guide to STAIR/MPE: Treatment for PTSD related to childhood abuse. *Cognitive and Behavioral Practice, 12,* 40–52.

Levitt, J. T., Malta, L. S., Martin, A., Davis, L., & Cloitre, M. (2007). The flexible application of a manualized treatment for PTSD symptoms and functional impairment related to the 9/11 World Trade Center attack. *Behaviour Research and Therapy, 45*(7), 1419–1433.

Lee, J. L., Nader, K., & Schiller, D. (2017). An update on memory reconsolidation updating. *Trends in Cognitive Sciences, 21,* 531–545.

Li, M., D'Arcy, C., & Meng, X. (2016). Maltreatment in childhood substantially increases the risk of adult depression and anxiety in prospective cohort studies: Systematic review, meta-analysis, and proportional attributable fractions. *Psychological Medicine, 46,* 717–730.

Lieberman, A. F., & Amaya-Jackson, L. (2005). Reciprocal influences of attachment and trauma: Using a dual lens in the assessment and treatment of infants, toddlers, and preschoolers. In L. Berlin, Y. Ziv, L. Amaya-Jackson, & M. T. Greenberg (Eds.), *Enhancing early attachments: Theory, research, intervention, and policy* (pp. 100–124). New York: Guilford Press.

Lifton, R. J. (1993). *The protean self: Human resilience in an age of fragmentation.* New York: Basic Books.

Lindy, J. (1996). Psychoanalytic psychotherapy of posttraumatic stress disorder: The nature of the therapeutic relationship. In B. van der Kolk, A. C. McFarlane, & I. Weisaeth (Eds.), *Traumatic stress: The effects of overwhelming experience on mind, body, and society* (pp. 525–536). New York: Guilford Press.

Linehan, M. M. (1993). *Cognitive-behavioral treatment of borderline personality disorder.* New York: Guilford Press.

Linehan, M. M. (2015). *DBT skills training manual* (2nd ed.). New York: Guilford Press.

Linehan, M. M., Korslund, K. E., Harned, M. S., Gallop, R. J., Lungu, A., Neacsiu, A. D., et al. (2015). Dialectical behavior therapy for high suicide risk in individuals with borderline personality disorder: A randomized clinical trial and component analysis. *JAMA Psychiatry, 72,* 475–482.

Lipschitz, D. S., Rasmusson, A. M., Anyan, W., Comwell, P., & Southwick, S. M. (2000). Clinical and functional correlates of posttraumatic stress disorder in urban adolescent girls at a primary care clinic. *Journal of the American Academy of Child and Adolescent Psychiatry, 39,* 1104–1111.

Lipschitz, D. S., Winegar, R. K., Hartnick, E., Foote, B., & Southwick, S. M. (1999a). Posttraumatic stress disorder in hospitalized adolescents: Psychiatric comorbidity and clinical correlates. *Journal of the American Academy of Child and Adolescent Psychiatry, 38,* 385–392.

Lipschitz, D. S., Winegar, R. K., Nicolaou, A. L., Hartnick, E., Wolfson, M., & Southwick, S. M. (1999b). Perceived abuse and neglect as risk factors for suicidal behavior in adolescent inpatients. *Journal of Nervous and Mental Disease, 187,* 29–32.

Litz, B. T., & Gray, M. J. (2002). Emotional numbing of posttraumatic stress disorder: Current and future research directions. *Australian and New Zealand Journal of Psychiatry, 36,* 198–204.

Liu, J., Fang, Y., Gong, J., Cui, X., Meng, T., Xiao, B., et al. (2017). Associations between suicidal behavior and childhood abuse and neglect: A meta-analysis. *Journal of Affective Disorders, 220,* 147–155.

Lorde, A. (1984). *Sister outsider: Essays and speeches.* Trumansburg, NY: Crossing Press.

Lyons-Ruth, K., Alpern, L., & Repacholi, B. (1993). Disorganized infant attachment classification and maternal psychosocial problems as predictors of hostile–aggressive behavior in the preschool classroom. *Child Development, 63,* 572–585.

MacIntosh, H. B., Cloitre, M., Kortis, K., Peck, A., & Weiss, B. J. (2018). Implementation and evaluation of the Skills Training in Affective and Interpersonal Regulation (STAIR) in a community setting in the context of childhood sexual abuse. *Research on Social Work Practice, 28*(5), 595–602.

MacKinnon, C. A. (2005, April 16). Who was afraid of Andrea Dworkin? *The New York Times,* p. 13.

Maercker, A., Brewin, C. R., Bryant, R. A., Cloitre, M., van Ommeren, M., Jones, L. M., et al. (2013). Diagnosis and classification of disorders specifically associated with stress: Proposals for ICD-11. *World Psychiatry, 12*(3), 198–206.

Main, M., Kaplan, N., & Cassidy, J. (1985). Security in infancy, childhood, and adulthood: A move to the level of representation. In I. Bretherton & E. Waters (Eds.), *Growing points of attachment theory and research. Monographs of the Society for Research in Child Development, 50*(1–2, Serial No. 209), 66–104.

Malatesta, C. Z., & Haviland, J. M. (1982). Learning display rules: The socialization of emotion expression in infancy. *Child Development, 53,* 991–1003.

Malmquist, C. P. (1986). Children who witness parental murder: Posttraumatic aspects. *Journal of the American Academy of Child and Adolescent Psychiatry, 25,* 320–325.

Maniglio, R. (2009). The impact of child sexual abuse on health: A systematic review of reviews. *Clinical Psychology Review, 29*(7), 647–657.

March, J. (1999). Assessment of pediatric posttraumatic stress disorder. In P. A. Saigh & J. D. Bremner (Eds.),

Postttraumatic stress disorder: A comprehensive text (pp. 199–218). Needham Heights, MA: Allyn & Bacon.

Martin, D. J., Garske, J. P., & Davis, M. K. (2000). Relation of the therapeutic alliance with outcome and other variables: A meta-analytic review. *Journal of Consulting and Clinical Psychology, 58,* 438–450.

Mathieu, F. (2012). *The compassion fatigue workbook: Creative tools for transforming compassion fatigue and vicarious traumatization.* New York: Routledge.

May, R. (1975). *The courage to create.* New York: Norton.

McCarthy, G., & Maughan, B. (2010). Negative childhood experiences and adult love relationships: The role of internal working models of attachment. *Attachment and Human Development, 12*(5), 445–461.

McDonagh, A., Friedman, M., McHugo, G., Ford, J., Sengupta, A., Mueser, K., et al. (2005). Randomized trial of cognitive behavioral therapy for chronic posttraumatic stress disorder in adult female survivors of childhood sexual abuse. *Journal of Consulting and Clinical Psychology, 73,* 515–524.

McFall, M. E., Marburg, M. M., Ko, G. N., & Veith, R., C. (1990). Autonomic responses to stress in Vietnam combat veterans with PTSD. *Biological Psychiatry, 27,* 1165–1175.

McLaughlin, K. A., Greif Green, J., Gruber, M. J., Sampson, N. A., Zaslavsky, A. M., & Kessler, R. C. (2012). Childhood adversities and first onset of psychiatric disorders in a national sample of US adolescents. *Archives of General Psychiatry, 69,* 1151–1160.

Messman, T. L., & Long, P. J. (1996). Child sexual abuse and its relationship to revictimization in adult women: A review. *Clinical Psychology Review, 5,* 397–420.

Messman-Moore, T. L., & Long, P. J. (2000). Child sexual abuse and revictimization in the form of adult sexual abuse, adult physical abuse, and adult psychological maltreatment. *Journal of Interpersonal Violence, 15,* 489–502.

Messman-Moore, T. L., Ward, R. M., & Zerubavel, N. (2013). The role of substance use and emotion dysregulation in predicting risk for incapacitated sexual revictimization in women: Results of a prospective investigation. *Psychology of Addictive Behaviors, 27,* 125–132.

Miron, L. R., & Orcutt, H. K. (2014). Pathways from childhood abuse to prospective revictimization: Depression, sex to reduce negative affect, and forecasted sexual behavior. *Child Abuse and Neglect, 38,* 1848–1859.

Monson, C. M., & Fredman, S. J. (2012). *Cognitive-behavioral conjoint therapy for PTSD: Harnessing the healing power of relationships.* New York: Guilford Press.

Muran, J. C., Segal, Z. V., Samstag, L. W., & Crawford, C. E. (1994). Patient pretreatment interpersonal problems in therapeutic alliance in short-term cognitive

therapy. *Journal of Consulting and Clinical Psychology, 62,* 185–190.

Nader, K., Schafe, G. E., & LeDoux, J. E. (2000). Reply—Reconsolidation: The labile nature of consolidation theory. *Nature Reviews Neuroscience, 1,* 216.

Nash, M. R., Hulsey, T. L., Sexton, M. C., Harralson, T. L., & Lambert, W. (1993). Perceived family environment, psychopathology, and dissociation. *Journal of Consulting and Clinical Psychology, 61,* 276–283.

Naughton, A. M., Maguire, S. A., Mann, M. K., Lumb, R. C., Tempest, V., Gracias, S., et al. (2013). Emotional, behavioral, and developmental features indicative of neglect or emotional abuse in preschool children: A systematic review. *JAMA Pediatrics, 167,* 769–775.

Nichols, K., Gergely, G., & Fonagy, P. (2001). Experimental protocols for investigating relationships among mother–infant interaction, affect regulation, physiological markers of stress responsiveness, and attachment. *Bulletin of the Menninger Clinic, 65*(3), 371–379.

Nickerson, A., Cloitre, M., Bryant, R. A., Schnyder, U., Morina, N., & Schick, M. (2016). The factor structure of complex posttraumatic stress disorder in traumatized refugees. *European Journal of Psychotraumatology, 7,* 33253.

Nickerson, A., Cloitre, M., & O'Donnell, M. (2018–2022). *Phase-based treatment for PTSD in traumatized refugees.* Grant from the Australian National Health and Medical Research Council.

Norman, R. E., Byambaa, M., De, R., Butchart, A., Scott, J., & Vos, T. (2012). The long-term health consequences of child physical abuse, emotional abuse, and neglect: A systematic review and meta-analysis. *PLOS Medicine, 9,* e1001349.

O'Dougherty Wright, M., Crawford, E., & Del Castillo, D. (2009). Childhood emotional maltreatment and later psychological distress among college students: The mediating role of maladaptive schemas. *Child Abuse and Neglect, 33,* 59–68.

Orth, U., Robins, R. W., & Soto, C. J. (2010). Tracking the trajectory of shame, guilt, and pride across the life span. *Journal of Personality and Social Psychology, 99,* 1061–1071.

Ortigo, K. M., & Cloitre, M. (2018, November 17). web-STAIR VA enterprise-wide initiative: A skills-based web program with coaching support targeting MST for rural veterans. In A. Edwards Stewart (Chair), *Technology for mental health in military and veteran populations.* Symposium conducted at the 52nd annual convention of the Association for Behavioral and Cognitive Therapies, Washington, DC.

Ortigo, K. M., Cloitre, M., Jackson, C., Weiss, B., & Schmidt, J. (2019). *webSTAIR: Skills Training in Affective and Interpersonal Regulation* [Online website]. Retrieved from *www.webSTAIR.org.*

Ortigo, K. M., Westen, D., DeFife, J. A., & Bradley, B. (2013). Attachment, social cognition, and posttraumatic stress symptoms in a traumatized, urban population: Evidence for the mediating role of object relations. *Journal of Traumatic Stress, 26,* 361–368.

Papa, A., & Bonanno, G. A. (2008). Smiling in the face of adversity: The interpersonal and intrapersonal functions of smiling. *Emotion, 8,* 1–12.

Parke, R. D., McDowell, D. J., Cladis, M., & Leidy, M. S. (2006). Family and peer relationships: The role of emotion regulatory processes. In D. K. Snyder, J. E. Simpson, & J. N. Hughes (Eds.), *Emotion regulation in couples and families: Pathways to dysfunction and health* (pp. 143–162). Washington, DC: American Psychological Association.

Pearlman, L. A., & Saakvitne, K. W. (1995). *Trauma and the therapist.* New York: Norton.

Pearlman, L. A., Wortman, C. B., Feuer, C. A., Farber, C. H., & Rando, T. A. (2014). *Treating traumatic bereavement: A practitioner's guide.* New York: Guilford Press.

Perepletchikova, F., & Kaufman, J. (2010). Emotional and behavioral sequelae of childhood maltreatment. *Current Opinion in Pediatrics, 22,* 610–615.

Perry, R. E., Blair, C., & Sullivan, R. M. (2017). Neurobiology of infant attachment: Attachment despite adversity and parental programming of emotionality. *Current Opinion in Psychology, 17,* 1–6.

Pitman, R. K., Orr, S. P., Forgue, D. F., de Jong, J. B., & Claiborn, J. M. (1987). Psychophysiologic assessment of post-traumatic stress disorder imagery in Vietnam combat veterans. *Archives of General Psychiatry, 44,* 970–975.

Platt, M. G., & Freyd, J. J. (2012). Trauma and negative underlying assumptions in feelings of shame: An exploratory study. *Psychological Trauma: Theory, Research, Practice, and Policy, 4,* 370–378.

Platt, M. G., & Freyd, J. J. (2015). Betray my trust, shame on me: Shame, dissociation, fear, and betrayal trauma. *Psychological Trauma: Theory, Research, Practice, and Policy, 7,* 398.

Platt, M. G., Luoma, J. B., & Freyd, J. J. (2017). Shame and dissociation in survivors of high and low betrayal trauma. *Journal of Aggression, Maltreatment and Trauma, 26*(1), 34–49.

Polusny, M., & Follette, V. (1995). Long-term correlates of child sexual abuse: Theory and review of the empirical literature. *Applied and Preventive Psychology: Current Scientific Perspectives, 4,* 143–166.

Pope, K. S., & Vasquez, M. J. T. (1998). *Ethics in psychotherapy and counseling: A practical guide* (2nd ed.). San Francisco: Jossey-Bass.

Putnam, F. W. (2004). *The costs and consequences of child abuse.* Paper presented at the annual meeting of the American Association for the Advancement of Science, Seattle, WA.

Pynoos, B., Frederick, C. J., Nader, K., Arroyo, W., Steinberg, A., Nunez, F., et al. (1987). Life threat and posttraumatic stress in school age children. *Archives of General Psychiatry, 44,* 1057–1063.

Quindlen, A. (1992). *Object lessons.* Branson, MO: Ivy Books.

Rapaport, M. H., Endicott, J., & Clary, C. M. (2002). Post-traumatic stress disorder and quality of life: Results across 64 weeks of sertraline treatment. *Journal of Clinical Psychiatry, 63,* 59–65.

Ray, K. C., Jackson, J. L., & Townsley, R. M. (1991). Family environments of victims of intrafamilial and extrafamilial child sexual abuse. *Journal of Family Violence, 6,* 365–374.

Riggs, S. A., Cusimano, A. M., & Benson, K. M. (2011). Childhood emotional abuse and attachment processes in the dyadic adjustment of dating couples. *Journal of Counseling Psychology, 58*(1), 126–138.

Roberts, N., Cloitre, M., Bisson, J. I., & Brewin, C. (2018). *The International Trauma Interview for ICD-11 PTSD.* Unpublished interview.

Rogers, C. R. (1951). *Client-centered therapy.* Boston: Houghton Mifflin.

Rosenberg, M. (1965). *Society and the adolescent self-image.* Princeton, NJ: Princeton University Press.

Rothbaum, B. O., & Foa, E. B. (1999). *Reclaiming your life after rape: Cognitive behavioral therapy for post-traumatic stress disorder.* New York: Oxford University Press.

Rothschild, B. (2006). *Help for the helper: The psychophysiology of compassion fatigue and vicarious trauma.* New York: Norton.

Safran, J. D. (1990a). Towards a refinement of cognitive therapy in light of interpersonal theory: I. Theory. *Clinical Psychology Review, 10,* 87–105.

Safran, J. D. (1990b). Towards a refinement of cognitive therapy in light of interpersonal theory: II. Practice. *Clinical Psychology Review, 10,* 107–121.

Safran, J. D., & Segal, Z. V. (1990). *Interpersonal process in cognitive therapy.* New York: Basic Books.

Santiago, A., Aoki, C., & Sullivan, R. M. (2017). From attachment to independence: Stress hormone control of ecologically relevant emergence of infants' responses to threat. *Current Opinion in Behavioral Sciences, 14,* 78–85.

Saraiya, T., & Lopez-Castro, T. (2016). Ashamed and afraid: A scoping review of the role of shame in post-traumatic stress disorder (PTSD). *Journal of Clinical Medicine, 5*(11), 94.

Schaef, A. W. (2000). *Meditations for living in balance: Daily solutions for people who do too much.* New York: HarperCollins.

Schauer, M., Neuner, F., & Elbert, T. (2011). *Narrative exposure therapy: A short-term treatment for traumatic stress disorders.* Boston: Hogrefe.

Scheier, M. F., & Carver, C. S. (1985). Optimism, coping and health: Assessment and implications of generalized outcome expectancies. *Health Psychology, 4,* 219–247.

Schwartz, D., & Proctor, L. J. (2000). Community violence exposure and children's social adjustment in the school peer groups: The mediating roles of emotion regulation and social cognition. *Journal of Consulting and Clinical Psychology, 68,* 670–683.

Scott, M. J., & Stradling, S. G. (1997). Client compliance with exposure treatments for posttraumatic stress disorder. *Journal of Traumatic Stress, 10,* 523–526.

Serretti, A., Cavallino, M. C., Macciardi, F., Namia, C., Franchni, L., Souery, D., et al. (1999). Social adjustment and self-esteem in remitted patients with mood disorders. *European Psychiatry, 14,* 137–142.

Shalev, A. Y. (1997). Discussion: Treatment of prolonged posttraumatic stress disorder—learning from experience. *Journal of Traumatic Stress, 10,* 415–423.

Shapiro, D. N., Kaplow, J. B., Amaya-Jackson, L., & Dodge, K. A. (2012). Behavioral markers of coping and psychiatric symptoms among sexually abused children. *Journal of Traumatic Stress, 25,* 157–163.

Shear, K., Frank, E., Houck, P., & Reynolds, C. F. (2005). Treatment of complicated grief: A randomized controlled trial. *Journal of the American Medical Association, 293*(21), 2601–2608.

Sheridan, M. J. (1995). A proposed intergenerational model of substance abuse, family functioning, and abuse/neglect. *Child Abuse and Neglect, 19,* 519–530.

Shields, A. M., & Cicchetti, D. (1998). Reactive aggression among maltreated children: The contributions of attention and emotion dysregulation. *Journal of Clinical Child Psychology, 27,* 381–395.

Shipman, K. L., & Zeman, J. (2001). Socialization of children's emotion regulation in mother–child dyads: A developmental psychopathology perspective. *Developmental Psychopathology, 13,* 317–336.

Shipman, K. L., Zeman, J., Penza, S., & Champion, K. (2000). Emotion management skills in sexually maltreated and nonmaltreated girls: A developmental psychopathology perspective. *Developmental Psychopathology, 12,* 47–62.

Solomon, J., George, C., & DeJong, A. (1995). Children classified as controlling at age six: Evidence of disorganized representational strategies and aggression at home and at school. *Developmental Psychopathology, 73,* 447–463.

Stedman's medical dictionary (27th ed.). (2000). Philadelphia: Lippincott Williams & Wilkins.

Steinem, G. (1992). *Revolution from within: A book of self-esteem.* Boston: Little, Brown.

Stern, D. N. (1985). *The interpersonal world of the infant.* New York: Basic Books.

Stiles, W. B., Agnew-Davis, R., Hardy, G. E., Barkman, M., & Shapiro, D. A. (1998). Relations of the alliance with psychotherapy outcome: Findings in the second Sheffield psychotherapy project. *Journal of Consulting and Clinical Psychology, 67,* 13–18.

Stith, S. M., Liu, T., Davies, L. C., Boykin, E. L., Alder, M. C., Harris, J. M., et al. (2009). Risk factors in child maltreatment: A meta-analytic review of the literature. *Aggression and Violent Behavior, 14,* 13–29.

Stuewig, J., Tangney, J. P., Kendall, S., Folk, J. B., Meyer, C. R., & Dearing, R. L. (2015). Children's proneness to shame and guilt predict risky and illegal behaviors in young adulthood. *Child Psychiatry and Human Development, 46,* 217–227.

Suglia, S. F., Koenen, K. C., Boynton-Jarrett, R., Chan, P. S., Clark, C. J., Danese, A., et al. (2018). Childhood and adolescent adversity and cardiometabolic outcomes: A scientific statement from the American Heart Association. *Circulation, 137*(5), e15–e28.

Tarrier, N., Pilgrim, H., Sommerfield, C., Faragher, B., Reynolds, M., Graham, E., et al. (1999). A randomized trial of cognitive therapy and imaginal exposure in the treatment of chronic posttraumatic stress disorder. *Journal of Consulting and Clinical Psychology, 67,* 13–18.

Teicher, M. H., & Samson, J. A. (2013). Childhood maltreatment and psychopathology: A case for ecophenotypic variants as clinically and neurobiologically distinct subtypes. *American Journal of Psychiatry, 170,* 1114–1133.

Tener, D., & Murphy, S. B. (2015). Adult disclosure of child sexual abuse: A literature review. *Trauma, Violence, and Abuse, 16,* 391–400.

Tilghman-Osborne, C., Cole, D. A., Felton, J. W., & Ciesla, J. A. (2008). Relation of guilt, shame, behavioral and characterological self-blame to depressive symptoms in adolescents over time. *Journal of Social and Clinical Psychology, 27,* 809–842.

Trappler, B., & Newville, H. (2007). Trauma healing via cognitive behavior therapy in chronically hospitalized patients. *Psychiatric Quarterly, 78,* 317–325.

Turner, S. W., McFarlane, A. C., & van der Kolk, B. (1996). The therapeutic environment and new explorations in the treatment of posttraumatic stress disorder. In B. A. van der Kolk, A. C. McFarlane, & L. Weisaeth (Eds.), *Traumatic stress: The effects of overwhelming experience on mind, body, and society* (pp. 537–596). New York: Guilford Press.

van der Kolk, B. (1996). The complexity of adaptation to trauma: Self-regulation, stimulus discrimination, and characterological development. In B. A. van der Kolk, A. C. McFarlane, & I. Weisaeth (Eds.), *Traumatic stress: The effects of overwhelming experience on mind, body, and society* (pp. 182–213). New York: Guilford Press.

van der Kolk, B., Roth, S., Pelcovitz, D., & Mandel, F. S. (1993). *Complex posttraumatic stress disorder: Results of the posttraumatic stress disorder field trials for DSM-IV.* Washington, DC: American Psychiatric Association.

Van Dernoot Lipsky, L. (2009). *Trauma stewardship: An everyday guide to caring for self while caring for others.* San Francisco: Berrett-Koehler.

van IJzendoorn, M. H., & Kroonenberg, P. M. (1988). Cross-cultural patterns of attachment: A meta-analysis of the Strange Situation. *Child Development, 59,* 147–156.

Vigil Dombeck, M. J., Hoffman, J. E., Ramsey, K. M., Jaworski, B. K., Ortigo, K. M., Weiss, B., et al. (2017). STAIR Coach (Version 1.0, iOS) [Mobile application software]. Retrieved from *http://myvaapps.com.*

Wachtel, P. (1997). *Psychoanalysis, behavior therapy, and the relational world.* Washington, DC: American Psychological Association.

Weathers, F. W., Blake, D. D., Schnurr, P. P., Kaloupek, D. G., Marx, B. P., & Keane, T. M. (2013a). Clinician-Administered PTSD Scale for DSM-5 (CAPS-5). Retrieved from *www.ptsd.va.gov/professional/assessment/adult-int/caps.asp.*

Weathers, F. W., Litz, B. T., Keane, T. M., Palmieri, P. A., Marx, B. P., & Schnurr, P. P. (2013b). PTSD Checklist for DSM-5 (PCL-5). Retrieved from *www.ptsd.va.gov/professional/assessment/adult-sr/ptsd-checklist.asp.*

Weiss, B. J., Azevedo, K., Webb, K., Gimeno, J., & Cloitre, M. (2018). Telemental health delivery of Skills Training in Affective and Interpersonal Regulation (STAIR) for rural women veterans who have experienced military sexual trauma. *Journal of Traumatic Stress, 31,* 620–625.

Westphal, M., Seivert, N. H., & Bonanno, G. A. (2010). Expressive flexibility. *Emotion, 10,* 92–100.

Widom, C. S., Czaja, S. J., & DuMont, K. A. (2015). Intergenerational transmission of child abuse and neglect: Real or detection bias? *Science, 347*(6229), 1480–1485.

Wolfe, J., & Kimerling, R. (1997). Gender issues in the assessment of posttraumatic stress disorder. In J. P. Wilson & T. M. Keane (Eds.), *Assessing psychological trauma and PTSD* (pp. 192–238). New York: Guilford Press.

World Health Organization (WHO). (2018). *International statistical classification of diseases and related health problems* (11th rev.). Geneva, Switzerland: Autthor. Retrieved February 2, 2019, from *https://icd.who.int/browse11/l-m/en.*

Wyatt, G. E., Guthrie, D., & Notgrass, C. M. (1992). Differential effects of women's child sexual abuse and subsequent sexual revictimization. *Journal of Consulting and Clinical Psychology, 60,* 167–173.

Wyatt, G. E., Loeb, T. B., Solis, B., & Carmona, J. V. (1999). The prevalence and circumstances of child sexual abuse: Changes across a decade. *Child Abuse and Neglect, 23,* 45–60.

Yang, Q., Khoury, M. J., Rodriguez, C., Calle, E. E., Tathan, L. M., & Flanders, W. D. (1998). Family history score as a predictor of breast cancer mortality: Prospective data from the Cancer Prevention Study II, United States, 1982–1991. *American Journal of Epidemiology, 147,* 652–659.

Yeomans, F. E., Clarkin, J. F., & Kernberg, O. F. (2015). *Transference-focused psychotherapy for borderline personality disorder: A clinical guide.* Arlington, VA: American Psychiatric Publishing.

Yeomans, F. E., Gutfreund, J., Selzer, M. A., Clarkin, J. F., Hull, S. W., & Smith, T. E. (1994). Factors related to drop-outs by borderline patients: Treatment contract and therapeutic alliance. *Journal of Psychotherapy Practice and Research, 3,* 16–24.

Young, J. C., & Widom, C. S. (2014). Long-term effects of child abuse and neglect on emotion processing in adulthood. *Child Abuse and Neglect, 38,* 1369–1381.

Zamir, O., Szepsenwol, O., Englund, M. M., & Simpson, J. A. (2018). The role of dissociation in revictimization across the lifespan: A 32-year prospective study. *Child Abuse and Neglect, 79,* 144–153.

Zhu, P. (2016). *100 creativity ingredients: Everyone's playbook to unlock creativity.* Pennsauken, NJ: Book Baby.

Zlotnick, C., Zakriski, A. L., Shea, T. M., Costello, E., Begin, A., Pearlstein, T., et al. (1996). The long-term sequelae of sexual abuse: Support for a complex posttraumatic stress disorder. *Journal of Traumatic Stress, 9,* 195–205.

Index

Note. f or *t* following a page number indicates a figure or a table.

448